Contemporary Management of

Acute Lymphoblastic Leukemia

Contemporary Management of

Acute Lymphoblastic Leukemia

Editor

Vinod Pullarkat MD MRCP

Associate Professor
Department of Hematology and Hematopoietic Cell Transplantation
City of Hope National Medical Center
Los Angeles, California, USA

Foreword

Dan Douer MD

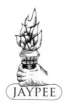

JAYPEE BROTHERS MEDICAL PUBLISHERS (P) LTD

New Delhi • London • Philadelphia • Panama

Jaypee Brothers Medical Publishers (P) Ltd

Headquarters

Jaypee Brothers Medical Publishers (P) Ltd
4838/24, Ansari Road, Daryaganj
New Delhi 110 002, India
Phone: +91-11-43574357
Fax: +91-11-43574314
Email: jaypee@jaypeebrothers.com

Overseas Offices

J.P. Medical Ltd
83 Victoria Street, London
SW1H 0HW (UK)
Phone: +44-2031708910
Fax: +02-03-0086180
Email: info@jpmedpub.com

Jaypee Medical Inc.
The Bourse
111 South Independence Mall East
Suite 835, Philadelphia, PA 19106, USA
Phone: +1 267-519-9789
Email: joe.rusko@jaypeebrothers.com

Jaypee Brothers Medical Publishers (P) Ltd
Bhotahity, Kathmandu, Nepal
Phone: +977-9741283608
Email: kathmandu@jaypeebrothers.com

Jaypee-Highlights Medical Publishers Inc.
City of Knowledge, Bld. 237, Clayton
Panama City, Panama
Phone: +1 507-301-0496
Fax: +1 507-301-0499
Email: cservice@jphmedical.com

Jaypee Brothers Medical Publishers (P) Ltd
17/1-B Babar Road, Block-B, Shaymali
Mohammadpur, Dhaka-1207
Bangladesh
Mobile: +08801912003485
Email: jaypeedhaka@gmail.com

Website: www.jaypeebrothers.com
Website: www.jaypeedigital.com

© 2014, Jaypee Brothers Medical Publishers

Inquiries for bulk sales may be solicited at: jaypee@jaypeebrothers.com

Contemporary Management of Acute Lymphoblastic Leukemia

First Edition: **2014**

ISBN: 978-93-5152-241-6

Printed at: Ajanta Offset & Packagings Ltd., New Delhi

Contents

Contributors

Editor

Vinod Pullarkat MD MRCP
Associate Professor
Department of Hematology and Hematopoietic Cell Transplantation
City of Hope National Medical Center
Los Angeles, California, USA

Contributing Authors

Ibrahim Aldoss MD
Clinical Instructor
Department of Hematology/
Hematopoietic Cell Transplantation
City of Hope National Medical Center
Los Angeles, California, USA

Patrick W Burke MD
Fellow, Hematology/Medical Oncology
Memorial Sloan-Kettering Cancer Center
New York, USA

Dario Campana MD PhD
Mrs. Lee Kong Chian Chair in Advanced
Cellular Therapy
Professor, Department of Paediatrics
Yong Loo Lin School of Medicine
National University of Singapore,
Singapore

Preeti Chaudhary MD
Fellow, Division of Hematology
University of Southern California
Los Angeles, California, USA

Wendy Cozen DO MPH
Professor
Departments of Preventive Medicine and
Pathology
Keck School of Medicine
University of Southern California
Los Angeles, California, USA

Lloyd E Damon MD
Professor of Clinical Medicine
University of California
San Francisco, California, USA

Dan Douer MD
Attending Physician
Leukemia Service
Memorial Sloan Kettering Cancer Center
New York, USA

Stéphanie Dulucq PharmD PhD
Biology Pharmacist
Bordeaux Hospital University Center
University Victor Ségalen Bordeaux 2
Inserm U876, Bordeaux, France

Kristen Eisenman MD
Assistant Professor
Department of Pediatrics
University of Colorado School of
Medicine
Aurora, Colorado, USA

Stephen J Forman MD
Chair, Department of Hematology and
Hematopoietic Cell Transplantation
City of Hope National Medical Center
Los Angeles, California, USA

Cynthia Hinh BS
Research Associate
Children's Hospital Los Angeles
University of Southern California
Los Angeles, California, USA

Stephen P Hunger MD
Professor, Department of Pediatrics
University of Colorado School of
Medicine
Aurora, Colorado, USA

Amie E Hwang PhD MPH
Research Associate
Department of Preventive Medicine
Keck School of Medicine
University of Southern California
Los Angeles, California, USA

Enzi Jiang MD PhD
Research Associate
Department of Pediatrics
Division of Hematology and Oncology
Children's Hospital Los Angeles
Los Angeles, California, USA

Sajad J Khazal MD
Clinical Fellow
Division of Pediatric Hematology and
Oncology
Children's Hospital Los Angeles
Los Angeles, California, USA

Yong-Mi Kim MD MPH PhD
Assistant Professor
Department of Pediatrics and Pathology
Children's Hospital Los Angeles
University of Southern California
Los Angeles, California, USA

Maja Krajinovic MD PhD
Professor
Departments of Pediatrics and
Pharmacology
University of Montreal
Montreal, Canada

Roberta McKean-Cowdin PhD
Associate Professor
Department of Preventive Medicine
Keck School of Medicine
University of Southern California
Los Angeles, California, USA

Rebecca L Olin MD
Assistant Professor of Clinical Medicine
University of California
San Francisco, California, USA

Sheeja T Pullarkat MD
Associate Professor
Department of Pathology and Laboratory
Medicine
David Geffen School of Medicine
University of California
Los Angeles, California, USA

Ashley E Rogers MD
Assistant Professor
Department of Pediatrics
University of Colorado School of Medicine
Aurora, Colorado, USA

Marilyn L Slovak PhD FACMG
Medical Director of Cytogenetics
Palo Verde Laboratory/Sonora Quest
Laboratories
Tempe, Arizona, USA

Martin S Tallman MD
Chief, Leukemia Service
Memorial Sloan-Kettering Cancer Center
New York, USA

Sandra H Thomas PhD
Research Scientist
Department of Hematology and
Hematopoietic Cell Transplantation
City of Hope National Medical Center
Los Angeles, California, USA

Kevin Y Urayama PhD MPH
Research Scientist
St. Luke's Life Science Institute
Center for Clinical Epidemiology
Chuo-ku, Tokyo, Japan

Justin M Watts MD
Clinical Fellow
Memorial Sloan-Kettering Cancer Center
New York, USA

Anna K Wong MD
Staff Pathologist
Diagnostic Pathology Medical Group Inc
Sacramento, California, USA

Allen EJ Yeoh MBBS MMed
Associate Professor
Department of Paediatrics
Yong Loo Lin School of Medicine,
National University of Singapore
Senior Consultant
Division of Paediatric, Haematology-
Oncology
Khoo Teck Puat - National University
Children's Medical Institute
National University Hospital, Singapore
Associate Professor, Cancer Science
Institute, Singapore

Foreword

Dan Douer MD
Attending Physician
Leukemia Service
Memorial Sloan Kettering Cancer Center
New York, USA

The classification of leukemias became technically possible once methods for staining blood films were developed, thus dividing the acute forms into acute myeloid leukemia (AML) and acute lymphocytic leukemia (ALL). It is remarkable that such a simple technique was able to recognize two distinct entities, derived from two functionally different hematopoietic cell pathways, at a time when the hierarchy of the hematopoietic stem cell growth and differentiation was yet not experimentally established. The clinical and biological characteristics of ALL, as distinct from AML, were firmly confirmed with contemporary methods for studying patient populations and leukemia cell biology. This volume provides a timely and up-to-date detailed review of different aspects of ALL.

Acute lymphocytic leukemia is more common in children, in whom it is the most common cancer and the majority of ALL patients are treated by pediatricians; although 40% of the patients are older than age 21. The development of well-defined sets of cellular (surface or cytoplasmic) markers have provided pathologists practical tools to rapidly and reliably, establish the diagnosis and phenotype of ALL. However, recurring cytogenetic abnormalities better define the different prognostic subgroups of ALL that occur at different rates in different age groups and partially explain the significantly better outcome in children. The rapid development in molecular genetics has further defined the molecular heterogeneity of ALL whereby patients can be lumped into different subgroups with similar outcomes. This work was mostly done in children, adolescents, and young adults but the question whether older adults, for the most part, have different molecular abnormalities, remains open.

The treatment of pediatric ALL has developed over the past 40 years by a series of large clinical trials each designed with the results of earlier trials in mind and as a result, currently 80% of children are cured. More recently, molecular testing can define at diagnosis those children who will have a worse outcome with the same treatment, such as those with Philadelphia (Ph) negative ALL but with a molecular signature of Ph positive ALL, carrying mutations in the *IKZF1*, *CRLF2*, *JAK2*, and other genes. Treatment of adults, on the other hand evolved empirically and much less systematically into multiple regimens, all with the same unfavorable outcome of approximately 40% long term survival. Due to this lack of an established standard of care, new directions are needed to improve the outcome in adult ALL. One approach is from realizing that separating pediatric from adult regimens at age 16–21 is arbitrary; pediatric regimens can be tolerated in older adults (at least until age 40–50) and preliminary studies show promising results. The use of pediatric approach in adults is more complex than the regimen itself due to compliance and psychosocial differences between children and young adults. A second general treatment concept that is not well recognized but is well supported by the distinct epidemiological, molecular, and other proprieties of ALL is that the general treatment principles of AML may not apply to ALL. For example, the mandatory central nervous system prophylaxis in all ages (rarely used in AML) has resulted in the greatest increment in survival. Also, the concept of short periods of very intense myelosuppressive AML-like chemotherapy may not apply so well in ALL but rather longer less myelosuppressive regimens may be more effective as exemplified by the long-term, low intensity maintenance phase of therapy that is unique for ALL. This concept is also highlighted by the critical role of a longer duration of therapy with the nonmyelosuppressive agent, L-asparaginase, that is so far used almost exclusively in ALL. With these changes in our chemotherapy approaches and introduction of novel and effective drugs (e.g., tyrosine kinase inhibitors in Ph+ ALL), the role of hematopoietic stem cell transplantation, especially as consolidation therapy in adult ALL, is continuously being defined.

Several other evolving topics are discussed comprehensively. First, several prognostic factors at diagnosis are highlighted in the different chapters on pathology, molecular biology, and cytogenetics. However, after treatment has begun, faster response with early lower disease burden measured by minimal residual disease (MRD) is critical in determining response and deciding on treatment changes. MRD is routinely monitored in children, but its application needs better standardization in adults. Second, dosing of drugs based on pharmacogenomic principles should allow better tailoring treatments for individual patients in the future. Finally, novel targeted approaches use antibodies either in their "naked" forms or more recently as drug conjugates as well as antibodies that are genetically engineered into normal autologous T cells in attempt to harness the patient's own immune system against ALL cells offer much promise.

Today, most children with ALL are cured. We hope that with the introduction of molecular stratification and new treatment approaches, the cure rate of adults will also increase. We need to pay particular attention to long term complications like therapy-related AML, within the much broader spectrum of survivorship problems, including quality of life and psychosocial issues that will become more prevalent as we anticipate more ALL survivors.

In this volume, Dr Pullarkat, an experienced investigator in the field of acute leukemia has brought together a panel of world renowned experts specializing in various aspects of the biology and therapy of ALL. Each chapter is a concise, yet comprehensive and up-to-date review of the developments in that field. This book would be a valuable reference for anyone involved in caring for patients with ALL.

Preface

Acute lymphoblastic leukemia (ALL), the commonest childhood leukemia, is now an eminently curable disease in children, thanks to developments in chemotherapy over the last 6 decades. However, adult ALL still remains a therapeutic challenge, particularly in older patients who are not candidates for intensive chemotherapy or hematopoietic stem cell transplantation (HSCT). Much work, therefore, remains to be done in order to improve outcomes of adult patients as well as patients with relapsed disease. This book is an attempt to compile the latest advances in the understanding of the pathogenesis of ALL as well as various aspects of its treatment.

The history of ALL therapy is fascinating and has important lessons for basic as well as clinical oncology research. In chapter 1, I have tried to briefly depict the evolution of ALL therapy from the remarkable efforts of early pioneers of cancer chemotherapy to the origin and development of modern oncology cooperative groups.

ALL is a heterogeneous disease with interesting epidemiologic features that differentiate childhood and adult ALL. Large scale epidemiologic studies as well as recent advances in genomic technology have provided interesting insights into the etiology of ALL, which for the most part still remains unclear. These data are discussed comprehensively in chapter 2.

The recent years have seen an explosion in knowledge regarding the cytogenetics, genomics, and molecular pathogenesis of ALL. These developments have led to the better classification as well as risk stratification of the disease which is critical for successful therapy. These topics are covered extensively in chapters 3 to 5.

Much of the advances in ALL therapy have come from systematic performance of large clinical trials by cooperative groups. Treatment of childhood and adult ALL are discussed in chapters 6 and 7. Although many aspects of treatment remain unclear, particularly in adult ALL, we have attempted to provide evidence based recommendations whenever possible. Chapter 8 deals with the use of asparaginase, a key drug in pediatric ALL therapy and discusses in detail its increasing role in adult ALL therapy.

Minimal residual disease monitoring has become an integral part of modern ALL therapy. However, it is technically challenging and requires standardization. These aspects are covered in chapter 9. Chapter 10 is devoted to prophylaxis and treatment of CNS disease, a critical component of ALL therapy. Advances in pharmacogenomics have the potential to allow tailoring of ALL therapy based on patient and disease characteristics in order to maximize efficacy and minimize toxicity. Pharmacogenomics of ALL therapy is discussed in chapter 11.

Allogeneic HSCT remains the only curative therapy for many ALL patients particularly those with relapsed disease. However, the role of HSCT in ALL therapy is continually evolving. As we gather molecular prognostic data, one can hope that we will be able to better select the patients who would benefit most from allogeneic HSCT. Use of HSCT in ALL is discussed in chapter 12.

As an increasing number of childhood ALL survivors enter adulthood; awareness of the long-term sequelae of therapy is critical in order to ensure quality of life and longevity of survivors. Long-term complications of ALL therapy and their management are considered in chapter 13.

In recent years, there has been tremendous excitement generated by the success of two immunologic approaches to ALL therapy, namely bispecific T-cell engaging antibodies and autologous chimeric antigen receptor expressing T-cells. These and other novel approaches hold promise to further improve outcomes of ALL therapy and are discussed in chapter 14.

Vinod Pullarkat MD MRCP
Associate Professor
Department of Hematology and
Hematopoietic Cell Transplantation
City of Hope National Medical Center
Los Angeles, California, USA

Acknowledgments

I wish to thank Dr Madhu Choudhary and Jaypee Brothers Medical Publishers for approaching me with the concept for this volume. I thank her as well as her editorial staff for providing me and my fellow contributors prompt assistance and support throughout the publishing process.

I am deeply indebted to all the contributors who despite their busy schedules took the time and effort to write the comprehensive and up-to-date chapters without which this book would not have been possible. Finally, I would like to thank all our patients for their trust and selfless participation in our clinical trials.

Treatment of Acute Lymphoblastic Leukemia: A Historical Perspective

Vinod Pullarkat

INTRODUCTION

Treatment of acute lymphoblastic leukemia (ALL) represents one of the triumphs of modern oncologic chemotherapy. Once a uniformly fatal cancer, childhood ALL currently has around a 90% cure rate and majority of these children can be expected to lead long and productive lives (Figure 1-1).[1] This remarkable success can be attributed to innovative drug design, rational combination of chemotherapeutic agents, astute clinical observations, and systematic performance of large clinical trials. These results become even more impressive when one considers the fact that most of this success was achieved before molecular pathogenesis of ALL was delineated using modern laboratory techniques.

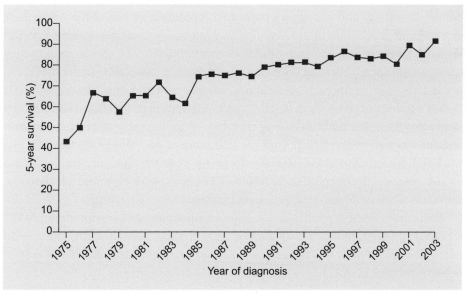

Figure 1-1 Five-year relative survival of patients with acute lymphoblastic leukemia diagnosed before 20 years of age (1975–2003).

DEVELOPMENT OF MODERN CHEMOTHERAPEUTIC AGENTS

A brief history of the development of agents that form the backbone of modern chemotherapy for ALL follows.

Methotrexate

Observations in folic acid deficiency as well as "acceleration" of acute leukemia by folic acid conjugate therapy led Sidney Farber, a pathologist at Children's Hospital in Boston to postulate that folic acid antagonists would be effective in acute leukemia.[2]

A true pioneer in cancer chemotherapy, Yellapragada Subbarow, already an accomplished biochemist at Harvard University had moved to Lederle Laboratories (a division of American Cynamid Company) in Pearl River, New York after he was denied a permanent appointment at Harvard. At Lederle, Subbarow developed a method to synthesize folic acid following which he worked on various folic acid conjugates. He provided Drs Farber and Louis Diamond with adequate quantities of various folate antagonists including 4-aminopteroyl glutamic acid (aminopterin) for clinical testing.[2,3] During the period from November 1947 to April 1948, these investigators treated 16 children with acute leukemia with various folate antagonists including aminopterin. Ten of these patients showed "clinical, hematologic, and pathological evidence of improvement" to aminopterin, a remarkable result at a time when no effective therapy existed and even temporary remissions were unheard of. Farber, Diamond, and colleagues published the details of five of the responders in a seminal publication in the *New England Journal of Medicine* on June 3, 1948.[4] Probably unaware of the magnitude of their contribution to ALL chemotherapy, they were cautious in interpreting their results and made it clear in the paper that these remissions were "temporary" and did not represent a "cure". It is a testament to Dr Farber's conviction in his ideas that he, a pathologist turned clinician persevered at a time when there was nihilism among clinicians about the value of treating pediatric leukemia as well as skepticism from his colleagues of the value of his findings. His work laid the foundation for specialized care for pediatric leukemia and led to the establishment of Children's Cancer Research Foundation which would later become the world renowned Dana Farber Cancer Institute.[2]

Eventually, the less toxic folate antagonist methotrexate (amethopterin, MTX) replaced aminopterin as a mainstay of ALL therapy. Subsequently, intrathecal administration of MTX was found to be effective in treating central nervous system (CNS) involvement of ALL.[5,6]

6-Mercaptopurine

Since around 1942, George Hitchings and co-workers at Wellcome Research Laboratories had been systematically studying the structure of purines and pyrimidines. Based on the hypothesis that malignant cells were different from normal cells in utilizing purines and pyrimidines for DNA synthesis, they synthesized various analogs of these compounds as potential chemotherapeutic agents. Research into antimetabolites had received a boost by the publication by Farber et al. on the activity of MTX. In collaboration with Hitchings' group, investigators at Sloan Kettering Institute (now Memorial Sloan Kettering Cancer Center) in New York initiated testing of various purine and pyrimidine analogs in mouse models of leukemia as well as patients. Of the various compounds, 6-mercaptopurine (6-MP) was found to be the most active in a screening program using transplanted mouse tumors.[7]

In a landmark paper published in 1953, Burchenal et al. reported results of treating various cancers including acute leukemia with 6-MP. The majority of patients in this study were children with acute leukemia. These children had the best responses to 6-MP with 15 of 45 achieving "hematologic remissions" including some who were resistant to folic acid antagonists. These investigators were particularly surprised by the lack of non-hematologic toxicity especially when 6-MP was used to treat childhood acute leukemia.[8] The pronounced antileukemic activity of 6-MP in ALL would soon be confirmed by other investigators (see below under Early Clinical Trials). It was also noted later that the antileukemic activity of different nucleoside analogs against acute leukemia was markedly different with agents like 6-azauracil showing no benefit.[9] Hitchings, Elion, and Black were awarded the Nobel Prize in 1988 for "discoveries of important principles for drug treatment".

Corticosteroids

The laboratory observations of Dougherty and White that increased adrenal cortical function in animals led to involution of lymphoid tissues[10] as well as observation by Heilman and Kendall that lymphoid tumors in mice regressed after administration of adrenal steroids[11] led Pearson and colleagues at Sloan Kettering Institute to investigate its activity in lymphoid tumors in man in the late 1940s. They observed regression of lymphadenopathy in patients with lymphoid tumors as well as clinical and hematologic remissions in patients with acute leukemia.[12] Subsequently, in 1954, Fessas, Wintrobe, and colleagues published their experience with cortisone therapy in acute leukemia. Remarkably, among 22 children with ALL aged below 10 years, a complete remission was observed in 18 after cortisone therapy. These investigators made the definite conclusion that corticosteroid therapy only benefited acute leukemias of the lymphoid lineage and emphasized the importance of differentiating acute lymphoid from acute myeloid leukemia based on careful morphologic examination and cytochemical staining. They also recognized the need for objective criteria for treatment response and defined "complete remission," principles that would be fundamental for later ALL studies.[13]

Vinca Alkaloids

The periwinkle plant had enjoyed a reputation as an oral hypoglycemic agent. While investigating its hypoglycemic properties, investigators at Lilly laboratories noticed survival prolongation in mice implanted with the ALL P-1534. Subsequently, various alkaloids active against this leukemia model including vinblastine and vincristine were characterized by Svoboda and colleagues at Lilly. Investigators at Lilly Clinic initially noticed responses to vincristine at low doses in lymphoid malignancies.[14] Subsequently, larger doses were tested in childhood acute leukemia by Karon and colleagues at the National Cancer Institute with impressive results. In a report published in 1962, they reported complete remissions after vincristine therapy in at least 7 of 13 children who had previously failed 6-MP and MTX therapy.[15] Unlike vincristine, the related vinca alkaloid vinblastine had minimal activity in acute leukemia.

EARLY CLINICAL TRIALS IN ALL

Once multiple agents with potent antileukemic activity against ALL were available, the need to conduct systematic clinical trials in a multicenter fashion was quickly recognized. These efforts were pioneered by the group of investigators at the Clinical Center of the National Cancer Institute (NCI) in Bethesda, Maryland led by Emil Frei III and Emil Freireich who conducted a series of clinical trials that would lay the foundation for modern clinical trials in oncology. Their earliest combination trial done in collaboration with Dr James Holland at Roswell Park Memorial Institute in Buffalo, New York and published in 1958 (Protocol 1) was a randomized study to test the effect of combining the two most active chemotherapeutic agents at that time, namely MTX and 6-MP. This study tested two dosing schedules of MTX (intermittent versus continuous) combined with 6-MP and concluded that these schedules were not significantly different.[16]

Soon other institutions would join this group which was named Acute Leukemia Cooperative Group B (ALGB), a precursor of the modern cooperative group Cancer and Leukemia Group B (CALGB).[17,18] In one of their earliest trials (Protocol 2), this group conducted a 318 patient trial from 13 institutions and conclusively proved that treatment with 6-MP and MTX together produced higher rate of complete remission than either agent alone.[19] The era of large cooperative group studies in acute leukemia had begun.

These early trials were limited in their use of modern statistical techniques. For the next trial (Protocol 3), however, the group with the assistance of statistician Edmund Gehan applied novel statistical techniques to the trial design.[17] This was a trial comparing 6-MP to placebo maintenance in patients who had achieved a complete remission with corticosteroids alone. Patients in complete remission were randomly assigned to 6-MP or placebo in a double-blind fashion and patients on placebo could cross over to 6-MP if they had a relapse. The duration of remission between the arms was compared using a restricted sequential procedure where patients at each institution were paired and randomly assigned one or the other therapy followed by assessment of preference for 6-MP or placebo based on remission duration. The trial had to be stopped early when a clear preference for 6-MP maintenance was noticed. After enrolment of 21 patient pairs, the median duration of remission was 33 weeks for 6-MP versus 9 weeks for placebo.[20] The statistical analytical techniques used in this study were truly novel at that time and in many ways this trial embodied much of the principles of a modern double-blind, randomized clinical trial.[17]

Drug screening in the 1950s was aided in large measure by the development of the carcinogen induced murine leukemia model L1210 by Lloyd Law at NCI which became the primary screening model for acute leukemia.[21] Cyclophosphamide was found to be active in ALL by Donald Fernbach and colleagues.[22] Subsequently, trials of multiagent combination chemotherapy would be conducted and were found to yield remissions of durations not achieved in ALL thus far. Notable in this regard are the NCI VAMP [vincristine, amethopterin (methotrexate), mercaptopurine, and prednisone) regimen and CALGB protocol 6313 (13th protocol of 1963) consisting of same agents as in VAMP plus cyclophosphamide and carmustine, both of which tested combination therapy with active agents available at that time.[23,24] These regimens were formulated based on the fundamental principles of combination chemotherapy, i.e., combining active agents with different mechanisms of action and non-overlapping toxicity. Development of combination regimens was also helped by the studies of Howard Skipper, a mathematical biologist at Southern Research Institute in Birmingham, Alabama who formulated the "cell kill" hypothesis based on kinetics of the L1210 mouse model.[23,25]

Based on outcomes of the various clinical trials done thus far, Donald Pinkel at St. Jude Children's Research Hospital in Memphis, Tennessee introduced the concept of "Total Therapy" consisting of phases of induction, consolidation, CNS directed therapy, and maintenance, of all which form the cornerstones of modern ALL regimens. By around 1965, this therapy was yielding survivals of 5 years or more in a significant number of treated children and "cure" in ALL had become a reality.[26,27] L-asparaginase was subsequently found to be active in ALL and added to pediatric ALL regimens (see chapter 8 for detailed history of its development). Over the next 4 decades or so, various cooperative groups including the Berlin-Frankfurt-Munster group formed in 1970 would obtain incremental improvements in survival by modifications of the concept of total therapy and achieve astounding success in the treatment of childhood ALL. It is important to note that the only major drug development during this period was the introduction of tyrosine kinase inhibitors which improved the outcome of Philadelphia chromosome positive ALL. The survival improvements in adult ALL have been very modest and painfully slow with long-term survival rates only around 50% at the present time. Various reasons have been attributed to this disparity between adults and children and are discussed in Chapter 7. Cooperative group trials also have made therapy better tolerated with less long-term side effects; the elimination of prophylactic CNS radiation is most notable in this regard.

IMMUNOTHERAPY FOR ALL

At a time when chemotherapy was making deep inroads into the therapy of ALL, Georges Mathé, initially at Institute Gustav Roussy and Hôpital Paul-Brousse in Villejuif, France took the unconventional approach of testing various forms of immunotherapy including adoptive immunotherapy for treatment of ALL in the late 1950s and 1960s. Mathé had observed antileukemic effect of allogeneic marrow grafted into mice with transplanted or spontaneous leukemia including virally induced leukemia. Another premise for trying immunotherapy was that some cases of childhood leukemia may have a viral origin and may be controlled by an immune response against viral antigens. This was based on Mathé's earlier observation in mice with leukemia induced by Charlotte Friend's virus that both the leukemia as well as the viral infection was controlled by grafting allogeneic bone marrow.[28]

E Donnall Thomas at University of Washington, Seattle who would later receive the Nobel prize for his pioneering work on bone marrow transplantation had done extensive studies in mice and dogs to define radiation doses for conditioning. In 1959, Thomas and colleagues performed syngeneic bone marrow transplants in two children with ALL who were conditioned with total body radiation. Although engraftment was achieved, both patients would succumb to disease relapse.[29] Mathé is credited with successfully performing the first sibling bone marrow transplant for acute leukemia in April 1963. This patient, a 26-year-old physician with refractory ALL was conditioned with total body irradiation and infused with bone marrow from six donors including four siblings and both parents. Hematopoietic engraftment from one of the brothers was demonstrated and so was tolerance to that donor. This patient remained in remission until December 1964 when he died of complications from herpetic encephalitis.[30] Although Mathé and colleagues had performed allogeneic bone marrow transplants in at least 21 ALL patients by 1965, there were very few long-term survivors with most patients succumbing to infections or graft-versus-host disease, the latter complication was well characterized in their reports and referred to as "secondary syndrome".[30,31] With knowledge of the genetics of human leukocyte antigens (HLAs) as well as refinements in HLA typing, developments in immunosuppression, and supportive care, allogeneic hematopoietic stem cell transplantation (HSCT) would become a widely used and effective therapy for ALL (see chapter 12).

Mathé and colleagues also tested other forms of immunotherapy in ALL including Bacillus Calmette-Guérin (BCG), irradiated allogeneic lymphoblasts, and even infusion of leukocytes collected by leukapheresis from patients with chronic myeloid leukemia.[28,32] In one controlled trial, they showed prolongation of remission duration by immunization with BCG or irradiated leukemic cells.[28] These therapies were clearly innovative at that time. However, interest in immunotherapy other than hematopoietic stem cell transplantation waned due to the high efficacy of chemotherapy in childhood ALL, lack of adequate technology, as well as the belief that ALL was not amenable to immune mediated therapy, probably based on the lack of efficacy of donor lymphocyte infusions in inducing remissions in patients who had relapsed after allogeneic HSCT. This was generally perceived as evidence for lack of potent graft versus leukemia effect in ALL.

THE FUTURE

"Prediction is very difficult, especially about the future."

—Niels Bohr

After decades of poor results with intensification of conventional chemotherapy in adult and encouraged by the success of tyrosine kinase inhibitors in Philadelphia chromosome-positive ALL, it was thought that agents targeting aberrant molecular pathways would provide the much awaited breakthroughs needed to improve results in adult ALL. Therefore, it came as tremendous surprise that two immune mediated therapies would hold the greatest promise for the future of ALL therapy, particularly in adults. These agents, namely, bispecific T-cell engaging (BiTE) antibodies and chimeric antigen receptor (CAR) modified T-cells targeting the CD19 antigen are highly active and have yielded unprecedented remission rates in relapsed ALL (discussed in detail in chapter 14). These agents have the potential to change the landscape of adult ALL therapy and salvage patients who have relapsed after chemotherapy or allogeneic hematopoietic stem cell transplantation.

Much progress needs to be made in adults to achieve results similar to childhood ALL. Paradoxically, in children, the current focus is to reduce or tailor therapy especially in good risk patients in order to minimize deleterious effects of therapy on a growing population of childhood ALL survivors. Assessment of minimal residual disease status and pharmacogenetic factors would be expected to allow such modifications of therapy (discussed in chapters 9 and 11, respectively).

The early history of ALL therapy is a remarkable story of successful collaboration between academia and industry as well as collaboration among clinical investigators to efficiently perform meaningful cooperative group clinical trials. Both of these aspects of clinical research have been the subject of much criticism recently. One can only hope that the current decade will see progress in adult ALL at a pace that is reminiscent of progress in childhood ALL therapy made in the 1950s.

REFERENCES

1. Diller L. Clinical practice. Adult primary care after childhood acute lymphoblastic leukemia. *N Engl J Med*. 2011;365:1417-24.
2. Miller DR. A tribute to Sidney Farber--the father of modern chemotherapy. *Br J Haematol*. 2006;134:20-6.
3. Hutchings BL, Mowat JH, Oleson JJ, et al. Pteroylaspartic acid, an antagonist for pteroyl glutamic acid. *J Biol Chem*. 1947;170:323-8.
4. Farber S, Diamond LK. Temporary remissions in acute leukemia in children produced by folic acid antagonist, 4-aminopteroyl-glutamic acid. *N Engl J Med*. 1948;238:787-93.
5. Whiteside JA, Philips FS, Dargeon HW, et al. Intrathecal amethopterin in neurological manifestations of leukemia. *AMA Arch Intern Med*. 1958;101:279-85.
6. Hyman CB, Bogle JM, Brubaker CA, et al. Central nervous system involvement by leukemia in children. II. Therapy with intrathecal methotrexate. *Blood*. 1965;25:13-22.
7. Clarke DA, Philips FS, Sternberg SS, et al. 6-mercaptopurine: effects on mouse sarcoma 180 and in normal animals. *Cancer Res*. 1953;13:593-604.
8. Burchenal JH, Murphy ML, Ellison RR, et al. Clinical evaluation of a new antimetabolite, 6-mercaptopurine in the treatment of leukemia and allied diseases. *Blood*. 1953;8:965-99.
9. Freireich EJ, Frei III E, Holland JF, et al. Evaluation of a new chemotherapeutic agent in patients with "Advanced Refractory" acute leukemia. Studies of 6-azauracil. *Blood*. 1960; 16:1268-78.
10. Dougherty TF, White A. Effect of pituitary adrenotropic hormone on lymphoid tissue. *Proc Soc Exp Biol Med*. 1943;53:132-3.
11. Hellman FR, Kendall EC. The influence of 11-dehydro-17-hydroxycorticosterone (compound E) on the growth of a malignant tumor in the mouse. *Endocrinology*. 1944;34:416-20.
12. Pearson OH, Eliel LP, Rawson RW, et al. Adrenocorticotropic hormone- and cortisone-induced regression of lymphoid tumors in man: a preliminary report. *Cancer*. 1949;2:943-5.
13. Fessas P, Wintrobe MM, Thompson RB, et al. Treatment of acute leukemia with cortisone and corticotropin. *AMA Arch Intern Med*. 1954;94:384-401.
14. Johnson IS, Armstrong JG, Gorman M, et al. The vinca alkaloids: a new class of oncolytic agents. *Cancer Res*. 1963;23:1390-427.
15. Karon MR, Freireich EJ, Frei III E. A preliminary report on vincristine sulfate-a new active agent for the treatment of acute leukemia. *Pediatrics*. 1962;30:791-6.
16. Frei E III, Holland JF, Schneiderman MA, et al. A comparative study of two regimens of combination chemotherapy in acute leukemia. *Blood*. 1958;13:1126-48.
17. Gehan EA, Freireich EJ. The 6-MP versus placebo clinical trial. *Clin Trials*. 2011;8:288-97.
18. Keating P, Cambrosio A. From screening to clinical research: the cure of leukemia and the early development of the cooperative oncology groups, 1955-1966. *Bull Hist Med*. 2002;76:299-334.
19. Frei E III, Freireich EJ, Gehan E, et al. Studies of sequential and combination antimetabolite therapy in acute leukemia: 6-mercaptopurine and methotrexate. *Blood*. 1961;18:431-54.
20. Freireich EJ, Gehan E, Frei III E, et al. The effect of 6-mercaptopurine on the duration of steroid-induced remissions in acute leukemia: a model for evaluation of other potentially useful therapy. *Blood*. 1963;21:699-716.
21. Law LW, Dunn TB, Boyle PJ, et al. Observations on the effect of a folic acid antagonist on transplantable lymphoid leukemias in mice. *J Natl Cancer Inst*. 1949;10:179-92.
22. Fernbach DJ, Sutow WW, Thurman WG, et al. Clinical evaluation of cyclophosphamide. A new agent for the treatment of children with acute leukemia. *JAMA*. 1962;182:30-7.
23. DeVita VT, Chu E. A history of cancer chemotherapy. *Cancer Res*. 2008;68:8643-53.
24. Larson RA, Stone RM, Mayer RJ, et al. Fifty years of clinical research by the leukemia committee of the Cancer and Leukemia Group B. *Clin Cancer Res*. 2006;12:3556s-63s.

25. Skipper HE, Schabel FM, Mellet LB, et al. Implications of biochemical, cytokinetic, pharmacologic and toxicologic relationships in the design of optimal therapeutic schedules. *Cancer Chemother Rep.* 1950;54:431-50.
26. Pinkel D. Five-year follow up of "total therapy" of childhood lymphocytic leukemia. *JAMA.* 1971;216:648-52.
27. Pinkel D. Total Therapy of acute lymphoblastic leukemia. *JAMA.* 1972;222:1170.
28. Mathé G, Amiel JL, Schwarzenberg L, et al. Active immunotherapy for acute lymphoblastic leukemia. *Lancet.* 1969;1:697-9.
29. Thomas ED, Lochte HL, Cannon JH, et al. Supralethal whole body irradiation and isologous marrow transplantation in man. *J Clin Invest.* 1959;38:1709-16.
30. Mathé G, Amiel JL, Schwarzenberg L, et al. Successful allogenic bone marrow transplantation in man: chimerism, induced specific tolerance and possible antileukemia effects. *Blood.* 1965;25:179-96.
31. Mathé G, Amiel JL, Schwarzenberg L, et al. Adoptive immunotherapy of acute leukemia: experimental and clinical results. *Cancer Res.* 1965;25:179-96.
32. Schwarzenberg L, Mathé G, Schneider M, et al. Attempted adoptive immunotherapy of acute leukemia by leucocyte transfusions. *Lancet.* 1966;2:365-8.

CHAPTER 2

Epidemiology and Etiology of Acute Lymphoblastic Leukemia

Amie E Hwang, Kevin Y Urayama, Roberta McKean-Cowdin, Wendy Cozen

INTRODUCTION

In this chapter, we present an overview of the epidemiology of acute lymphoblastic leukemia (ALL), including descriptive epidemiology, genetic risk factors, and environmental risk factors. The evidence for early childhood infectious exposure as a determinant for childhood ALL (defined as diagnosis from 0 years to 15 of years of age) is discussed, in the context of the two prevailing hypotheses, Kinlen's population mixing hypothesis and Greaves' delayed infection hypothesis. The two-hit or multi-hit model of leukemogenesis now widely accepted is described, e.g., that a preleukemic clone occurs *in utero* and that other exposures are necessary to permit the expansion of the clone to frank leukemia. A brief review of other accepted (e.g., ionizing radiation) and controversial [e.g., electromagnetic fields (EMF)] risk factors is also presented. Criteria for manuscripts included in this review include a reasonable sample size for a rare cancer (at least 100 cases), well-conducted case-control and registry-based studies, and recent meta-analyses. Several very large population-based studies of childhood ALL have been conducted in order to examine a number of different hypotheses; the largest of these are described in table 2-1.[1-3]

DESCRIPTIVE EPIDEMIOLOGY

Incidence and Mortality

Acute lymphoblastic leukemia is a rare cancer, with 6,000 cases diagnosed annually in the United States overall.[4] ALL derived from B-cell precursors comprises about 85% of childhood ALL, with the remainder comprised of T-cell precursors. At older ages, the proportion of B-cell ALL decreases to 75%. There is a geographically consistent bimodal incidence pattern with a peak in early childhood before 5 years of age of about 7/100,000 person-years at risk, and a gradual increase in older ages to approximately 3/100,000 person-years at risk (Figure 2-1). Mortality has dropped dramatically among children to about 0.5/100,000 person-years at risk in young children and 1/100,000 person-years of risk in older children (Figure 2-1). However, among the elderly, the mortality rate is high relative to incidence, approaching or surpassing the incidence rate.

Table 2-1	Brief Description of Large Population Based Case-control Studies of Childhood ALL[1-3]				
Study name	Acronym	Number of ALL cases	Period of recruitment	Case ascertainment	Control ascertainment	Exposure assessment
UKCCS	United Kingdom Childhood Cancer Study	1,403	1991–1998	Age 0–14 years, diagnosed with childhood leukemia in England, Scotland, and Wales	1:2 matched on month and year of birth, and residence	Parental interview, biospecimen from cases and parents, medical records, radon/gamma/EMF measurements
NCCLS	Northern California Childhood Leukemia Study	839	1995–present	Age 0–14 years, California residents diagnosed with childhood leukemia, ascertained from hospitals	Randomly selected from birth registry matched on date of birth, sex, maternal residence	Parental interview, biospecimen from cases and mothers, environmental home sampling
ESCALE	Etude Sur les Cancers et les Leucémies de l'Enfant (Study on Environmental and Genetic Risk Factors of Childhood Cancers and Leukemia)	648	2003–2004	Age 0–14 years, diagnosed with childhood leukemia	Randomly selected population based controls	Parental interview, biospecimen from cases and parents, medical records

ALL, acute lymphoblastic leukemia; EMF, electromagnetic field.

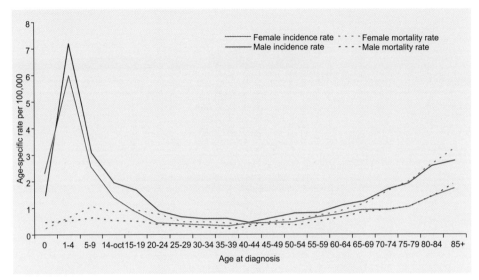

Figure 2-1 Average annual age-specific incidence and mortality rates for acute lymphoblastic leukemia, 1973–2009 [US National Cancer Institute Surveillance Epidemiology and End-Results (SEER) program]. *Source:* www.SEER.cancer.gov.

Males of all ages have a 50% higher incidence rate than females. Globally, the highest incidence rates among males are seen in Los Angeles Hispanics and Israeli Jews born in Asia or Africa (each 3.4/100,000 person-years), followed by San Francisco Hispanic males, and those in various Central and South American countries, and Israeli male Jews born in Europe or the United States (Figure 2-2). Los Angeles Hispanic females have the highest incidence rates among females at 2.7/100,000 person-years followed by Quito, Ecuador (2.5/100,000 person-years), and Costa Rica (2.4/100,000 person-years) (Figure 2-2). Incidence rates for Israeli females born in Africa/Asia or Europe/United States were low, indicating a large sex-disparity. African-Americans and Africans in Zimbabwe have among the lowest incidence rates, which may be related to a lower prevalence of a risk allele (ARIDB5) in this population.[5,6]

Between 1975 and 2009, ALL incidence rates increased by 25% and 62% among male and female children under 5 years old, respectively, while mortality rates decreased by 33% and 79% over the same time period (Figure 2-3A). In contrast, both incidence and mortality rates increased for persons 5 years of age and older, by 34% and 90%, respectively (Figure 2-3B).

For males and females of all races diagnosed less than 5 years old, 10-year relative survival rates were 79% and 83%, respectively (Figure 2-4A). Ten year relative survival rates dropped precipitously for males and females diagnosed

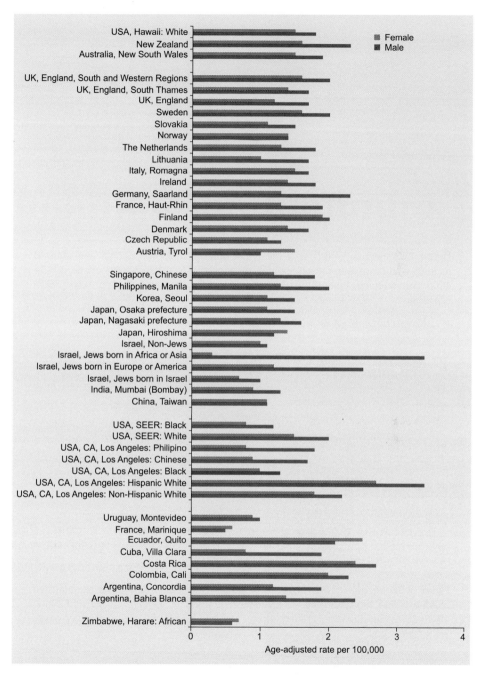

Figure 2-2 Age-adjusted incidence rates for acute lymphoblastic leukemia worldwide.
Source: Cancer Incidence in Five Continent, IARC. www.IARC.WHO.org.

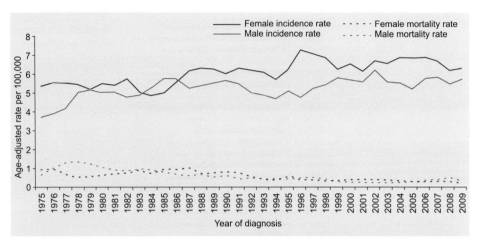

Figure 2-3A Secular trends of acute lymphoblastic leukemia annual age-adjusted incidence and mortality rates in patients diagnosed at less than 5 years of age, 1975–2009 (Surveillance, Epidemiology, and End-Results Program). *Source:* www.SEER.cancer.gov.

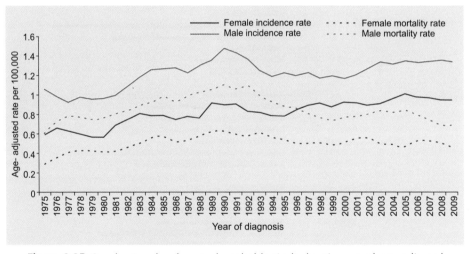

Figure 2-3B Secular trends of acute lymphoblastic leukemia annual age-adjusted incidence and mortality rates in patients diagnosed at 5 years of age and older, 1975–2009 (Surveillance, Epidemiology, and End-Results Program). *Source:* www.SEER.cancer.gov

from 5 years to 54 years of age, to 51% and 57%, respectively (Figure 2-4B); even more for patients diagnosed at 55 years and older at 10% and 11%, respectively (Figure 2-4C). African-American males and females had the poorest relative

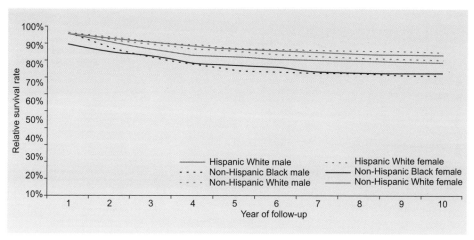

Figure 2-4A Secular trends of acute lymphoblastic leukemia annual relative survival rates in patients diagnosed at less than 5 years of age, 1973–2009 (Surveillance, Epidemiology, and End-Results Program). *Source:* www.SEER.cancer.gov.

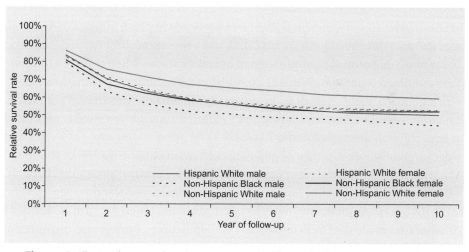

Figure 2-4B Secular trends of acute lymphoblastic leukemia annual relative survival rates in patients diagnosed at 5–54 years of age, 1973–2009 (Surveillance, Epidemiology, and End-Results Program). *Source:* www.SEER.cancer.gov.

survival over time in early childhood and adulthood (Figures 2-4A and B). African-American and Hispanic males diagnosed at older ages had marginally poorer survival relative to other gender/ethnic groups (Figure 2-4C).

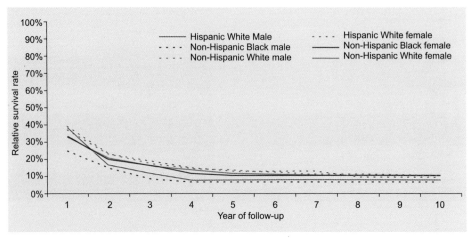

Figure 2-4C Secular trends of acute lymphoblastic leukemia annual relative survival rates in patients diagnosed at 55+ years of age, 1973-2009 (Surveillance, Epidemiology, and End-Results Program). *Source:* www.SEER.cancer.gov.

Socioeconomic Status

In Los Angeles County, there is a slight trend towards higher incidence of ALL at all ages and lower socioeconomic status (SES), more pronounced for females, based on an income/education algorithm assigned by census tract.[7] When childhood cancers were examined separately, with ALL comprising the majority, a positive association with higher SES was observed, again, especially for females. More recent population data from both Los Angeles County and California state show a weaker SES trend in both children diagnosed under 5 years old and persons diagnosed at 5 years and older (unpublished). A review of population-based ecological studies of childhood ALL from the US, UK, and Australia showed mainly a positive association between father's occupational status, family income, and income/education categorization of census tracts.[8] An analysis of more recent studies concluded that firm associations could not be made due to heterogeneity in populations, timing, and measures of SES, although there was some evidence for a positive association between risk of ALL and parents' SES at the time of birth.[9] Case-control and cohort studies cannot reliably be used to assess an association because of potential selection bias. Thus, at this time, there is no conclusive evidence regarding an association between SES and risk of ALL.

GENETIC RISK FACTORS

The vast majority of research on genetic risk factors for ALL is confined to childhood disease, due to the extreme rarity of this leukemia in adults. There does not appear to be a strong familial risk of ALL, siblings are variably reported to have a marginal increased risk.[5] The excess risk observed in young monozygotic twins is likely due to direct twin-twin transfusion of malignant cells and is thus not inherited.[5] Nevertheless, excess ALL risk is associated with some very rare heritable conditions, including Down's syndrome/trisomy 21, ataxia telangiectasia, Li-Fraumeni syndrome, Klinefelter syndrome, Fanconi anemia, Wiskott-Aldrich syndrome, and Bloom syndrome, suggesting some genetic contribution.[10]

Increasing evidence suggests that common genetic variants associated with modest levels of risk may contribute to a substantial proportion of ALL etiology.[11,12] As in many chronic diseases, the relationship between genetic risk variants and ALL are modified by environmental and lifestyle factors. Our current understanding of genetic susceptibility factors in childhood ALL is a result of numerous epidemiological studies, mostly case-control in design that have utilized one of two complementary strategies, the candidate gene or genome-wide association (GWA) approach. Genetic variation in the form of single nucleotide polymorphisms (SNPs) is most commonly used in these types of studies. Other potentially useful markers also include insertion/deletions, microsatellite markers, and copy number variations. Candidate gene studies are initiated with specific *a priori* hypotheses based on known biological functions of the genes that have relevance to proposed disease pathology. Specific genetic variants with known correlations with gene expression and/or function are usually targeted, but a haplotype tagging approach utilizing a panel of genetic variants within a candidate gene region is also commonly employed. The premise is that disease susceptibility may be identified without directly knowing the causal locus since segments of the genome are arranged into distinct haplotype blocks defined by the level of linkage disequilibrium (LD) exhibited between neighboring genetic markers.[13] The genome-wide approach is similarly based around this concept of LD between loci, but hypothesis testing is completely agnostic in that a large number of variants that represent the genetic diversity of the entire genome, regardless of candidate genes status, are assembled and evaluated in one study.

Candidate Gene Association Studies

There are numerous candidate gene studies examining the genetic susceptibility to childhood ALL and the numbers continue to increase. A previous review conducted in 2008 identified 59 articles[14] and a current search of the literature in 2013 showed greater than double this number.[12] The majority of these studies were based on small sample sizes conducted across different ethnic populations, factors which may have contributed to the general view that study results are widely inconsistent. The genes most commonly examined belong to biological pathways involving folate metabolism and transport, xenobiotic metabolism and transport, immune function, DNA repair, and cell cycle control. More than 400 candidate gene loci belonging to these pathways have been examined in relation to childhood ALL risk in at least one study; there is growing evidence suggesting a relationship with several of these loci. The following is not a comprehensive description of all studies, but summarizes the results for candidate loci that are currently supported by the most consistent evidence to date.

Folate and its bioactive metabolic substrates are essential for numerous bodily functions, particularly for their role in DNA methylation and synthesis that aid the rapid cell division and growth requirements associated with pregnancy and early infancy.[15,16] Folate deficiency may contribute to carcinogenesis via hypomethylation of important regulatory genes as well as induction of DNA damage through uracil misincorporation during DNA replication.[15] Variants in more than a dozen genes, including those encoding methylene tetrahydrofolate reductase (MTHFR), may alter folate metabolism and contribute to the risk of childhood leukemia. Two functional SNPs associated with reduced MTHFR enzymatic activities, C677T and A1298C have been examined in numerous case-control studies.[7-9] Recent meta-analyses have consistently shown a likely inverse relationship between C677T and childhood ALL risk,[17-19] but no association with A1298C. Consistent evidence is emerging for 5-methyltetrahydrofolate-homocysteine methyltransferase (MTR) A2756G, 5-methyltetrahydrofolate-homocysteine MTR reductase A66G, serine hydroxymethyltransferase 1(SHMT1) C1420T, and solute carrier family 19 member 1 (SLC19A1) G80A, genetic variants residing in other key genes of the folate pathway.

Another presumptive causal pathway involves xenobiotics, which are harmful but naturally occurring chemicals. These must gain entry into target cells via membrane transporters and undergo cellular metabolic processes that alter their activity. The complete metabolism of xenobiotic compounds is divided into two phases, each utilizing different sets of metabolic enzymes. The metabolic activation performed by the phase I (bioactivation) enzymes are usually necessary in order for the phase II (detoxification) enzymes to convert the activated intermediate into a detoxified water-soluble compound that is eliminated from the cell. Genetic polymorphisms that disrupt the equilibrium between these two phases may compromise the hosts' ability to detoxify xenobiotics and thus may potentially increase the hosts' susceptibility to developing cancer. Genetic variants of the membrane transporter gene, ATP-binding cassette subfamily B member 1 (ABCB1/MDR1), has received attention as a locus that may be involved in both ALL risk and response to therapy due to its ability to interact with both environmental carcinogens and chemotherapeutic agents. Results of two meta-analyses[20,21] are both suggestive of an increased risk of childhood ALL associated with homozygous carriers of C3435T, but when considered with two subsequent studies showing nonsignificant associations,[22,23] interpretation remains inconclusive. Combined results for another functional ABCB1 SNP, G2677T/A, does not show evidence of a statistically significant association.

Genetic variants in other pathways have also been evaluated. Among the several variants examined within the phase I metabolism cytochrome P450 (CYP) family of genes, a statistically significant increased risk of childhood ALL associated with T6235C was reported based on a meta-analysis of 7 studies,[20] which has recently been replicated in another meta-analysis including 12 studies.[24] Variants in the phase II metabolic gene pathway have been evaluated, with results suggesting an association with the widely studied deletion of GSTM1, a member within the family of glutathione S-transferase genes. A meta-analysis of 15 studies showed a statistically significant increased risk associated with the GSTM1 deletion,[20] and an additional 3 of 5 subsequent studies reported a statistically significant elevated risk.[22,23,25-27] Recently, an increasing number of studies have evaluated the effect of the slow NAT2 acetylator genotype on childhood leukemia risk. The class of slow acetylator alleles is represented by combinations of polymorphic sites (C282T, T341C, C481T, G590A, A803G, and G857A). While previous studies have used slightly varying classifications of acetylation status for NAT2, three studies have reported statistically significant increased ALL risk associated with slow acetylator alleles,[28-30] and two studies observed elevated but nonsignificant risk estimates.[22,31] The NAD(P)H dehydrogenase quinone type 1 (NQO1) gene is another widely studied phase II locus. While a previous meta-analysis of 6 studies indicated a marginally significant association for NQO1 C609T, results from a large number of studies published more recently appear inconsistent, with significant result reported in both directions.[22,23,25,26,28,32-34]

Childhood ALL results from chromosomal alterations and somatic mutations that disrupt the normal process by which lymphoid progenitor cells differentiate and senesce.[35] These are the result of unrepaired DNA damage, such as double strand breaks (DSB).[36] Among the few established risk factors for childhood ALL are exposure to ionizing radiation and certain chemotherapeutic agent,[37] both of which are well-known genotoxic exposures. Repair of DNA damage is critical,[38] thus alterations in innate DNA repair pathways including nucleotide excision repair, mismatch repair (MMR), and DSB repair may play a role in leukemia development. Two independently conducted meta-analyses have recently reported statistically significant increased risks associated with XRCC1 G28152A.[39,40] Subgroup analyses indicated an effect predominantly in Asians. No associations with childhood ALL were found for the two other widely studied XRCC1 variants: C26304T, which showed heterogeneity in results across six studies,[39,40] and G27466A examined in fewer studies.[39]

Exposure to common infections and the role of immune-related processes have emerged as strong candidate risk factors for childhood ALL.[41] An immune response to a foreign antigen involves a complex cascade of events beginning with the activation of T lymphocytes and accompanied by vast production/secretion of cytokines and recruitment of other immune cells. Genetic variation influencing immunological pathways including innate and adaptive immunity may affect ALL susceptibility. Due to its highly polymorphic nature and central role in immune response, the human leukocyte antigen (HLA) genes were one of the first loci to be examined in childhood leukemia. HLA is polygenic and broadly classified into class I (HLA-A, B, and C) and II (HLA-DR, DQ, and DP) genes that encode cell surface glycoproteins that bind and present processed antigens to T lymphocytes crucial to both cellular and humoral immune response.[42] To date, evidence has emerged suggesting association with several HLA class II genetic variants but not class I. The HLA-DR53 antigen encoded by the HLA-DRB4 locus which exists only on haplotypes possessing HLA-DRB1*04, *07, and *09 has been associated with increased risks for the major types of leukemia in adults and children,[43] including evidence from two studies of childhood ALL indicating a male-specific increase in HLA-DRB4 alleles in cases compared to controls.[43,44] More recently, two additional studies show increased risks associated with HLA-DRB1*04 in an Iranian[45] and European American population.[46] The HLA-DRB1*15 allele was also identified as a risk locus in two studies.[47,48] A second HLA gene, HLA-DPB1, has also emerged as a potential ALL-associated locus based on results from three studies.[49-51]

Genome-wide Association Studies

Collectively based on seven previous GWA studies and various follow-up analyses, strong evidence of an association with ALL overall and/or specific ALL subtypes is available for four independent loci implicating a role for the Ikaros family zinc finger 1 (*IKZF1*, 7p12.2), AT-rich interactive domain 5B (ARID5B, 10q21.2), CCAAT/enhancer-binding protein epsilon (CEBPE, 14q11.2), and cyclin-dependent kinase inhibitor 2A (CDKN2A, 9p21.3) genes.[52-59] Strong evidence is also available for another five loci around the tumor protein p63 (TP63, 3q28) and loci in or near protein tyrosine phosphatase receptor type J (PTPRJ, 11p11.2), olfactory receptor family 8 subfamily U member 8 (*OR8U8*, 11q11), integrator complex subunit 10 (INTS10, 8p21.3), and BMI1 polycomb ring finger oncogene (BMI1) and phosphatidylinositol-5-phosphate 4-kinase 2A (BMI1-PIPK2A, 10p12);[52,59] many of these results still require additional confirmation. The IKAROS transcription factor encoded by IKZF1 is a regulator of lymphocyte differentiation. In germline mutant, mice exhibiting loss of IKZF1 expression, lymphocyte development is inhibited and leads to an aggressive form of lymphoblastic leukemia.[55,60] In humans, chromosomal deletions involving IKZF1 are observed in about a third of high-risk B-cell precursor ALL and a large proportion of BCR-ABL1-positive ALL patients.[61,62] ARID5B is involved in embryogenesis and growth retardation, animal studies have shown defects in the B lymphoid compartment in ARID5B knockout mice,[63] and ARID5B expression is up-regulated in acute promyelocytic leukemia.[64] However, the specific contribution to leukemogenesis is less understood. A third gene involved in lymphoid development and/or leukemogenesis, CEBPE, is a known target of translocations in B-cell precursor ALL.[65] CDKN2A is a tumor suppressor gene that encodes p16, a negative regulator of cyclin-dependent kinases, and p14, an activator of p53. Deletion of CDKN2A is among the most common genetic events in childhood B- and T-lineage ALL.[56,66] The potential role for OR8U8 and INTS10 annotated to SNPs found to be associated with TEL-AML1 positive ALL is less clear. The direct mechanisms for an involvement of TP63 and PTPRJ in leukemogenesis are not well understood, but TP63 has been shown to possess features of a tumor suppressor, and PTPRJ involvement has been described in a number of cancers.[52] In addition, mice with impaired protein tyrosine phosphatase encoded by PTPRJ have been shown to display a partial peripheral B-cell developmental block.[67] The most recently identified putative risk locus, PIP4K2A, encodes an enzyme involved in the formation of an important second messenger molecule, PIP3, a pathway that is initiated upon activation of the B-cell receptor.[59] While PIP4K2A may plausibly be involved in the regulation of lymphoid cell differentiation, further mechanistic studies are required to clarify its potential involvement in leukemogenesis.

While the current state of evidence regarding the identification of risk loci for childhood ALL appear promising, these observations have not yet translated into tangible clinical applications. However, the expectations are that these studies will advance our understanding of the detailed causal pathways leading to disease, and eventually contribute to the development of novel therapeutics, identification of biomarkers for refined disease prediction, and monitoring of disease progression and treatment response.[68] Indeed, this improved knowledge of causal pathways may also reveal clues about modifiable environmental and lifestyle risk factors that can be used to develop public health-based prevention measures.

Translocations

Recurrent abnormalities in chromosomal integrity, such as hyperdiploidy, translocations, deletions, and other rearrangements, are a hallmark of ALL. Translocations in patients with childhood leukemia are closely associated with the molecular and biological subtypes of ALL, and serve as an independent prognostic marker for choice of therapy (Table 2-2). Genetic abnormalities involved in other malignancies lead to subsequent chromosomal instability, however, translocations commonly seen in leukemia patients are stable and result in chimeric or fusion genes and hybrid proteins with altered properties, such as transcriptional regulation or kinase activity.[69]

Studies of twins and of neonatal blood spots indicate that the chromosomal rearrangements for childhood ALL occur *in utero* with an exception of E2A-PBX1 fusion which occurs postnatally. These changes most likely arise from a single

Table 2-2	ALL Translocations by Subtype					
Subtype	Translocation	Fusion gene	Frequency of infant ALL	Frequency of comman ALL	Frequency of adult ALL	Prognosis
Pro-B-monocytic phenotype	MLL at 11q23 with multiple partner chromosomes	MLL-AF4, MLL-ENL, MLL-AF8	85%	8%	10%	Poor
B cell precursor	t(12;21) (p13;q22)	TEL-AML1		20%	2%	Good
	t(1;19) (q23;p13)	TCF3-PBX1		5%	3%	Poor
	t(9;22) (q34;q11)	BCR-ABL		5%	25%	Poor

MLL, mixed lineage leukemia; ALL, acute lymphoblastic leukemia.

causative event, and occur early in hematopoietic stem cells in the fetal liver or bone marrow.[69] To date, over 200 translocations have been identified in childhood leukemia. The most commonly occurring translocations, mixed lineage leukemia (MLL) (infant ALL) and TEL-AML1 (cALL) are discussed in further detail. In adult ALL, the cytogenetic subgrouping is mainly dependent on the presence or absence of Philadelphia chromosome, arising from t(9;22)(q34;q11), which comprises 25% of adult ALL. Due to the rarity of this disease in adults, cytogenetic profiling has not yet been extensively established.[69]

Specific Translocations: Mixed-lineage Leukemia

The very high concordance rate of ALL diagnosed at less than 1 year old in mono-zygotic twins is likely due to transfusion of the preleukemic clone from one twin to the other via the fetal blood supply,[70] and is comprised mainly of cases with the MLL translocation. ALL occurring in the first year after birth carries a distinct molecular genetic profile. It is the B-cell progenitor monocytic phenotype and a chromosomal translocation of the MLL gene at the 11q23 location is demonstrable in over 85% of cases. MLL translocations partner with more than 40 other chromosomes,[71] most commonly with the AF4 gene at chromosome 4, forming a MLL-AF4 fusion protein.[72] Patients with MLL translocations have poor prognosis and are more likely to have early relapse after chemotherapy.[71] MLL translocations are associated with the use of chemotherapeutic drugs that function as DNA topoisomerase II inhibitors.[72] Infant ALL cases with MLL translocations are significantly associated with maternal exposure to pesticides and "DNA-damaging" drugs.[73] The concordance rate among twins with infant ALL is close to 100% if twins are monochorionic monozygotic, however, the concordance rate among older twins with common acute lymphoblastic leukemia (cALL) is only about 10%. This suggests that the MLL gene arrangement alone in a B-cell clone may be sufficient to cause infant leukemia, but for ALL in older children, additional postnatal events may be necessary.[69] Thus, infant ALL is likely to have a different etiology than ALL diagnosed at older ages 2–15.

Children harboring one of the three most common MLL translocation partners (AF4, ENL, and AF9) experience a 22–30% 5-year event free survival (EFS), whereas those with less common MLL rearrangements have twice as favorable EFS (53%).[72] Such a disparity is not observed in infant acute myeloid leukemia (AML) patients.

Specific Translocations: TEL-AML1

The majority of chromosomal translocations in childhood ALL patients involve either TEL or AML1 genes, each of which forms rearrangement with other genes, although the two genes partner with each other most frequently. The translocation between the short arm of chromosome 12 and the long arm of chromosome 21, t(12;21) (9p13;q22) occurs in 25–30% of B-lineage patients. Patients with this translocation have a good prognosis, with EFS close to 90% independent of age, leukocyte count and treatment protocols.[71,74] TEL is a member of the class of transcriptional factor genes and AML1 encodes a DNA binding component for a transcription factor. The TEL-AML1 fusion protein inhibits transcriptional activity that is otherwise initiated by AML1 when it binds to a specific region of DNA. This switch from a normal enhancer function protein to an inhibitor protein by chromosomal translocation frequently occurs in translocation involving AML1 among ALL and AML patients. The fusion proteins target to modify various transcriptional activities involving a family of HOX genes that encode important transcription factors for differentiation of embryonic and hematopoietic stem cells.

A study of cord blood samples of 567 healthy newborns detected TEL-AML1 fusion gene in about 1% of all tested samples, a frequency 100 times greater than the incidence of ALL with TEL-AML1 translocation.[75] Thus, a large proportion of the population carries the preleukemic clone yet do not develop the disease, and that subsequent events may be required for leukemogenesis. Based on this evidence, Greaves' proposed that this first translocation occurs *in utero* but that a "second-hit" is necessary for development of ALL. To date, epidemiologic studies have not yet identified a specific exposure during pregnancy that results in TEL-AML1 translocation.

INFECTION AND IMMUNOLOGICAL EXPOSURES

Viral infection ranks high as a possible cause of ALL due to the documented viral cause of leukemia in chickens, cats and cattle, the evidence from surrogate measures of infection, and clusters with no other explanation.[5,76] However, after decades of research, a causal infectious agent has not been identified.[5] In 1988, two non-mutually exclusive hypotheses were proposed to describe how infections generally may be involved in the etiology of ALL; Kinlen's population mixing hypothesis and Greave's delayed infection hypothesis.

Kinlen's Population Mixing Hypothesis

Kinlen examined characteristics of leukemia and non-Hodgkin lymphoma clusters near two of Britain's nuclear reprocessing plants in Sellafield and Dounreay, and in the New Town of Glenrothes in Scotland. A report on the clusters found that radiological exposure did not account for the excess cases near the nuclear plants in the clusters in Britain.[77] Kinlen demonstrated that in the New Town of Glenrothes, an isolated region in Scotland which had experienced a large influx people in 1950s, a marked increase of leukemia was observed (10 observed, 3.6 expected), especially in those under 5 years of age (7 observed, 1.5 expected).[78] Kinlen then proposed that these clusters could be explained by an influx of an immigrants to the local area bringing infection into a relatively isolated community with low herd immunity,[78] with leukemia as a rare outcome. A recent ecological study of 107 rural villages in France reported that rural regions with high levels of population mixing experienced significantly higher incidence of childhood leukemia compared to rural regions with low population mixing [incidence rate ratio (IRR) = 2.67, 95% confidence interval (CI) = 1.16-5.87], and the effect estimate was markedly higher among children under age 6 (IRR = 5.46, 95% CI = 1.35–23.34).[79] A recent meta-analysis of 18 independent studies of childhood leukemia and population mixing also found that a significant excess risk of childhood leukemia was associated with rural population mixing [meta relative risk (RR meta) = 1.57, 95% CI = 1.44–1.72] and that the risk was consistently observed across ages 0–14.[80] Of the 18 studies, 3 studies specifically examined the effect of population mixing in ALL patients,[81-83] but showed mixed results. Wartenberg et al. using United States SEER data, found that the changes in rural county population sizes in US were associated with increased incidence of ALL from 1980 to 1989,[83] while Alexander et al. and Koushilk et al. found no evidence of increased risk of ALL in areas of high population mixing in Hong Kong[81] and in Canada,[82] respectively. A well-documented cluster of childhood leukemia in Fallon, Nevada between 1997 and 2003 triggered several successive and comprehensive examinations of possible causes for the cluster. The lack of evidence implicating chemical or radiation, and an unusual space-time pattern of cases suggest that a transmissible infectious agent may be another possible culprit.[76,84] However, the United Kingdom Childhood Cancer Study (UKCCS), a large scale population-based case-control study of nearly 1,400 ALL cases and 3,000 matched controls, found no association between ALL and population mixing.[85] This study also examined 17 published reports on population mixing and concluded that they do not provide consistent evidence for population mixing hypothesis.[85] Nevertheless, this hypothesis remains an attractive explanation for observed space-time clusters of childhood ALL.

Greaves' Delayed Infection Hypothesis

As above, Greaves' proposed that a minimal "two-hits" are necessary for cALL. The first event, the formation of preleukemic clone via chromosomal translocation or hyperdiploidy, occurs *in utero* and is already present at birth, documented by studies of neonatal blood spot samples and studies of twins concordant for childhood ALL.[86] The factors that lead to the development of the preleukemic clone are not known. However, twin studies suggest that the prenatal genetic events are sufficient to cause leukemia in the youngest patients, with a secondary postnatal event is also required for the rest.[87] Elevated levels of interleukin (IL)-10 at birth measured from neonatal birth spots was significantly and inversely associated with subsequent development of ALL [odds ratio (OR) = 0.12, 95% CI = 0.06–0.27], suggested that children with ALL may have dysregulated immune function at birth.[88]

Greaves' hypothesized that the second hit involved an altered immune response. Based on epidemiological data discussed below, he posited that delayed exposure to common infections usually acquired early in life could result in a permissive immune response which would permit the development of leukemia from a preleukmic clone, a model relevant especially to the common pre-B cell ALL that occurs in 2–5 year olds.[89] This hypothesis predates the "hygiene hypothesis"[90] which similarly posited that a lack of childhood infectious exposures associated with increasing economic development and smaller family size would prevent the normal maturation of the immune response and lead to an increased risk of atopy. During infancy, a repertoire of immune challenges is expected and essential for adaptive immune system's efficient response to future challenges. Infectious isolation early in life followed by subsequent infectious challenge may result in aberrant immune response and to trigger overt formation of cALL. Of interest, there is similar evidence of a deficit of early childhood infectious exposures and risk of adolescent/young adult Hodgkin lymphoma, another cancer derived primarily from B-lymphocytes.[91]

Kinlen's population mixing and Greaves' delayed infection hypotheses are not mutually exclusive and share key commonalities. Both include a mechanism for delayed exposure to common infections. Subsequent exposure to as yet unidentified but possibly common and subclinical infectious agents in the setting of an immature or subclinically deficient immune response may then trigger inappropriate B-cell activation and expansion of a preleukemic clone. A study based on 3,150 ALL patients aged 0–14 years of age obtained from the UK National Tumor Registry and population census data found an excess risk of ALL to be associated with a higher degree of population mixing, but only in the young age group between 1 year and

5 years, whose subtype, cALL is hypothesized to occur due to delayed exposure to infection as suggested by Greaves'.[92]

Measures of Early Exposure to Infection

The measurement of exposure to infection directly through medical records or prospective or banked samples is challenging due to the length of time between the exposures and development of the cancer, even when the majority of cancers occur in young children. Prospective cohort studies are impractical due to the rarity of the cancer. Epidemiologic studies have employed a variety of methods to evaluate this association. The studies evaluating these exposures discussed below are generally limited to childhood ALL unless otherwise specified.

The inherent difficulty in measuring such exposures has been well documented.[93] Because direct measurement of early childhood illness in a retrospective study design is subject to substantial bias and misclassification, proxy measures, such as daycare attendance, social exposure to other children, and number of siblings and birth order have also been used.[94] Responses are more reliable using these surrogate measures than questioning parents about specific infections, but the disadvantage is misclassification. There are inherent strengths and flaws in each method, and here we review the literature according to the method of exposure ascertainment.

Studies using Medical Records or Serology to Document Infection

Several studies have used the mothers' obstetrics records or neonatal medical records to assess early life infection history. Findings from these studies are mostly limited to illnesses that occur very early in life. The most recent report from the UKCCS, a national population-based case-control study (Table 2-1), found that cases of ALL had significantly more clinically recorded infections in the first year of life, especially during the neonatal period (defined as less than 1 month old), than the age-matched control children without cancer.[95] Furthermore, the number of neonatal infectious episodes was correlated with age at diagnosis, with more episodes correlated with younger age diagnosis.[96] In a population-based study using administrative and health claims in Taiwan's National Health Insurance Program, any infection in the first year of life or in the year prior to diagnosis was positively associated with ALL.[97] However, the UK General Practice Research Database of 112 ALL cases and 2,240 controls, one of the world's largest longitudinal medical records database, showed no evidence of recorded infection being associated with ALL (OR = 1.05, 95% CI = 0.64–1.74).[98] Using mothers' obstetrics hospital records, McKinney and colleagues reported that neonatal infection was inversely associated with ALL (OR = 0.49, 95% CI = 0.26–0.95), especially for those diagnosed under 4 years of age.[99] However, neonatal factors associated with physiological stress, such as low Apgar score or asphyxia at birth, were positively associated with ALL risk.[99]

Past exposure to common infections has also been examined using serological markers. A serological study of 94 incident ALL cases and 94 matched hospital controls found that ALL was inversely associated with evidence of EBV, HHV-6, mycoplasma pneumonia, and parvovirus infections among those children diagnosed greater than 5 years of age.[100]

Studies Based on Parental Reports

Parental reports of children's past illness history are often used in retrospective case-control studies examining risk factors for childhood ALL. With a few exceptions, the majority report an inverse association suggesting protection. The Northern California Childhood Leukemia Study (NCCLS) reported that ear infection, especially occurring before 6 months of age, was significantly protective for ALL among both non-Hispanic white (OR = 0.39, 95% CI = 0.17–0.91) and Hispanic (OR = 0.48, 95% CI = 0.27–0.83) populations.[101] In France, two studies, one population-based case-control study (ESCALE)[3] and one hospital based case-control study both found evidence that early common infections were protective for ALL on the order of 30–40%.[102]. Other studies have found similar protective effects from early childhood infection.[103-105] The Children's Oncology Group conducted a case-control study among Down's syndrome children with 158 incident ALL cases and 173 controls and found that any type of infection in the first 2 years of life was protective for ALL.[106] However, the German Childhood Cancer Registry population-based case-control study consisting of over 1,000 cases and 2,000 controls, found no association between the number of infections reported by mothers and risk of ALL,[107] and an increased risk of ALL in children with history of tonsillectomy or appendectomy prior to the diagnosis (unspecified length of time) (OR = 1.4, 95% CI = 1.1–1.9). Two other studies also have reported null associations.[108,109] Only one very small study conducted in New Zealand reported a large positive effect of early childhood infection on all childhood leukemia risk,[110] but ALL was not specifically examined and the wide confidence intervals suggest instability of the effect measure due to small numbers.

Family Structure

Birth order and sibship size (number of siblings) may serve as proxies for exposure to infection via other children, and/or may reflect the prenatal environment *in utero*. The UKCCS reported a modest 14% significant increased risk of ALL in first or second-born compared to third or later-born children.[95] Two other studies found a similar risk of ALL with earlier birth order.[104,111] The ESCALE study in France found a protective effect from having shorter interval to birth of the next older sibling and late birth order.[3] The NCLLS study reported that having an older sibling was protective for ALL (OR = 0.68, 95% CI = 0.5–0.92).[101] The German Childhood Cancer Registry study also reported a small but significant protective effect of being second or later born children for cALL.[107] An inverse association between the number of siblings and ALL risk in 1–4 year olds has also been reported.[112] However, a few studies reported no association between birth order, number of siblings, and risk of ALL.[102,103,113] Thus, there the preponderance of evidence suggests that few siblings and early birth order increase the risk of childhood ALL.

Daycare

Daycare attendance has been measured as a surrogate for early childhood exposure to infection in a number of studies. A large population-based Danish study composed of 599 ALL cases and 5,590 matched controls found a consistent significant protective effect of daycare attendance on childhood ALL incidence by lineage subtype, karyotype, and age at diagnosis (overall OR = 0.68, 95% CI = 0.48–0.95).[114] The UKCCS found a similar protective effect of daycare attendance across different subtypes of ALL with stronger protection among children who attended formal daycare compared to informal daycare. A protective effect was also found for children who had regular social contact with other children without daycare attendance suggesting that the protective effect of daycare attendance is likely due to exposure to other children.[113] Several other studies have also found similar protective effect of daycare attendance.[3,102,115,116] A meta-analysis of 14 studies, including those cited here, showed an overall inverse association between daycare attendance and ALL (meta OR = 0.76, 95% CI = 0.67–0.87).[117]

However, a few studies have reported no association between daycare attendance and ALL.[103,105,118] Chan et al. found that daycare attendance in first year of life was not statistically associated with ALL (OR = 0.96, 95% CI = 0.70–1.32).[105] However, results from the NCCLS suggest that ethnicity could modify the effect of daycare, especially if children of certain cultural backgrounds are routinely exposed to other children at an early age. A protective effect was observed in non-Hispanic whites, but not in Hispanics, who typically have larger families with more social interaction.[101,119] A German Children's Cancer Registry study with 600 cALL cases reported no association between social contacts with cALL risk among children older than 18 months.[107] In this study, social contact was measured by parental employment status because it was assumed that children were likely to attend daycare and have more social contact if both parents work, however, other childcare options other than daycare, such as grandparent babysitting, may have been used.

Thus, the evidence suggests a protective effect of daycare on childhood ALL, consistent with Greaves' delayed exposure to infection hypothesis.

Vaccinations

In 1986, a large-scale population based study of childhood cancer patients and matched controls found that cases had a deficit of all types of immunizations relative to controls, but the protective effect was more pronounced for solid tumors than leukemias, and for adolescents than for children.[120] Since then, a number of studies have reported an inverse relationship between vaccination and childhood leukemia specifically[107,121-126] while a few have reported no association.[110,127] The majority of the studies were based on self-reports from the parents, with the exception of three most recent studies,[124-126] which were based solely on vaccination record; all found a consistent protective effect. Two of these studies, each independently conducted in the United States, reported that conjugate *Haemophilus influenza* type B (Hib) vaccine was significantly protective against ALL (OR = 0.57–0.81),[124,125] and one showed a significant dose-response effect.[125] A recent study using county-wide and public health region vaccination rates also reported that Hib (OR = 0.58, 95% CI = 0.42–0.82), hepatitis B virus, inactivated polio virus (IPV), and the toddler age vaccination series with diphtheria, tetanus, and pertussis (DTaP), IPV, and MMR were all inversely associated with ALL.[126] Thus, most studies examining this issue have found an inverse association between vaccination and ALL risk. The specificity of the result for a specific vaccine, conjugate Hib, lends some credibility. Although these two studies adjusted for maternal education and income, there may be unmeasured factors correlated with vaccination use (i.e., healthier lifestyle) that may account for the observed effect.

Maternal Illness

Maternal illness and medication use during pregnancy have been suspected as possible causes of ALL, most likely with respect to *in utero* development of the preleukemic clone. Studies evaluating these factors have shown fairly consistent results. Two case-control studies using mothers' medical records found that mothers who reported illnesses during pregnancy were at higher risk of having children who would later develop ALL. A history of lower genital infection increased the risk of ALL in children by 66% (95% CI = 1.04–2.53),[128] and having anemia during pregnancy was also significantly associated with childhood leukemia by over twofold (95% CI = 1.2–5.0).[129] Other studies that relied on the self-reported history of illness have also shown increased risk. A recent study of 365 case-control pairs reported that a self-reported history of influenza or pneumonia during pregnancy was significantly associated with ALL (OR = 1.89, 95% CI = 1.24–2.89), and the subset of cALL (OR = 1.41, 95% CI = 0.75–2.89).[130]

Results for medication use for maternal illnesses, however, are not as consistent. A German study of 650 ALL patients found almost a twofold increased risk associated with the use of diuretics and antihypertensive medications, but no association with pain relievers, antinausea agents, or cold medications was observed.[131] A study of 789 ALL cases in Canada reported that risk of ALL was increased in offspring of mothers who reported using any medication (OR = 1.3, 95% CI = 1.0–1.6) or teratogenic medications (OR = 1.4, 95% CI = 1.1–1.9) during pregnancy, but no associations were found with specific types of medication.[132]

Breastfeeding

Breast milk has long been recognized to provide antimicrobial and immune modulating agents and to protect against many infant illnesses.[133] The protective effects of breastfeeding on infectious illnesses and associated conditions in infants have been extensively reported and used as a basis for the recommended practice of breastfeeding by American Academy of Pediatrics.[134] Studies of breastfeeding and ALL have been inconsistent, some reporting no significant association and others protective association, and two comprehensive reviews recently conducted also had equivocal results. A meta-analysis of 14 studies in 2004 found a modest but significantly protective effect from both short (<6 months, meta OR = 0.88, 95% CI = 0.80–0.97) and long (> 6 months, OR = 0.76, 95% CI = 0.68–0.84) term breastfeeding.[133] In 2007, an Evidence Report from the Agency for Healthcare Research and Quality in US Department of Health and Human Services reported a similar protective effect based on a high quality subset of the papers previously included in the 2004 meta-analysis and found similar effects (meta OR = 0.80, 95% CI = 0.71–0.91).[135] Several independent studies have since reported similar protective effects.[3,95] Overall, the evidence is consistent for modest protection against ALL associated with breast feeding.

Allergy

The "hygiene hypothesis" proposed by Strachan in 1989 to explain the rising incidence of allergies in Western countries, states that relatively more hygienic living conditions results in fewer opportunities to infectious exposure in young children, which may in turn prevent the immune system from developing normally resulting in an increased risk of allergies. Because ALL and allergy share an association with relative childhood isolation from infectious exposures, a positive correlation would be expected. However, ALL and atopy have generally been inversely associated in most studies.

The German Children's Cancer Registry reported inverse associations from parental report of allergy in children with cALL (OR = 0.6, 95% CI = 0.5–0.9) and in their mothers (OR = 0.7, 95% CI = 0.6–0.9, respectively).[107] The UKCCS conducted an extensive examination of allergy and ALL using mothers' reports on allergic symptoms from birth to diagnosis verified by general practitioner, specialist referral, and prescription history, and found consistent protective effects from having at least one allergy (OR = 0.77, 95% CI = 0.60–0.98), eczema (OR = 0.70, 95% CI = 0.51–0.97), and hay fever (OR = 0.47, 95% CI = 0.26–0.85).[136] The ESCALE study in France reported inverse associations with farm visits (OR = 0.4, 95%CI = 0.3–0.6), asthma (OR = 0.7, 95%CI = 0.4–1.0), and eczema (OR = 0.7, 95% CI = 0.6–0.9) based on parental interview.[3] In a meta-analysis of atopy and leukemia based on 10 case-control studies, including the studies previously mentioned, a consistent pattern of reduced risk for ALL, but not for overall CL or AML was observed for a history any atopy/allergies, as well as specific atopic conditions. However, a large population-based case-control study of the National Health Insurance Database in Taiwan with 846 ALL cases and 3,374 controls reported significant excess risk of ALL with record based history of allergy during first year of life (OR = 1.36, 95% CI = 1.11–1.67), in less than (OR = 1.72, 95% CI = 1.46–2.03) and more than 1 year prior to diagnosis (OR = 1.29, 95% CI = 1.08–1.53).[137] The NCCLS conducted in California also reported a positive association between ALL and maternal serum total/specific immunoglobulin E (IgE), a serological predictor for allergy, especially among Hispanics.[138]

Overall, the majority of the studies report an inverse association with allergy. Considering that delayed or lack of early exposure to infections is linked to an increased risk of both allergy and ALL, a positive association between allergy and ALL would be expected. This paradigm is further complicated by a finding that mothers of children with ALL have higher levels of IgE, often an indicator of allergy, than mothers of children without ALL.[138] While the exact mechanism between allergy and ALL has not yet been clearly postulated, it is clear that the relationship may be an indirect one in which both allergies and ALL may share some underlying mechanism related to infectious etiology.[139] It is worth noting that atopy is inversely associated with non-Hodgkin lymphoma consistently to about the same degree as ALL.[140] Non-Hodgkin lymphoma is also a cancer originating from mainly B lymphocytes, but it occurs predominantly in older adults.[141] An alternative explanation for the consistent inverse association is reverse causality, i.e., that the developing neoplasia in B lymphocytes causes a decreased ability to produce IgE antibodies that manifests as a deficit of allergies in cases.[142]

SUMMARY

The overall data suggest that medically documented, early infections are associated with an increased ALL risk, while overall infections, including more mild infections, ascertained by parental report, are largely protective. The different trends in the results of studies based on medical records and parental reports highlight two issues. First, differential parental recall bias between cases and controls is not likely here as cases or parents of cases are usually more likely to report past exposures than controls, not less likely. Thus, the inverse association lends some credibility to the effect. The overt clinically symptomatic illnesses requiring physician visits may not necessarily reflect the infectious exposures implied by the delayed infection hypothesis but instead may indicate a subclinical immune deficiency (such as the decreased cord blood IL-10 levels in children destined to develop ALL relative to controls).[88] In addition, only a small proportion of infectious illnesses lead to a physician visit,[143] and if higher SES groups preferentially participate as controls (relative to cases), the more frequent infections may reflect better access to care rather than a biological mechanism.

As final evidence of an effect of childhood exposures, one study examined interactions between proxies for exposure to infections in early childhood (i.e. birth order, daycare attendance, ear infections in the first year of life and breastfeeding) with the observed DP1 supertype association (*see* Genetic Risk Factors).[51] Statistically significant interactions were detected between HLA-DPB1 and two proxies for early immune modulation, having an older sibling and breastfeeding. This finding suggests that HLA-DPB1 genetic variation combined with an insufficiently modulated immune system may trigger an adverse immune response that contributes to childhood ALL risk and adds additional credibility to Greaves' delayed infection hypothesis.

ENVIRONMENTAL EXPOSURES

Pesticide Exposure

Pesticides include a broad classification of chemicals that are used to kill or control insects, molds, plants, or animals.[144] The relationship between pesticides and childhood leukemia strongly suggest that parental exposure to pesticides before or during pregnancy is associated with elevated risk; however, the specific chemical agent, dose, or route of exposure has not been clarified. A summary of epidemiologic studies through 2007 found that use of household insecticide during preconception or *in utero* periods was most strongly associated with childhood ALL.[145] Limitations of past studies included crude exposure assessment, recall bias of parents, small numbers of exposed cases, and heterogeneity of study leukemia types.[145] More recent studies have included detailed exposure assessment including dose-response gradients.[146,147] A recent meta-analysis of household exposure to pesticides and childhood leukemia using 13 case-control studies (1987–2009) found a positive association (meta OR = 1.74, 95% CI = 1.37–2.21). This association was elevated for exposures during or after pregnancy (meta OR = 2.19), for acute non-lymphocytic leukemia (ANLL) (meta OR = 2.30, 95% CI = 1.53–3.45) and ALL (meta OR = 2.17, 95% CI = 1.83–2.56). The association was strongest for insecticides and exposures inside the house;[148] however, associations also have been reported for herbicides. Meta-analyses have found associations between childhood leukemia and maternal occupational prenatal exposure to pesticides,[149] but not with paternal occupational exposure.[149,150] A population-based case-control study of childhood ALL conducted in Australia found no association between paternal occupational exposure to pesticides before or near conception and childhood ALL. The authors reported that the prevalence of occupational exposure to pesticides among women was less than 2%, therefore, the study was not statistically powered to evaluate maternal occupational exposure and ALL.[151]

Benzene

Benzene is an established cause of AML or ANLL and is classified as a group 1 carcinogen by the International Agency for Research on Cancer, largely based on 30 years of epidemiologic occupational data.[152,153] Exposure to benzene can occur occupationally through exposure to solvents from the chemical industry, petroleum refineries, oil pipelines, autorepair shops, as well as environmentally from vehicle emissions and cigarette smoke.[154] Multiple genes and biologic pathways are the target of benzene which can result in chromosomal, genetic, and epigenetic abnormalities in hematopoietic stem cells.[154] While more recent reports have provided evidence of an association between benzene and other types of leukemia, including ALL, the evidence for these associations is not considered as strong as that of ANLL.[155] A recent meta-analysis of occupational exposure to benzene and risk of ALL, largely in the petroleum or chemical industry, found an approximate 40% increase in risk for benzene exposed workers with ALL (meta OR = 1.44, 95% CI = 1.03–2.02) based on a random-effects model and a 14% increase in risk for chronic lymphocytic leukemia (CLL) that was not statistically significant.[153] The effect for both subtypes was stronger and statistically significant when investigators restricted to studies conducted in or after 1970, when the diagnostic and classification methods for leukemia and the exposure assessment methods for benzene would be more similar. A separate meta-analysis of 15 studies concluded that the data was insufficient to evaluate ALL, but found an increased risk of CLL and the expected strong dose-response increased risk of AML.[156]

Smoking

Tobacco smoke contains over 60 known carcinogens.[157] The major groups of chemicals are volatile hydrocarbons (i.e., benzene), aldehydes, aromatic amines, polycyclic aromatic hydrocarbons, and nitrosamines. Benzene is a volatile hydrocarbon, is one of the major carcinogen, and the only established leukemogen.[157] An active smoker is exposed to about 2 mg of benzene per day. Studies have shown a consistent and strong association between occupational exposure to benzene and risk of AML, but not with risk of ALL. Extensive studies of smoking and risk of adult and childhood leukemia have been conducted in the last 20 years. Because adult acute leukemia mostly consists of the myeloid type, there are few studies on adult acute lymphoid leukemia. One of the few studies to address the issue, conducted by National Institute of Environmental Health Services, reported a three-fold borderline significant increase in risk for ALL among patients aged 60 or older (OR = 3.4, 95% CI = 0.97–11.9).[158]

Research on parental smoking and risk of childhood leukemia has also been extensively conducted, with inconsistent results. To date, more than 20 studies have investigated the association between maternal smoking before or during pregnancy and risk of childhood ALL; most found no significant association. Several meta-analyses showed that paternal smoking may be slightly more consistently associated. A recent meta-analysis based on 18 studies on paternal smoking and childhood ALL indicated found significant and time specific relationships; preconception meta OR = 1.24, during pregnancy meta OR = 1.24, after birth meta OR = 1.25, overall anytime meta OR =1.11.[159] A study in Australia showed that paternal smoking of 15 or more cigarettes per day around the time of child's conception increased the risk of ALL by 35% while maternal smoking was not associated.[160] NCCLS also found that paternal preconception smoking combined with maternal postnatal smoking conferred a greater risk for ALL, compared to paternal preconception smoking alone (p = 0.004). There was no association with maternal smoking alone.[161] A recent meta-analysis based on 18 studies examining paternal smoking and childhood ALL found a consistent ~24% increase in ALL risk with paternal smoking over preconception, during pregnancy, and after birth.[159]

Ionizing Radiation

Ionizing radiation is considered one of the few established environmental causes of childhood ALL and AML.[162,163] The evidence for increased childhood cancer and leukemia risk due to diagnostic X-rays was first described in 1956 from a case-control study of postnatal exposure of the child or prenatal exposure of the mother to diagnostic X-rays[164,165] and confirmed in subsequent studies.[166-169] Several studies also have shown that radiotherapy for benign diseases, such as ankylosing spondylitis, ringworm, and enlarged thymus increase the risk of childhood leukemia or death due to leukemia.[163,170,171] Strong evidence has been amassed that Japanese children exposed to ionizing radiation from the World War II atomic bombs were at significantly elevated risk of leukemia; exposure to 1 Gray of radiation or higher resulted in a seven-fold increased risk of leukemia.[172]

Recent studies of diagnostic X-rays have been less conclusive. One case-control study found no association with ALL overall (OR = 1.2, 95% CI = 1.0–1.6) for exposure to three or more diagnostic X-rays, but did find a statistically significant increase in risk specifically for B-cell ALL (OR = 3.2, 95% CI = 1.5–7.2).[173] A population-based case-control study of children 14 years of age and younger at diagnosis found that children were at increased risk of ALL after receiving three or more postnatal X-rays (OR = 1.85, 95% CI = 1.12–2.29) and for B-cell ALL after receiving one or more postnatal X-rays (OR = 1.4, 95% CI = 1.06–1.56).[174] The absence of associations between prenatal X-ray exposure and childhood leukemia in some recent studies may be due to the use of lower dose in recent years.[173] Concern over use of modern radiographic techniques on children that involve relatively high doses of radiation, such as computed tomography scans, is a source of risk of ongoing concern.[175] A dose of a few milligray to the bone marrow of a small child has been estimated to potentially double their risk of leukemia, although the absolute risk of leukemia would remain low.[176] While the use of radiographic diagnostics remains important, the potential risk associated with their use, especially among children, remains an important consideration.

Electromagnetic Fields

Extremely Low-frequency

Extremely low-frequency (ELF) magnetic fields (>0 to ~300 Hz) have been classified as possibly carcinogenic to humans, largely based on epidemiological studies that consistently have shown associations between long-term average exposures to magnetic fields above 0.3/0.4 mT and the risk of childhood leukemia.[177] More than 20 epidemiologic studies have been conducted on the topic. Three pooled analyses of case-control studies have shown a 1.4- to 1.7-fold increased risk of childhood leukemia for ELF-EMF exposure levels above 0.3 μT or 0.4 μT.[178-180] Data on high dose exposure to magnetic fields greater than 0.4 μT remains limited and the shape of any dose-response curve remains unspecified.[177] Proposed biological mechanisms by which ELF-EMF might cause ALL include indirect action through induction of currents in cells or tissue heating, however, animal studies provide little support that exposure to EMF alone would induce cancer.[181,182] An estimated population attributable risk for childhood leukemia based on summary relative risks was 1.9%, suggesting the potential impact of EMF exposure on the absolute number of childhood leukemia cases may be limited.[180] Other confounding factors, including pesticides, parental smoking, and traffic density, have been suggested as potential alternative explanations for the observed ELF-EMF childhood leukemia association, however, no studies have shown this in their data.[183] The consistency of results for a variety of exposure methods including self-report, wire-coding, and dosimetry suggests that differential misclassification of exposure is unlikely to explain the positive association. The consistent, positive associations remain interesting, but the absence of a clear biological explanation supporting the ELF-EMF and childhood leukemia association, limits our ability to conclude the ELF-EMF is a cause of childhood leukemia.

Radio Towers and Mobile Phones

Radio frequency (RF) fields (~3 × 10^3–10^9 Hz) have not been as thoroughly investigated as ELF-EMF and childhood leukemia, but several studies have provided data on RF from transmission towers or mobile phone use. A pooled estimate from 2 large case-control studies found no evidence of association between RF fields and childhood ALL risk.[177] The first study included 1,928 cases diagnosed between 1993 and 1999 and an equal number of hospital-based controls. RF fields were modeled based on residential distance from amplitude modulation (AM) radio transmission towers. The study found an excess of leukemias within 2 km of the AM towers (OR = 2.15, 95% CI = 1.00–4.67), however, no association was found based on predicted field strength or peak exposure estimates.[184] Similarly, a separate case-control study of AM and FM radio and television broadcast transmitters and childhood ALL found no overall association (OR = 0.86, 95% CI = 0.67–1.11).[185] This study included 1,959 ALL cases and three population-based controls per case using estimated field exposure based on modeling.[185] More recently, concern for exposure to RF fields through mobile phone use with respect to leukemia and brain cancer has been growing. One case-control study in South East England explored the relationship between mobile phone use and adult leukemia, overall and by subtype. Mobile phone history was obtained by interview from 806 cases of leukemia (ages 18–59 years) and 585 non-biological relatives. No association was found between mobile phone use and leukemia risk (OR = 1.06, 95% CI = 0.76–1.46) overall, or by years since first use, lifetime years of use, cumulative number of calls. Further, no pattern of increased risk was observed for acute myeloid, acute lymphoblastic, or chronic myclogenous leukemia (CML).[186]

Obesity and Nutrition

Obesity

According to Center for Disease Control and Prevention report from 2009–2010, 36% of US adults and 17% of US children aged 2–19 are obese[187] and this proportion is rapidly rising. Non-Hodgkin lymphoma, Hodgkin lymphoma, and multiple myeloma have been linked to obesity.[188] A study based on a cohort of 2 million Norwegian adults found a significant and consistent increase in risk of ALL with increasing in body mass index among men.[189] A multisite Canadian case-control study with 51 incident cases of ALL and 5,039 controls also found a significant association between obesity and ALL.[190] A meta-analysis of nine studies on obesity and incidence of leukemia, including the Norwegian study mentioned here, found that obesity was associated with increase in risk of ALL (RR = 1.65, 95% CI = 1.16–2.35), AML (RR = 1.52, 1.19–1.95), CLL (RR = 1.25, 95% CI = 1.11–1.41), and CML (RR = 1.26, 95% CI = 1.09–1.46).[191]

Nutrition

Studies on diet have focused on childhood ALL as the outcome. A nationwide study in Greece based on 131 matched pairs of ALL cases and controls found that several components of maternal diet during pregnancy were associated with risk of ALL in their offspring. Relatively greater consumption of fruits (OR = 0.72, 95%

CI = 0.57–0.91), vegetables (0.76, 95% CI = 0.60–0.95), and fish and seafood (OR = 0.72, 95% CI = 0.59–0.89) intake was inversely associated with ALL; whereas relatively greater intake of sugars and syrup (OR = 1.32, 95% CI = 1.05–1.57) and meat and meat products (OR = 1.25, 95% CI = 1.00–1.57) was positively associated.[192]

Maternal diet pattern prior to conception may also impact the risk of childhood ALL.[193,194] The NCCLS study found a protective effect of vegetables and fruits (OR = 0.64, 95% CI = 0.48–0.85), protein sources (OR = 0.55, 95% CI = 0.32–0.96), and legume (OR = 0.75, 95% CI = 0.59–0.95) food groups regularly consumed 1 year before pregnancy.[194] Specific food items that conferred the most significant protection were oranges, cantaloupe, green beans, beans, carrots, and beef. Macro, and micronutrient analysis showed that consumption of fiber from fruits and vegetables and vitamin A carotenoids were significantly protective for ALL in their offspring.[194] A population based study of 145 incident ALL cases and 370 matched controls in Taiwan reported that children with ALL tend to eat cured meat and fish more frequently (OR = 1.74, 95% CI = 1.15–2.64), and vegetable (OR = 0.55, 95% CI = 0.37–0.83) and bean curd (OR = 0.55, 95% CI = 0.34–0.89) less frequently than children without ALL.[195]

Supplement Intake

Taking folic acid before and during pregnancy reduced the risk of ALL in offspring by 60% (OR = 0.4, 95% CI = 0.3–0.6), as reported by the French ESCALE.[196] A population-based multicenter study in Australia based on 393 cases and 1,249 controls found a small protective effect of folate supplementation before pregnancy (OR = 0.71, 95% CI = 0.51–0.98) but not during pregnancy.[197] A study in New Zealand, however, showed no association between folic acid supplementation before and during pregnancy and ALL risk in offspring.[198] Dietary intake of folic acid also did not show any association with ALL according to the NCCLS study.[193,194] The Pediatric Oncology Group of Ontario also reported that the incidence rate of ALL did not significantly decline after the implementation of mandatory Canadian folic acid flour fortification in mid-1997.[199] A meta-analysis based on 5 case-control or cohort studies found that any vitamin supplementation during pregnancy decreases the risk of ALL in the offspring by 17% (meta OR = 0.83, 95% CI = 0.73–0.94).[197] A German study of 650 ALL patients also showed marginally significant protection from any vitamin, folate, or iron supplements (OR = 0.84, 95% CI = 0.69–1.01).[131] A smaller study in Western Australia based on 83 cases and 166 matched controls found a significant protective effect of taking either iron or folate supplements during pregnancy (OR = 0.37, 95% CI = 0.21–0.65).[200] Thus, the majority of the evidence suggests a protective effect of maternal use of folate, especially for those taken prior to conception, but further studies are necessary to clarify the optimal timing and the effect of supplements other than folate.

SUMMARY

The risk pattern of ALL has a distinct bimodal incidence curve and ethnic disparity (higher in Hispanics, lower in Asians, relative to Whites). Much progress has been made on understanding the etiology for childhood leukemia, while little has been elucidated for leukemia in adults. A multi-hit model of causation is accepted, with the first hit likely occurring *in utero* and other triggers occurring after birth. For infant ALL, the *in utero* lesion may be sufficient. Several genetic translocations classically occur, with the most common being MLL and TEL-AML1. It is clear that both genetic and environmental exposures play a role in ALL etiology. Multiple genetic variants in several pathways have been identified as associated with ALL risk, including folate metabolism and transport, xenobiotic metabolism and transport, immune function, including HLA alleles, DNA repair, and cell cycle control. There is evidence infection plays a role in childhood etiology, either via an altered, permissive immune response due to a delayed childhood infection (Greaves' hypothesis) or exposure to infection through population mixing (Kinlen's hypothesis). Other environmental exposures, such as ionizing radiation, obesity, pesticide exposure, and paternal smoking seem to be consistently associated with ALL risk, while the evidence for EMF, cell phone use, and benzene remains unconvincing. A diet with relatively more fruits, vegetables and fish, and less red meat and sugar appears to have a protective effect, but the studies are heterogeneous in design and measurement thus firm conclusions about the benefit specific to ALL risk cannot be made at this time. The evidence for a protective effect associated with maternal intake of folate supplements is relatively consistent. Future studies should continue to elucidate pathways and gene-environment interaction for childhood leukemia and attempt to make further progress on causation in adults.

ACKNOWLEDGMENTS

We wish to thank Niquelle Brown, MS, and Yang Yu, MS, for their assistance in preparing this chapter.

GLOSSARY OF TERMS

- *Age-adjusted incidence rate*: Occurrence of new cases over a given time period (incidence) per population at risk, adjusted for age distribution of a standard population or source population
- *Age-specific incidence rate*: Occurrence of new cases over a given time period (incidence) per a population a risk within a specific age range
- *Case-control study*: An epidemiologic method in which cases (disease) and controls (unaffected) are recruited at the time of or after diagnosis (of cases) with exposures ascertained retrospectively

- *Cohort study*: An epidemiologic method in which participants are recruited based on exposure status (exposed vs. non-exposed) and are prospectively followed for onset of disease
- *Confidence interval*: An interval indicating a reliability of a parameter estimate (i.e., 95% CI indicates 95% reliability that a parameter is a true estimate for a given population).
- *Incidence*: Frequency of newly diagnosed cases of disease within a given time period.
- *Incidence rate*: The rate at which newly diagnosed cases occur within a given time period per a population at risk
- *Population-based*: Refers to ascertainment of cases and controls from an identifiable population source, usually geographic.

REFERENCES

1. The United Kingdom Childhood Cancer Study: objectives, materials and methods. UK Childhood Cancer Study Investigators. *Br J Cancer*. 2000;82(5):1073-102.
2. Metayer C, Milne E, Clavel J, et al. The Childhood Leukemia International Consortium. *Cancer Epidemiol*. 2013;37(3):336-47.
3. Rudant J, Orsi L, Menegaux F, et al. Childhood acute leukemia, early common infections, and allergy: The ESCALE Study. *Am J Epidemiol*. 2010;172(9):1015-27.
4. Siegel R, Naishadham D, Jemal A. Cancer statistics, 2012. *CA Cancer J Clin*. 2012;62(1):10-29.
5. Inaba H, Greaves M, Mullighan CG. Acute lymphoblastic leukaemia. *Lancet*. 2013;381(9881): 1943-55.
6. Curado MP, Edwards B, Shin HR, et al. Cancer Incidence in Five Continents. IARC Scientific Publications No. 160, Lyon, IARC. 2007;(6).
7. Mack TM, Cancers in the Urban Environment; Patterns of Malignant Disease in Los Angeles County and its Neighborhoods, 1 edition. Calofornia: Academic Press; 1998.
8. Poole C, Greenland S, Luetters C, et al. Socioeconomic status and childhood leukaemia: a review. *Int J Epidemiol*. 2006;35(2):370-84.
9. Adam M, Rebholz CE, Egger M, et al. Childhood leukaemia and socioeconomic status: what is the evidence? *Radiat Prot Dosimetry*. 2008;132(2):246-54.
10. Ziino O, Rondelli R, Micalizzi C, et al. Acute lymphoblastic leukemia in children with associated genetic conditions other than Down's syndrome. The AIEOP experience. *Haematologica*. 2006;91(1):139-40.
11. Enciso-Mora V, Hosking FJ, Sheridan E, et al. Common genetic variation contributes significantly to the risk of childhood B-cell precursor acute lymphoblastic leukemia. *Leukemia*. 2012;26(10):2212-5.
12. Urayama KY, Chokkalingam AP, Manabe A, et al. Current evidence for an inherited genetic basis of childhood acute lymphoblastic leukemia. *Int J Hematol*. 2012;97(1):3-19.
13. Wall JD, Pritchard JK. Haplotype blocks and linkage disequilibrium in the human genome. *Nat Rev Genet*. 2003;4(8):587-97.
14. Chokkalingam AP, Buffler PA. Genetic susceptibility to childhood leukaemia. *Radiat Prot Dosimetry*. 2008;132(2):119-29.
15. Blount BC, Mack MM, Wehr CM, et al. Folate deficiency causes uracil misincorporation into human DNA and chromosome breakage: implications for cancer and neuronal damage. *Proc Natl Acad Sci U S A*. 1997;94(7):3290-5.
16. Das PM, Singal R. DNA methylation and cancer. *J Clin Oncol*. 2004;22(22):4632-42.

17. Wang H, Wang J, Zhao L, et al. Methylenetetrahydrofolate Reductase Polymorphisms and Risk of Acute Lymphoblastic Leukemia-Evidence from an updated meta-analysis including 35 studies. *BMC Med Genet.* 2012;13(1):77.
18. Yan J, Yin M, Dreyer ZE, et al. A meta-analysis of MTHFR C677T and A1298C polymorphisms and risk of acute lymphoblastic leukemia in children. *Pediatr Blood Cancer.* 2012;58(4):513-8.
19. Zintzaras E, Doxani C, Rodopoulou P, et al. Variants of the MTHFR gene and susceptibility to acute lymphoblastic leukemia in children: a synthesis of genetic association studies. *Cancer Epidemiol.* 2012;36(2):169-76.
20. Vijayakrishnan J, Houlston RS. Candidate gene association studies and risk of childhood acute lymphoblastic leukemia: a systematic review and meta-analysis. *Haematologica.* 2010;95(8):1405-14.
21. Wang J, Wang B, Bi J, et al. MDR1 gene C3435T polymorphism and cancer risk: a meta-analysis of 34 case-control studies. *J Cancer Res Clin Oncol.* 2012;138(6):979-89.
22. Chokkalingam AP, Metayer C, Scelo GA, et al. Variation in xenobiotic transport and metabolism genes, household chemical exposures, and risk of childhood acute lymphoblastic leukemia. *Cancer Causes Control.* 2012;23(8):1367-75.
23. Yeoh AE, Lu Y, Chan JY, et al. Genetic susceptibility to childhood acute lymphoblastic leukemia shows protection in Malay boys: results from the Malaysia-Singapore ALL Study Group. *Leuk Res.* 2010;34(3):276-83.
24. Zhuo W, Zhang L, Qiu Z, et al. Does cytochrome P450 1A1 MspI polymorphism increase acute lymphoblastic leukemia risk? Evidence from 2013 cases and 2903 controls. *Gene.* 2012;510(1):14-21.
25. Chan JY, Ugrasena DG, Lum DW, et al. Xenobiotic and folate pathway gene polymorphisms and risk of childhood acute lymphoblastic leukaemia in Javanese children. *Hematol Oncol.* 2011;29(3):116-23.
26. Rimando MG, Chua MN, Yuson Ed, et al. Prevalence of GSTT1, GSTM1 and NQO1 (609C>T) in Filipino children with ALL (acute lymphoblastic leukaemia). *Biosci Rep.* 2008;28(3):117-24.
27. Suneetha KJ, Nancy KN, Rajalekshmy KR, et al. Role of GSTM1 (Present/Null) and GSTP1 (Ile105Val) polymorphisms in susceptibility to acute lymphoblastic leukemia among the South Indian population. *Asian Pac J Cancer Prev.* 2008;9(4):733-6.
28. Bonaventure A, Goujon-Bellec S, Rudant J, et al. Maternal smoking during pregnancy, genetic polymorphisms of metabolic enzymes, and childhood acute leukemia: the ESCALE study (SFCE). *Cancer Causes Control.* 2012;23(2):329-45.
29. Krajinovic M, Richer C, Sinnett H, et al. Genetic polymorphisms of N-acetyltransferases 1 and 2 and gene-gene interaction in the susceptibility to childhood acute lymphoblastic leukemia. *Cancer Epidemiol Biomarkers Prev.* 2000;9(6):557-62.
30. Zanrosso CW, Emerenciano M, Faro A, et al. Genetic variability in N-acetyltransferase 2 gene determines susceptibility to childhood lymphoid or myeloid leukemia in Brazil. *Leuk Lymphoma.* 2012;53(2):323-7.
31. Silveira VS, Canalle R, Scrideli CA, et al. CYP3A5 and NAT2 gene polymorphisms: role in childhood acute lymphoblastic leukemia risk and treatment outcome. *Mol Cell Biochem.* 2012;364(1-2):217-23.
32. de Aguiar Goncalves BA, Vasconcelos GM, Thuler LC, et al. NQO1 rs1800566 (C609T), PON1 rs662 (Q192R), and PON1 rs854560 (L55M) polymorphisms segregate the risk of childhood acute leukemias according to age range distribution. *Cancer Causes Control.* 2012;23(11):1811-9.
33. Silveira Vda S, Canalle R, Scrideli CA, et al. Role of the CYP2D6, EPHX1, MPO, and NQO1 genes in the susceptibility to acute lymphoblastic leukemia in Brazilian children. *Environ Mol Mutagen.* 2010;51(1):48-56.

34. Yamaguti GG, Lourenço GJ, Silveira VS, et al. Increased risk for acute lymphoblastic leukemia in children with cytochrome P450A1 (CYP1A1)- and NAD(P)H:quinone oxidoreductase 1 (NQO1)-inherited gene variants. *Acta Haematol.* 2010;124(3):182-4.

35. Pui CH. Childhood leukemias. *N Engl J Med.* 1995;332(24):1618-30.

36. Gillert E, Leis T, Repp R, et al. A DNA damage repair mechanism is involved in the origin of chromosomal translocations t(4;11) in primary leukemic cells. *Oncogene.* 1999; 18(33):4663-71.

37. Buffler PA, Kwan ML, Reynolds P, et al. Environmental and genetic risk factors for childhood leukemia: appraising the evidence. *Cancer Invest.* 2005;23(1):60-75.

38. Lindahl T, Wood RD. Quality control by DNA repair. *Science.* 1999;286(5446):1897-905.

39. Wang L, Yin F, Xu X, et al. X-ray repair cross-complementing group 1 (XRCC1) genetic polymorphisms and risk of childhood acute lymphoblastic leukemia: a meta-analysis. *PLoS One.* 2012;7(4):e34897.

40. Wang R, Hu X, Zhou Y, et al. XRCC1 Arg399Gln and Arg194Trp polymorphisms in childhood acute lymphoblastic leukemia risk: a meta-analysis. *Leuk Lymphoma.* 2013;54(1):153-9.

41. McNally RJ, Eden TO. An infectious aetiology for childhood acute leukaemia: a review of the evidence. *Br J Haematol.* 2004;127(3):243-63.

42. Shiina T, Inoko H, Kulski JK. An update of the HLA genomic region, locus information and disease associations: 2004. *Tissue Antigens.* 2004;64(6):631-49.

43. Dorak MT, Oguz FS, Yalman N, et al. A male-specific increase in the HLA-DRB4 (DR53) frequency in high-risk and relapsed childhood ALL. *Leuk Res.* 2002;26(7):651-6.

44. Dorak MT. Lawson T, Machulla HK, et al. Unravelling an HLA-DR association in childhood acute lymphoblastic leukemia. *Blood.* 1999;94(2):694-700.

45. Yari F, Sobhani M, Sabaghi F, et al. Frequencies of HLA-DRB1 in Iranian normal population and in patients with acute lymphoblastic leukemia. *Arch Med Res.* 2008;39(2):205-8.

46. Klitz W, Gragert L, Trachtenberg E. Spectrum of HLA associations: the case of medically refractory pediatric acute lymphoblastic leukemia. *Immunogenetics.* 2012;64(6):409-19.

47. Morrison BA, Ucisik-Akkaya E, Flores H, et al. Multiple sclerosis risk markers in HLA-DRA, HLA-C, and IFNG genes are associated with sex-specific childhood leukemia risk. *Autoimmunity.* 2010;43(8):690-7.

48. Wang XJ, Ai XF, Sun HY, et al. [Relation of HLA-DRB1*15 with pathogenesis in 162 childhood cases of acute lymphoblastic leukemia]. Zhongguo Shi Yan Xue Ye Xue Za Zhi. 2009;17(6):1507-10.

49. Urayama KY, Chokkalingam AP, Metayer C, et al. HLA-DP genetic variation, proxies for early life immune modulation and childhood acute lymphoblastic leukemia risk. *Blood.* 2012;120(15):3039-47.

50. Taylor GM, Dearden S, Ravetto P, et al. Genetic susceptibility to childhood common acute lymphoblastic leukaemia is associated with polymorphic peptide-binding pocket profiles in HLA-DPB1*0201. *Hum Mol Genet.* 2002;11(14):1585-97.

51. Taylor GM, Robinson MD, Binchy A, et al. Preliminary evidence of an association between HLA-DPB1*0201 and childhood common acute lymphobastic leukaemia supports an infectious aetiology. *Leukemia.* 1995;9(3):440-3.

52. Ellinghaus E, Stanulla M, Richter G, et al. Identification of germline susceptibility loci in ETV6-RUNX1-rearranged childhood acute lymphoblastic leukemia. *Leukemia.* 2012;26(5):902-9.

53. Han S, Lee KM, Park SK, et al. Genome-wide association study of childhood acute lymphoblastic leukemia in Korea. *Leuk Res.* 2010;34(10):1271-4.

54. Orsi L, Rudant J, Bonaventure A, et al. Genetic polymorphisms and childhood acute lymphoblastic leukemia: GWAS of the ESCALE study (SFCE). *Leukemia.* 2012;26(12):2561-4.

55. Papaemmanuil E, Hosking FJ, Vijayakrishnan J, et al. Loci on 7p12.2, 10q21.2 and 14q11.2 are associated with risk of childhood acute lymphoblastic leukemia. *Nat Genet.* 2009;41(9):1006-10.

56. Sherborne AL, Hosking FJ, Prasad RB, et al. Variation in CDKN2A at 9p21.3 influences childhood acute lymphoblastic leukemia risk. *Nat Genet.* 2010;42(6):492-4.

57. Treviño LR, Yang W, French D, et al. Germline genomic variants associated with childhood acute lymphoblastic leukemia. *Nat Genet.* 2009;41(9):1001-5.

58. Walsh KM, Chokkalingam AP, Hsu LI, et al. Associations between genome-wide Native American ancestry, known risk alleles and B-cell ALL risk in Hispanic children. *Leukemia.* 2013.

59. Xu H, Yang W, Perez-Andreu V, et al. Novel susceptibility variants at 10p12.31-12.2 for childhood acute lymphoblastic leukemia in ethnically diverse populations. *J Natl Cancer Inst.* 2013;105(10):733-42.

60. Georgopoulos K, Bigby M, Wang JH, et al. The Ikaros gene is required for the development of all lymphoid lineages. *Cell.* 1994;79(1):143-56.

61. Mullighan CG, Miller CB, Radtke I, et al. BCR-ABL1 lymphoblastic leukaemia is characterized by the deletion of Ikaros. *Nature.* 2008;453(7191):110-4.

62. Mullighan CG, Su X, Zhang J, et al. Deletion of IKZF1 and prognosis in acute lymphoblastic leukemia. *N Engl J Med.* 2009;360(5):470-80.

63. Lahoud MH, Ristevski S, Venter DJ, et al. Gene targeting of Desrt, a novel ARID class DNA-binding protein, causes growth retardation and abnormal development of reproductive organs. *Genome Res.* 2001;11(8):1327-34.

64. Chang LW, Payton JE, Yuan W, et al. Computational identification of the normal and perturbed genetic networks involved in myeloid differentiation and acute promyelocytic leukemia. *Genome Biol.* 2008;9(2):R38.

65. Akasaka T, Balasas T, Russell LJ, et al. Five members of the CEBP transcription factor family are targeted by recurrent IGH translocations in B-cell precursor acute lymphoblastic leukemia (BCP-ALL). *Blood.* 2007;109(8):3451-61.

66. Mullighan CG, Downing JR. Genome-wide profiling of genetic alterations in acute lymphoblastic leukemia: recent insights and future directions. *Leukemia.* 2009;23(7):1209-18.

67. Zhu JW, Brdicka T, Katsumoto TR, et al. Structurally distinct phosphatases CD45 and CD148 both regulate B cell and macrophage immunoreceptor signaling. *Immunity.* 2008;28(2):183-96.

68. McCarthy MI, Abecasis GR, Cardon LR, et al. Genome-wide association studies for complex traits: consensus, uncertainty and challenges. *Nat Rev Genet.* 2008;9(5):356-69.

69. Greaves MF, Wiemels J. Origins of chromosome translocations in childhood leukaemia. *Nat Rev Cancer.* 2003;3(9):639-49.

70. Greaves MF, Maia AT, Wiemels JL, et al. Leukemia in twins: lessons in natural history. *Blood.* 2003;102(7):2321-33.

71. Armstrong SA, Look AT. Molecular genetics of acute lymphoblastic leukemia. *J Clin Oncol.* 2005;23(26):6306-15.

72. Zweidler-McKay PA, Hilden JM. The ABCs of infant leukemia. *Curr Probl Pediatr Adolesc Health Care.* 2008;38(3):78-94.

73. Alexander FE, Patheal SL, Biondi A, et al. Transplacental chemical exposure and risk of infant leukemia with MLL gene fusion. *Cancer Res.* 2001;61(6):2542-6.

74. Harrison CJ, Foroni L. Cytogenetics and molecular genetics of acute lymphoblastic leukemia. *Rev Clin Exp Hematol.* 2002;6(2):91-113.

75. Mori H, Colman SM, Xiao Z, et al. Chromosome translocations and covert leukemic clones are generated during normal fetal development. *Proc Natl Acad Sci U S A.* 2002;99(12):8242-7.

76. Francis SS, Selvin S, Yang W, et al. Unusual space-time patterning of the Fallon, Nevada leukemia cluster: Evidence of an infectious etiology. *Chem Biol Interact.* 2012;196(3):102-9.

77. Urquhart JD, Black RJ, Muirhead MJ, et al. Case-control study of leukaemia and non-Hodgkin's lymphoma in children in Caithness near the Dounreay nuclear installation. *BMJ.* 1991;302(6778):687-92.

78. Kinlen L. Evidence for an infective cause of childhood leukaemia: comparison of a Scottish new town with nuclear reprocessing sites in Britain. *Lancet.* 1988;2(8624):1323-7.
79. Boutou O, Guizard AV, Slama R, et al. Population mixing and leukaemia in young people around the La Hague nuclear waste reprocessing plant. *Br J Cancer.* 2002;87(7):740-5.
80. Kinlen LJ. An examination, with a meta-analysis, of studies of childhood leukaemia in relation to population mixing. *Br J Cancer.* 2012;107(7):1163-8.
81. Alexander FE, Chan LC, Lam TH, et al. Clustering of childhood leukaemia in Hong Kong: association with the childhood peak and common acute lymphoblastic leukaemia and with population mixing. *Br J Cancer.* 1997;75(3):457-63.
82. Koushik A, King WD, McLaughlin JR. An ecologic study of childhood leukemia and population mixing in Ontario, Canada. *Cancer Causes Control.* 2001;12(6):483-90.
83. Wartenberg D, Schneider D, Brown S. Childhood leukaemia incidence and the population mixing hypothesis in US SEER data. *Br J Cancer.* 2004;90(9):1771-6.
84. Rubin CS, Holmes AK, Belson MG, et al. Investigating childhood leukemia in Churchill County, Nevada. *Environ Health Perspect.* 2007;115(1):151-7.
85. Law GR, Parslow RC, Roman E. Childhood cancer and population mixing. *Am J Epidemiol.* 2003;158(4):328-36.
86. Wiemels JL, Cazzaniga G, Daniotti M, et al. Prenatal origin of acute lymphoblastic leukaemia in children. *Lancet.* 1999;354(9189):1499-503.
87. Buckley JD, Buckley CM, Breslow NE, et al. Concordance for childhood cancer in twins. *Med Pediatr Oncol.* 1996;26(4):223-9.
88. Chang JS, Zhou M, Buffler PA, et al. Profound deficit of IL10 at birth in children who develop childhood acute lymphoblastic leukemia. *Cancer Epidemiol Biomarkers Prev.* 2011;20(8):1736-40.
89. Greaves MF. Speculations on the cause of childhood acute lymphoblastic leukemia. *Leukemia.* 1988;2(2):120-5.
90. Strachan DP. Hay fever, hygiene, and household size. *BMJ.* 1989;299(6710):1259-60.
91. Cozen W, Hamilton AS, Zhao P, et al. A protective role for early oral exposures in the etiology of young adult Hodgkin lymphoma. *Blood.* 2009;114(19):4014-20.
92. Stiller CA, Kroll ME, Boyle PJ, et al. Population mixing, socioeconomic status and incidence of childhood acute lymphoblastic leukaemia in England and Wales: analysis by census ward. *Br J Cancer.* 2008;98(5):1006-11.
93. Roman E, Simpson J, Ansell P, et al. Infectious proxies and childhood leukaemia: findings from the United Kingdom Childhood Cancer Study (UKCCS). *Blood Cells Mol Dis.* 2009;42(2):126-8.
94. Hwang AE, Mack TM, Hamilton AS, et al. Childhood infections and adult height in monozygotic twin pairs. *Am J Epidemiol.* 2013;178(4):551-8.
95. Crouch S, Lightfoot T, Simpson J, et al. Infectious illness in children subsequently diagnosed with acute lymphoblastic leukemia: modeling the trends from birth to diagnosis. *Am J Epidemiol.* 2012;176(5):402-8.
96. Roman E, Simpson J, Ansell P, et al. Childhood acute lymphoblastic leukemia and infections in the first year of life: a report from the United Kingdom Childhood Cancer Study. *Am J Epidemiol.* 2007;165(5):496-504.
97. Chang JS, Tsai CR, Tsai YW, et al. Medically diagnosed infections and risk of childhood leukaemia: a population-based case-control study. *Int J Epidemiol.* 2012;41(4):1050-9.
98. Cardwell CR, McKinney PA, Patterson CC, et al. Infections in early life and childhood leukaemia risk: a UK case-control study of general practitioner records. *Br J Cancer.* 2008; 99(9):1529-33.
99. McKinney PA, Juszczak E, Findlay E, et al. Pre- and perinatal risk factors for childhood leukaemia and other malignancies: a Scottish case control study. *Br J Cancer.* 1999;80(11):1844-51.

100. Petridou E, Dalamaga M, Mentis A, et al. Evidence on the infectious etiology of childhood leukemia: the role of low herd immunity (Greece). *Cancer Causes Control.* 2001;12(7):645-52.
101. Urayama KY, Ma X, Selvin S, et al. Early life exposure to infections and risk of childhood acute lymphoblastic leukemia. *Int J Cancer.* 2011;128(7):1632-43.
102. Perrillat F, Clavel J, Auclerc MF, et al. Day-care, early common infections and childhood acute leukaemia: a multicentre French case-control study. *Br J Cancer.* 2002;86(7):1064-9.
103. Neglia JP, Linet MS, Shu XO, et al. Patterns of infection and day care utilization and risk of childhood acute lymphoblastic leukaemia. *Br J Cancer.* 2000;82(1):234-40.
104. Jourdan-Da Silva N, Perel Y, Méchinaud F, et al. Infectious diseases in the first year of life, perinatal characteristics and childhood acute leukaemia. *Br J Cancer.* 2004;90(1):139-45.
105. Chan LC, Lam TH, Li CK, et al. Is the timing of exposure to infection a major determinant of acute lymphoblastic leukaemia in Hong Kong? *Paediatr Perinat Epidemiol.* 2002;16(2):154-65.
106. Canfield KN, Spector LG, Robison LL, et al. Childhood and maternal infections and risk of acute leukaemia in children with Down syndrome: a report from the Children's Oncology Group. *Br J Cancer.* 2004;91(11):1866-72.
107. Schuz J, Kaletsch U, Meinert R, et al. Association of childhood leukaemia with factors related to the immune system. *Br J Cancer.* 1999;80(3-4):585-90.
108. Rosenbaum PF, Buck GM, Brecher ML. Allergy and infectious disease histories and the risk of childhood acute lymphoblastic leukaemia. *Paediatr Perinat Epidemiol.* 2005;19(2):152-64.
109. MacArthur AC, McBride ML, Spinelli JJ, et al. Risk of childhood leukemia associated with vaccination, infection, and medication use in childhood: the Cross-Canada Childhood Leukemia Study. *Am J Epidemiol.* 2008;167(5):598-606.
110. Dockerty JD, Skegg DC, Elwood JM, et al. Infections, vaccinations, and the risk of childhood leukaemia. *Br J Cancer.* 1999;80(9):1483-9.
111. Ou SX, Han D, Severson RK, et al. Birth characteristics, maternal reproductive history, hormone use during pregnancy, and risk of childhood acute lymphocytic leukemia by immunophenotype (United States). *Cancer Causes Control.* 2002;13(1):15-25.
112. Westergaard T, Andersen PK, Pedersen JB, et al. Birth characteristics, sibling patterns, and acute leukemia risk in childhood: a population-based cohort study. *J Natl Cancer Inst.* 1997;89(13):939-47.
113. Gilham C, Peto J, Simpson J, et al. Day care in infancy and risk of childhood acute lymphoblastic leukaemia: findings from UK case-control study. *BMJ.* 2005;330(7503):1294.
114. Kamper-Jorgensen M, Woodward A, Wohlfahrt J, et al. Childcare in the first 2 years of life reduces the risk of childhood acute lymphoblastic leukaemia. *Leukemia.* 2008;22(1):189-93.
115. Ma X, Buffler PA, Selvin S, et al. Daycare attendance and risk of childhood acute lymphoblastic leukaemia. *Br J Cancer.* 2002;86(9):1419-24.
116. Infante-Rivard C, Fortier I, Olson E. Markers of infection, breast-feeding and childhood acute lymphoblastic leukaemia. *Br J Cancer.* 2000;83(11):1559-64.
117. Urayama KY, Buffler PA, Gallagher ER, et al. A meta-analysis of the association between day-care attendance and childhood acute lymphoblastic leukaemia. *Int J Epidemiol.* 2010;39(3):718-32.
118. Rosenbaum PF, Buck GM, Brecher ML. Early child-care and preschool experiences and the risk of childhood acute lymphoblastic leukemia. *Am J Epidemiol.* 2000;152(12):1136-44.
119. Ma X, Buffler PA, Wiemels JL, et al. Ethnic difference in daycare attendance, early infections, and risk of childhood acute lymphoblastic leukaemia. *Cancer Epidemiol Biomarkers Prev.* 2005;14(8):1928-34.
120. Kneale GW, Stewart AM, Wilson LM. Immunizations against infectious diseases and childhood cancers. *Cancer Immunol Immunother.* 1986;21(2):129-32.
121. McKinney PA, Cartwright RA, Saiu JM, et al. The inter-regional epidemiological study of childhood cancer (IRESCC): a case control study of aetiological factors in leukaemia and lymphoma. *Arch Dis Child.* 1987;62(3):279-87.

122. Nishi M, Miyake H. A case-control study of non-T cell acute lymphoblastic leukaemia of children in Hokkaido, Japan. *J Epidemiol Community Health.* 1989;43(4):352-5.
123. Kaatsch P, Kaletsch U, Krummenauer F, et al. Case control study on childhood leukemia in Lower Saxony, Germany. Basic considerations, methodology, and summary of results. *Klin Padiatr.* 1996;208(4):179-85.
124. Groves FD, Gridley G, Wacholder S, et al. Infant vaccinations and risk of childhood acute lymphoblastic leukaemia in the USA. *Br J Cancer.* 1999;81(1):175-8.
125. Ma X, Does MB, Metayer C, et al. Vaccination history and risk of childhood leukaemia. *Int J Epidemiol.* 2005;34(5):1100-9.
126. Pagaoa MA, Okcu MF, Bondy ML, et al. Associations between vaccination and childhood cancers in Texas regions. *J Pediatr.* 2011;158(6):996-1002.
127. Salonen T, Saxen L. Risk indicators in childhood malignancies. *Int J Cancer.* 1975;15(6):941-6.
128. Naumburg E, Bellocco R, Cnattingius S, et al. Perinatal exposure to infection and risk of childhood leukemia. *Med Pediatr Oncol.* 2002;38(6):391-7.
129. Roman E, Ansell P, Bull D. Leukaemia and non-Hodgkin's lymphoma in children and young adults: are prenatal and neonatal factors important determinants of disease? *Br J Cancer.* 1997;76(3):406-15.
130. Kwan ML, Metayer C, Crouse V, et al. Maternal illness and drug/medication use during the period surrounding pregnancy and risk of childhood leukemia among offspring. *Am J Epidemiol.* 2007;165(1):27-35.
131. Schuz J, Weihkopf T, Kaatsch P. Medication use during pregnancy and the risk of childhood cancer in the offspring. *Eur J Pediatr.* 2007;166(5):433-41.
132. Shaw AK, Infante-Rivard C, Morrison HI. Use of medication during pregnancy and risk of childhood leukemia (Canada). *Cancer Causes Control.* 2004;15(9):931-7.
133. Kwan ML, Buffler PA, Abrams B, et al. Breastfeeding and the risk of childhood leukemia: a meta-analysis. *Public Health Rep.* 2004;119(6):521-35.
134. Eidelman AI. Breastfeeding and the use of human milk. *Pediatrics.* 2012;129(3):e827-41.
135. Ip S, Chung M, Raman G, et al. Breastfeeding and maternal and infant health outcomes in developed countries. *Evid Rep Technol Assess (Full Rep).* 2007;(153):1-186.
136. Hughes AM, Lightfoot T, Simpson J, et al. Allergy and risk of childhood leukaemia: results from the UKCCS. *Int J Cancer.* 2007;121(4):819-24.
137. Chang JS, Tsai YW, Tsai CR, et al. Allergy and risk of childhood acute lymphoblastic leukemia: a population-based and record-based study. *Am J Epidemiol.* 2012;176(11):970-8.
138. Chang JS, Buffler PA, Metayer C, et al. Maternal immunoglobulin E and childhood leukemia. *Cancer Epidemiol Biomarkers Prev.* 2009;18(8):2221-7.
139. Chang JS, Wiemels JL, Buffler PA. Allergies and childhood leukemia. *Blood Cells Mol Dis.* 2009;42(2):99-104.
140. Vajdic CM, Falster MO, de Sanjose S, et al. Atopic disease and risk of non-Hodgkin lymphoma: an InterLymph pooled analysis. *Cancer Res.* 2009;69(16):6482-9.
141. Morton LM, Wang SS, Devesa SS, et al. Lymphoma incidence patterns by WHO subtype in the United States, 1992-2001. *Blood.* 2006;107(1):265-76.
142. Melbye M, Smedby KE, Lehtinen T, et al. Atopy and risk of non-Hodgkin lymphoma. *J Natl Cancer Inst.* 2007;99(2):158-66.
143. Hedin K, Andre M, Mölstad S, et al. Infections in families with small children: use of social insurance and healthcare. *Scand J Prim Health Care.* 2006;24(2):98-103.
144. Roberts JR, Karr CJ. Pesticide exposure in children. *Pediatrics.* 2012;130(6):e1765-88.
145. Infante-Rivard C, Weichenthal S. Pesticides and childhood cancer: an update of Zahm and Ward's 1998 review. *J Toxicol Environ Health B Crit Rev.* 2007;10(1-2):81-99.
146. Infante-Rivard C, Labuda D, Krajinovic M, et al. Risk of childhood leukemia associated with exposure to pesticides and with gene polymorphisms. *Epidemiology.* 1999;10(5):481-7.

147. Ma X, Buffler PA, Gunier RB, et al. Critical windows of exposure to household pesticides and risk of childhood leukemia. *Environ Health Perspect.* 2002;110(9):955-60.

148. Van Maele-Fabry G, Lantin AC, Hoet P, et al. Residential exposure to pesticides and childhood leukaemia: a systematic review and meta-analysis. *Environ Int.* 2011;37(1):280-91.

149. Wigle DT, Turner MC, Krewski D. A systematic review and meta-analysis of childhood leukemia and parental occupational pesticide exposure. *Environ Health Perspect.* 2009; 117(10):1505-13.

150. Vinson F, Merhi M, Baldi I, et al. Exposure to pesticides and risk of childhood cancer: a meta-analysis of recent epidemiological studies. *Occup Environ Med.* 2011;68(9):694-702.

151. Glass DC, Reid A, Bailey HD, et al. Risk of childhood acute lymphoblastic leukaemia following parental occupational exposure to pesticides. *Occup Environ Med.* 2012;69(11):846-9.

152. IARC, Overall evaluations of carcinogenicity: an updating of IARC Monographs volumes 1 to 42. *IARC Monogr Eval Carcinog Risks Hum Suppl.* 1987;7:1-440.

153. Vlaanderen J, Lan Q, Kromhout H, et al. Occupational benzene exposure and the risk of lymphoma subtypes: a meta-analysis of cohort studies incorporating three study quality dimensions. *Environ Health Perspect.* 2011;119(2):159-67.

154. McHale CM, Zhang L, Smith MT. Current understanding of the mechanism of benzene-induced leukemia in humans: implications for risk assessment. *Carcinogenesis.* 2012;33(2): 240-52.

155. Baan R, Grosse Y, Straif K, et al. A review of human carcinogens—Part F: chemical agents and related occupations. *Lancet Oncol.* 2009;10(12):1143-4.

156. Khalade A, Jaakkola MS, Pukkala E, et al. Exposure to benzene at work and the risk of leukemia: a systematic review and meta-analysis. *Environ Health.* 2010;9:31.

157. Chang JS. Parental smoking and childhood leukemia. *Methods Mol Biol.* 2009;472:103-37.

158. Sandler DP, Shore DL, Anderson JR, et al. Cigarette smoking and risk of acute leukemia: associations with morphology and cytogenetic abnormalities in bone marrow. *J Natl Cancer Inst.* 1993;85(24):1994-2003.

159. Liu R, Zhang L, McHale CM, et al. Paternal smoking and risk of childhood acute lymphoblastic leukemia: systematic review and meta-analysis. *J Oncol.* 2011;2011:854584.

160. Milne E, Greenop KR, Scott RJ, et al. Parental prenatal smoking and risk of childhood acute lymphoblastic leukemia. *Am J Epidemiol.* 2012;175(1):43-53.

161. Chang JS, Selvin S, Metayer C, et al. Parental smoking and the risk of childhood leukemia. *Am J Epidemiol.* 2006;163(12):1091-100.

162. Mahoney MC, Moysich KB, McCarthy PL, et al. The Chernobyl childhood leukemia study: background & lessons learned. *Environ Health.* 2004;3(1):12.

163. Ron E. Ionizing radiation and cancer risk: evidence from epidemiology. *Radiat Res.* 1998; 150(5 Suppl):S30-41.

164. Doll R, Wakeford R. Risk of childhood cancer from fetal irradiation. *Br J Radiol.* 1997;70: 130-9.

165. Giles D, Hewitt D, Stewart A, et al. Malignant disease in childhood and diagnostic irradiation in utero. *Lancet.* 1956;271(6940):447.

166. Hewitt D, Sanders B, Stewart A. Oxford Survey of Childhood Cancers: progress report. IV. Reliability of data reported by case and control mothers. *Mon Bull Minist Health Public Health Lab Serv.* 1966;25:80-5.

167. Knox E, et al. Prenatal irradiation and childhood cancer. *J Soc Radiol Prot.* 1987;7(4):177.

168. Macmahon B. Prenatal x-ray exposure and childhood cancer. *J Natl Cancer Inst.* 1962; 28:1173-91.

169. Mole RH. Childhood cancer after prenatal exposure to diagnostic X-ray examinations in Britain. *Br J Cancer.* 1990;62(1):152-68.

170. Darby SC, Doll R, Gill SK, et al. Long term mortality after a single treatment course with X-rays in patients treated for ankylosing spondylitis. *Br J Cancer.* 1987;55(2):179-90.

171. Murray R, Heckel P, Hempelmann LH. Leukemia in children exposed to ionizing radiation. *N Engl J Med*. 1959;261:585-9.
172. Boice JD. Cancer following irradiation in childhood and adolescence. *Med Pediatr Oncol Suppl*. 1996;1:29-34.
173. Shu XO, Potter JD, Linet MS, et al. Diagnostic X-rays and ultrasound exposure and risk of childhood acute lymphoblastic leukemia by immunophenotype. *Cancer Epidemiol Biomarkers Prev*. 2002;11(2):177-85.
174. Bartley K, Metayer C, Selvin S, et al. Diagnostic X-rays and risk of childhood leukaemia. *Int J Epidemiol*. 2010;39(6):1628-37.
175. Brenner DJ, Hall EJ. Computed tomography—an increasing source of radiation exposure. *N Engl J Med*. 2007;357(22):2277-84.
176. Wakeford R, Little MP, Kendall GM. Risk of childhood leukemia after low-level exposure to ionizing radiation. *Expert Rev Hematol*. 2010;3(3):251-4.
177. Schuz J, Ahlbom A. Exposure to electromagnetic fields and the risk of childhood leukaemia: a review. *Radiat Prot Dosimetry*. 2008;132(2):202-11.
178. Ahlbom A, Day N, Feychting M, et al. A pooled analysis of magnetic fields and childhood leukaemia. *Br J Cancer*. 2000;83(5):692-8.
179. Greenland S, Sheppard AR, Kaune WT, et al. A pooled analysis of magnetic fields, wire codes, and childhood leukemia. Childhood Leukemia-EMF Study Group. *Epidemiology*. 2000;11(6):624-34.
180. Teepen JC, van Dijck JA. Impact of high electromagnetic field levels on childhood leukemia incidence. *Int J Cancer*. 2012;131(4):769-78.
181. Wertheimer N, LeeperE. Electrical wiring configurations and childhood cancer. *Am J Epidemiol*. 1979;109(3):273-84.
182. Kavet R. EMF and current cancer concepts. *Bioelectromagnetics*. 1996;17(5):339-57.
183. Kheifets L, Repacholi M, Saunders R, et al. The sensitivity of children to electromagnetic fields. *Pediatrics*. 2005;116(2):e303-13.
184. Ha M, Im H, Lee M, et al. Radio-frequency radiation exposure from AM radio transmitters and childhood leukemia and brain cancer. *Am J Epidemiol*. 2007;166(3):270-9.
185. Merzenich H, Schmiedel S, Bennack S, et al. Childhood leukemia in relation to radio frequency electromagnetic fields in the vicinity of TV and radio broadcast transmitters. *Am J Epidemiol*. 2008;168(10):1169-78.
186. Cooke R, Laing S, Swerdlow AJ. A case-control study of risk of leukaemia in relation to mobile phone use. *Br J Cancer*. 2010;103(11):1729-35.
187. Ogden CL, Carroll MD, Kit BK, et al. Prevalence of obesity in the United States, 2009–2010. *NCHS Data Brief*. 2012;(82):1-8.
188. Lichtman MA. Obesity and the risk for a hematological malignancy: leukemia, lymphoma, or myeloma. *Oncologist*. 2010;15(10):1083-101.
189. Engeland A, Tretli S, Hansen S, et al. Height and body mass index and risk of lympho-hematopoietic malignancies in two million Norwegian men and women. *Am J Epidemiol*. 2007;165(1):44-52.
190. Kasim K, Levallois P, Abdous B, et al. Lifestyle factors and the risk of adult leukemia in Canada. *Cancer Causes Control*. 2005;16(5):489-500.
191. Larsson SC, Wolk A. Overweight and obesity and incidence of leukemia: a meta-analysis of cohort studies. *Int J Cancer*. 2008;122(6):1418-21.
192. Petridou E, Ntouvelis E, Dessypris N, et al. Maternal diet and acute lymphoblastic leukemia in young children. *Cancer Epidemiol Biomarkers Prev*. 2005;14(8):1935-9.
193. Jensen CD, Block G, Buffler P, et al. Maternal dietary risk factors in childhood acute lymphoblastic leukemia (United States). *Cancer Causes Control*. 2004;15(6):559-70.
194. Kwan ML, Jensen CD, Block G, et al. Maternal diet and risk of childhood acute lymphoblastic leukemia. *Public Health Rep*. 2009;124(4):503-14.

195. Liu CY, Hsu YH, Wu MT, et al. Cured meat, vegetables, and bean-curd foods in relation to childhood acute leukemia risk: a population based case-control study. *BMC Cancer.* 2009;9:15.
196. Amigou A, Rudant J, Orsi L, et al. Folic acid supplementation, MTHFR and MTRR polymorphisms, and the risk of childhood leukemia: the ESCALE study (SFCE). *Cancer Causes Control.* 2012;23(8):1265-77.
197. Milne E, Royle JA, Miller M, et al. Maternal folate and other vitamin supplementation during pregnancy and risk of acute lymphoblastic leukemia in the offspring. *Int J Cancer.* 2010;126(11):2690-9.
198. Dockerty JD, Herbison P, Skegg DC, et al. Vitamin and mineral supplements in pregnancy and the risk of childhood acute lymphoblastic leukaemia: a case-control study. *BMC Public Health.* 2007;7:136.
199. Grupp SG, Greenberg ML, Ray JG, et al. Pediatric cancer rates after universal folic acid flour fortification in Ontario. *J Clin Pharmacol.* 2011;51(1):60-5.
200. Thompson JR, Gerald PF, Willoughby ML, et al. Maternal folate supplementation in pregnancy and protection against acute lymphoblastic leukaemia in childhood: a case-control study. *Lancet.* 2001;358(9297):1935-40.

Diagnosis and Classification of Acute Lymphoblastic Leukemia

Anna K Wong, Sheeja T Pullarkat

INTRODUCTION

Acute lymphoblastic leukemia (ALL) is a neoplasm of progenitor lymphoid cells and is the most common cancer among children in the United States.[1,2] Based on the cell of origin, ALL can be subdivided into two main categories, namely; B-acute lymphoblastic leukemia/lymphoma (B-ALL) and T-acute lymphoblastic leukemia/lymphoma (T-ALL).[3] The distinction between lymphoma and leukemia is based on the predominant site of involvement. The term lymphoblastic lymphoma (LBL) is used if the neoplasm primarily involves extramedullary sites with minimal blood or bone marrow (BM) involvement. When the neoplastic cells involve more than 25% of the nucleated cellular composition in the blood or BM, the term lymphoblastic leukemia is more applicable. B-ALL and T-ALL are termed B-lymphoblastic leukemia/lymphoma and T-lymphoblastic leukemia/lymphoma, respectively, in the current World Health Organization classification. These terms will be used interchangeably throughout this chapter.

B-LYMPHOBLASTIC LEUKEMIA/LYMPHOMA

Definition

B-lymphoblastic leukemia/lymphoma is a clonal hematopoietic stem cell neoplasm characterized by a predominance of progenitor B-cells with minimal morphologic evidence of differentiation and lacking the capability for maturation.

Epidemiology

B-lymphoblastic leukemia/lymphoma is primarily a disease of children with 75% of cases occurring in children under 6 years of age.[4] The incidence decreases thereafter with a second peak at around 50 years of age.[5] Population-based studies in children and adults have consistently reported a higher incidence of B-ALL among Hispanics in the United States.[5,6] Among the lymphoblastic leukemias, approximately 80–85% are of the precursor B-cell phenotype.[5-7]

Etiology

Recent studies have suggested prenatal genetic events leading to leukemogenesis as the etiology of B-ALL. This theory has been exemplified by the presence of leukemia-specific translocations and antigen receptor gene rearrangements that have been documented in monozygotic twins with B-ALL.[8] A higher incidence of ALL in certain diseases, such as ataxia telangiectasia and Down syndrome supports an underlying genetic predisposition for B-ALL.[9-12] Environmental factors, namely; ionizing radiation has also been documented in ALL and chemotherapy has been rarely reported to be associated with ALL with chromosome 11q23 (MLL) gene rearrangements.[12]

Clinical Features

The clinical manifestations of B-ALL are primarily a result of BM infiltration by leukemic blasts leading to replacement of normal hematopoietic elements thereby decreasing normal hematopoiesis. These patients can present with cytopenias including anemia leading to weakness and pallor, thrombocytopenia causing petechiae and bruising, and neutropenia leading to infections and fever. The leukemic blasts cause expansion of the marrow cavity leading to bone pain which is a common complaint. In addition, hepatosplenomegaly and lymphadenopathy may be seen at presentation and organ dysfunction can occur as a result of leukemic infiltration.

Morphologic Findings

In BM smears and imprint preparations, the lymphoblasts vary from small- to medium-sized cells with high nuclear to cytoplasmic ratio, round to convoluted nuclear contours, coarsely reticular/homogeneous chromatin, and indistinct nucleoli to cells with dispersed chromatin and multiple prominent nucleoli and moderate amounts of light blue to blue grey cytoplasm (Figure 3-1). Cytoplasmic vacuoles are occasionally found and correspond to lipid and glycogen. In addition, cytoplasmic granules have been reported in about 10% of lymphoblasts; however, Auer rods are never observed in lymphoblasts. Rarely, lymphoblasts can display cytoplasmic projections resembling pseudopods which have been referred to as "hand mirror" cells.

Bone marrow core biopsy sections are usually hypercellular but may be normocellular and rarely hypocellular. Normal trilineage hematopoiesis is markedly decreased and the normal BM elements are replaced by diffuse sheets of lymphoblasts. Cytologically, the blasts appear monotonous and chromatin is evenly dispersed to moderately dense with inconspicuous nucleoli and in most cases the cytoplasm is barely discernible. Generally, in lymph nodes, the normal architecture is effaced by sheets of lymphoblast that often invade the capsule into the soft tissue in a single-file pattern. Due to the high proliferative rate, numerous tingible body macrophages can be identified within the sheets of lymphoblasts that can impart a "starry sky" appearance and mitotic figures are always easy to find (Figure 3-2).

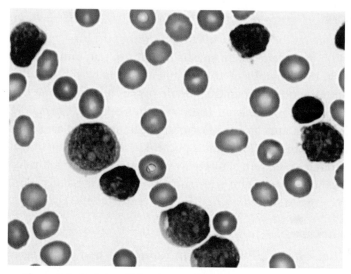

Figure 3-1 Peripheral blood smear illustrates many circulating lymphoblasts from a patient with B-lymphoblastic leukemia. Note size variation with scant to moderate cytoplasm, convoluted nuclear contours and distinct nucleoli (Wright-Giemsa stain, 1000× magnification).

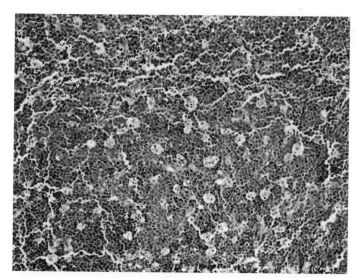

Figure 3-2 Bone marrow biopsy section diffusely involved by lymphoblasts with finely dispersed chromatin and increased mitotic activity. Note the tingible body macrophages imparting a "starry sky" appearance (H&E stain, 1000× magnification).

Cytochemistry

Cytochemistry detects the presence of enzymes within the blast cytoplasm and can be performed on peripheral blood smears or BM aspirate samples. The utility of cytochemistry in the diagnosis of ALL is limited especially with the advent of flow cytometry and immunohistochemistry. Some of the more common cytochemical stains include periodic acid-Schiff (PAS) and non-specific esterase (NSE). PAS stains glycogen which appears as coarse granules in the cytoplasm and is positive in 70–75% of lymphoblasts. NSE stain is positive in a small subset of lymphoblasts with a focal or punctate pattern of reactivity within the cytoplasm. Myeloperoxidase (MPO) is a myeloid enzyme found in primary granules and is useful in distinguishing myeloblasts (positive MPO) from lymphoblasts (negative MPO).

Immunophenotype

Normal B-cell maturation: B-cell antigen expression profile during maturation is depicted in figure 3-3. Briefly, precursor B-cells (normal, non-clonal B-lymphoblasts) arise from pluripotent stem cells in the BM and can variably express precursor as well as lineage-specific antigens, such as CD34, CD10, CD19, CD79a, terminal deoxynucelotidyl transferase (TdT), and human leukocyte antigen during their maturation. Once these precursor B-cells undergo heavy chain immunoglobulin, *VDJ* gene rearrangement and acquire surface immunoglobulin (sIg), they represent mature naïve B-lymphocytes and are no longer considered precursor B-cells. These naïve B-cells that have a distinctive immunophenotypic profile characterized by expression of CD5, IgM, and IgD circulate in peripheral blood and occupy the primary follicles and mantle zones in the lymph nodes. On encountering an antigen, the naïve B-cells undergo transformation and selection within the germinal center. Some B-cells further mature into antibody-producing plasma cells and memory cells, which is the final differentiation step for B-cells (Figure 3-3).

Historically, B-lymphoblastic leukemias were further subclassified based on the immunophenotype of the neoplastic B-lymphoblasts as they parallel the immunophenotypic profile of normal precursor B-cells during their development. Terms, such as early precursor B-ALL, common precursor B-ALL, and pre B-ALL are no longer used since they have no significant treatment or prognostic implications.

The diagnostic modality critical to establishing an accurate diagnosis of ALL is immunophenotyping which includes multicolor flow cytometry and immuno-histochemistry. Multicolor flow cytometry is performed on live cells (i.e., fresh peripheral blood, BM aspirates, BM cores, and unfixed tissues) and is by far the best and most commonly used modality for establishing a diagnosis of ALL. Immunohistochemistry is performed on formalin/B5 fixed BM core biopsies and soft tissue biopsies. A list of commonly used immunophenotypic markers in ALL is

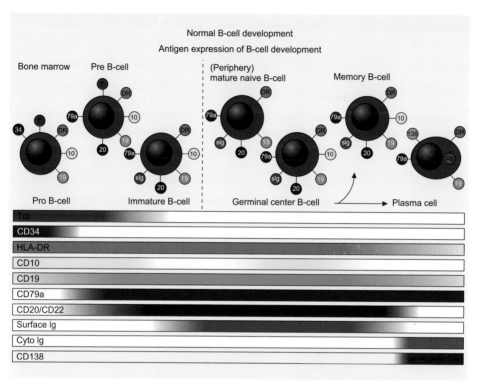

Figure 3-3 Normal B-lymphocyte development. B-cells are derived from the bone marrow and undergo various stages of antigen expression during the course of maturation. The antigens expressed can help differentiate between immature (B-lymphoblasts or hematogones) from mature B-cells. Note the figure depicts the antigenic expression of B-cells during maturation from left to right with the amount of antigen expression reflected by the color intensity (for instance, surface immunoglobulin begins its weak surface expression on immature B-cells and is strongest during the mature and activated stages). *Courtesy:* Dr. John Nguyen, University of California, San Diego.

described in table 3-1. The profile of antigen expression on the leukemic blasts not only helps in establishing the diagnosis of lymphoblastic leukemia but also serves as an important and unique fingerprint for later assessment for minimal residual disease by multicolor flow cytometry (see Chapter 9). B-lymphoblasts express various combinations of antigens including these common antigens: CD10, CD19, cytoplasmic CD22, CD34, CD38, CD45, cytoplasmic CD79a, TdT, PAX5, and HLA-DR (Table 3-1). Of the immunomarkers listed above, expression of CD19, cytoplasmic CD22, and cytoplasmic CD79a in combination or at a high intensity strongly supports B-lineage. CD19 is specific for precursor B lineage and is expressed in 98% of cases. Cytoplasmic CD22 is a highly sensitive marker and is present in nearly

Table 3-1	Commonly Used Immunophenotypic Markers in ALL	
Marker	*Lineage*	*Function*
CD34	Hematopoietic progenitor cells (blasts), endothelial cells, mesenchymal tumors	Intercellular adhesion protein
Terminal deoxynucelotidyl transferase	B- and T-cell blasts, aberrant expression may occur in myeloblasts	DNA polymerase active during immunoglobulin and T-cell gene rearrangement
CD1a	Cortical thymocytes, Langerhans cells	Associated with beta-2 microglobulin
CD99	Not lineage specific (lymphoblastic leukemias, myeloid leukemias, lymphomas, solid tumors)	MIC2 gene product regulating intercellular adhesion molecules
CD3	T-cell (very specific)	Binds to T-cell receptor
CD4	T-cell (helper), monocytes	Interacts with HLA class II
CD8	T-cell (suppressor/cytotoxic)	Recognize antigens displayed by antigen presenting cells
CD2	T-cell, natural killer cell	Signal transduction molecule
CD5	T-cell, naïve B-cells, B-cell lymphomas	Signal transduction molecule
CD7	T-cell (frequent loss in malignancy), natural killer cell, aberrant expression may occur on myeloblasts	T- and B-cell development
CD10	Common ALL antigen; early lymphoid progenitors especially B-ALL, hematogones, germinal center B-cells	Zinc metallopeptidase
CD19	B-cell (early marker)	B-cell development and differentiation
CD20	B-cell (late marker)	Calcium ion channel (proposed)
CD22	B-cell	Inhibits B-cell receptor signaling
CD38	Not lineage specific, activation marker	ADP-ribosyl cyclase 1
CD45	Pan leukocyte antigen (RA = B-cell; RO = myeloid and T-cells)	Tyrosine phosphatase with various isoforms
CD79a	B-cell	Associated with immunoglobulin molecule

ALL, acute lymphoblastic leukemia; CD, cluster of differentiation; HLA, human leukocyte antigen.

Source: Adapted from Dabbs D. Diagnostic Immunohistochemistry, 2nd edition. Philadelphia: Elsevier; 2006.

all cases of precursor B-ALL;[13] CD79a expression although initially thought to be specific for precursor B-ALL, can be seen in some cases of acute myeloid leukemia (AML) and T-ALL.[14] Expression of CD10 is seen in about 90% of cases of precursor B-ALL in children, however, is frequently absent in the majority of infantile ALL as well as adult ALL with MLL gene rearrangement.[12] CD20 is expressed relatively late in B-cell differentiation and is present in approximately 30% of cases. PAX5 is generally considered a specific and sensitive marker for B lineage on tissue sections, however, it is now known that it can be aberrantly expressed on myeloblasts in t(8;21) AML.[14] CD34, a progenitor cell/blast associated antigen, is expressed in 75% of ALL. TdT is useful in differentiating ALL from lymphoproliferative disorders of mature lymphocytes, which are TdT negative. It must be noted that TdT is also expressed in a small subset of normal B-lymphocyte precursors (hematogones), which are commonly found in pediatric as well as regenerating BM and hence is not a specific marker of leukemic blasts. Cytoplasmic immunoglobulin heavy chains (cIg) are present in 20% of precursor B-ALL, but lymphoblasts typically lack surface immunoglobulin expression. Gene rearrangement studies are rarely necessary for the initial diagnosis of B-ALL but may be valuable in the assessment of minimal residual disease. Clonal IgH can be detected in 90% of B-ALLs by polymerase chain reaction (PCR) (see also Chapter 9). Immunophenotypic asynchrony and aberrancy are detected in nearly all cases of B-ALL wherein the lymphoblasts deviate from the normal pattern of antigen expression characteristic of normal B-lymphocyte stages of maturation. B-lymphoblasts coexpress blends of early and late antigens not present on normal B-cell precursors (asynchronous antigen expression) and frequently demonstrate aberrant antigen expression whereby they coexpress one or more myeloid associated antigens, such as CD15, CD13, and CD33 (Figure 3-4). These differences in expression of antigens as well as specific patterns can be very useful in evaluation of follow-up BM specimens for minimal residual disease.

Although antigen expression on lymphoblasts is not an independent prognostic factor, in some instances, their immunoprofile correlates with distinct clinical or cytogenetic subtypes of B-ALL.[15] For example, B-ALL with MLL gene rearrangement typically lacks CD10 expression and is often CD19 positive. Lymphoblasts in B-ALL with t(9;22)(q34;q11.2) typically express CD19, TdT, as well as CD10 and frequently coexpress myeloid associated antigens CD13 and CD33. Correlation of immunophenotype with cytogenetics is further discussed in chapter 5.

Immunophenotype switch occur in about 50–75% of cases of B-ALL at first relapse.[16] These changes include both loss and gain of antigen expression. Major phenotypic switches or lineage switches are rare and when this occurs it is usually due to therapy rather than clonal evolution and these phenotypic shifts have not been reported to affect outcome.[16]

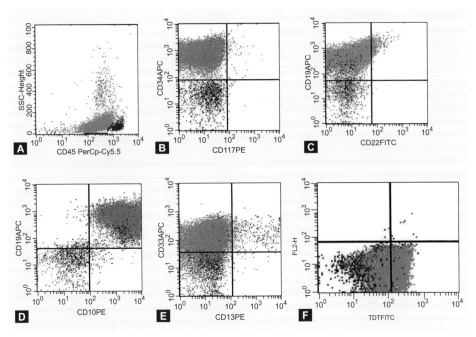

Figure 3-4 B-lymphoblastic leukemia/lymphoma. Flow cytometric immuno-phenotypic studies demonstrate a population of immature B-lymphoid cells (green) that are: **A,** dim CD45 positive; **B,** CD34 positive; **C,** CD19 positive; **D,** CD10 bright positive; **E,** CD33 aberrant positive; and **F,** TdT positive.

Cytogenetics

Cytogenetics plays a pivotal role in ALL diagnosis and has great prognostic and therapeutic implications. The various cytogenetic abnormalities define various categories of B-ALL in the current World Health Organization (WHO) classification.[17] More than 80–90% of precursor B-ALL has demonstrable chromosome abnormalities by conventional cytogenetic analysis and this incidence is even higher when advanced cytogenetic techniques are used to supplement conventional studies.[17] This is further discussed in chapter 5.

Diagnostic Criteria for B-ALL

General consensus dictates that 20% blast count on a manual differential count either on a peripheral blood smear (200 cell leukocyte differential count) or BM aspirate smear (500 cell count) is necessary for a diagnosis of B-ALL.[17] Blast quantitation may also be performed on an adequate BM core biopsy by immunostaining using the CD34 immunostain. In addition, TdT staining will demonstrate lymphoblasts in clusters of more than five cells as compared to hematogones where these TdT-positive cells occur as single cells. Flow cytometry, a valuable tool for qualitative assessment of blasts is generally not recommended for blast enumeration due to the fact that the specimen for flow cytometry may be hemodilute and quantification may be affected by other preanalytical processing variables.[18]

T-LYMPHOBLASTIC LEUKEMIA/LYMPHOMA
Definition

T-lymphoblastic leukemia/lymphoma is a malignant clonal neoplasm of immature T-cells that corresponds to any maturational stage prior to the medullary thymocyte stage of T-cell development. Unlike AML, there is no agreement upon percentage of lymphoblasts that defines T-ALL; however, the general recommendation is that at least 20% lymphoblasts be present for this diagnosis.[17]

Epidemiology

T-lymphoblastic leukemia/lymphoma represents between 15 and 25% of childhood and adult lymphoblastic leukemia/lymphoma, respectively (WHO). This neoplasm is most common during late childhood in male patients who classically presents with a mediastinal mass.[18]

Etiology

The etiology of T-ALL is unknown.

Clinical Features

T-lymphoblastic neoplasms can have a leukemic (T-ALL) or lymphomatous (T-LBL) presentation, both with high tumor burden. T-LBL classically involves the mediastinum and may also involve lymph nodes and extranodal sites, such as skin, tonsil, testes, central nervous system, liver, and spleen.[18,19] Mediastinal involvement may be bulky leading to compression of the regional anatomic structures resulting in symptoms, such as dyspnea, dysphagia, or superior venacaval syndrome.[20] In patients with a leukemic presentation, the white blood cell count is elevated with typically more than 25% BM involvement.[19] Other blood findings include blood cytopenias and bone pain which may present as an initial symptom prior to the development of significant abnormalities in the blood counts.[21]

Morphology

The morphologic characteristics of T-lymphoblasts are not unique as they can mimic B-ALL, AML, lymphoma, and some non-hematolymphoid tumors. T-lymphoblasts can have variable morphology which does not correlate with immunophenotype or clinical behavior. Some blasts can display high nuclear to cytoplasmic ratios, scanty cytoplasm, condensed chromatin, and inconspicuous nucleoli. Other blasts can have more blue-gray cytoplasm, irregular nuclear contours, and multiple nucleoli (Figure 3-5). Cytoplasmic vacuoles may also be occasionally seen.

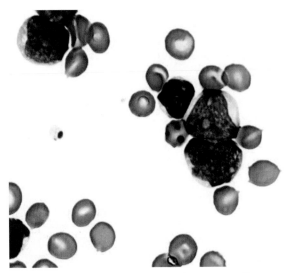

Figure 3-5 Peripheral blood smear illustrates many circulating lymphoblasts from a patient with T-lymphoblastic leukemia/lymphoma. The cells range from medium to large with scant to moderate cytoplasm, convoluted nuclear contours and distinct nucleoli (Wright-Giemsa stain, 1000× magnification).

Bone marrow, when involved by T-ALL, is often hypercellular and shows a diffuse sheet-like proliferation of blasts which can overtake the normal elements of the BM. When T-lymphoblasts involve the lymph nodes or thymus, it presents as either an interfollicular infiltrate or may have a more diffuse pattern of infiltration (Figure 3-6). The mitotic activity can be brisk with tumor cells undergoing apoptosis thus imparting a "starry sky" appearance, mimicking Burkitt lymphoma.[22]

Cytochemistry

Over the years, the role of cytochemistry has diminished as many laboratories utilize flow cytometry and immunohistochemistry as tools to immunophenotype blasts. Some commonly used cytochemistry stains include TdT, MPO, Sudan black, non-specific esterase, alpha naphthyl butyrate, chloroacetate esterase, and PAS.[17] Of these cytochemical stains, TdT may show positive staining in lymphoblasts but it is not unique to lymphoblasts as it can be aberrantly expressed in myeloblasts.

Immunophenotype

Normal T-cell development: T-lymphoblasts are immunophenotypically defined by the expression of T-cell markers corresponding to stages of normal T-cell maturation (Figure 3-7). The earliest stage is the progenitor T-cell (prothymocyte)

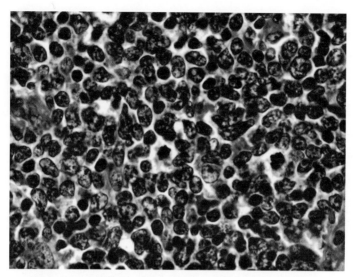

Figure 3-6 Mediastinal mass biopsy section showing diffuse involvement by T-lymphoblasts in a patient with T-lympho-blastic leukemia/lymphoma. The lymphoblasts are closely packed with irregular nuclear contours, finely dispersed chromatin, prominent nucleoli and increased mitotic activity (H&E stain, 1000× magnification).

that resides in the BM and expresses CD34, but is negative for CD3, CD4, and CD8. This T-cell progenitor traverses to the thymus where it undergoes the remainder of its maturation.[17] As a prothymocyte, these cells express CD7—the earliest T-cell marker along with TdT. Within the thymus, the prothymocyte undergoes antigen selection and T-cell receptor (TCR) gene rearrangement as it matures into a T-cell.[23] Cortical thymocytes express CD1a, CD2, CD3, CD5, CD7, and TdT.[24] Initially, cortical thymocytes are negative for both CD4 and CD8 and subsequently become positive for both CD4 and CD8.[24] The expression of CD3 is seen mainly in the cytoplasm but upon complete TCR gene rearrangement, CD3 is expressed on the surface in association with the surface expression of TCR beta.[21] TCR gene rearrangement is a multistep process that begins with gamma and delta genes followed by alpha and beta genes. The cortical thymocyte undergoes positive and negative antigen selection as it enters the thymic medulla where it becomes committed to being either a CD4+ T-cell (helper T-cell) or CD8+ T-cell lineage (cytotoxic T-cell).[21] Medullary thymocytes have an immunophenotype similar to mature T-cells.

As mentioned previously, immunophenotyping of acute leukemia is quintessential and is commonly performed by flow cytometry in conjunction with immunohistochemistry. Markers of immaturity include CD34, CD1a, CD99, and TdT. CD34 is a marker of hematopoietic progenitor cells and is expressed on

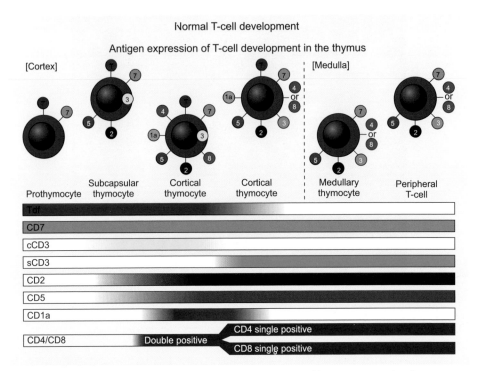

Normal T-cell development

Antigen expression of T-cell development in the thymus

[Cortex]   [Medulla]

Prothymocyte	Subcapsular thymocyte	Cortical thymocyte	Cortical thymocyte	Medullary thymocyte	Peripheral T-cell

| Tdt |
| CD7 |
| cCD3 |
| sCD3 |
| CD2 |
| CD5 |
| CD1a |
| CD4/CD8 | Double positive | CD4 single positive / CD8 single positive |

Figure 3-7 T-cells are derived from the bone marrow and leave to enter the thymus. Various antigens are expressed in the cytoplasm (c) and surface (s) of T-cells as they mature. T-cells with an antigen profile to the left of the dotted line have an immature immunophenotype while those to the right of the dotted line have a mature T-cell immunophenotype. Some markers of immaturity include TdT and CD1a. Note the divergent expression of surface markers CD4 and CD8 on the developing T-cells, they are doubly expressed within the cortex and eventually T-cells become either CD4 positive or CD8 negative. The amount of antigen expression is reflected by the color intensity. *Courtesy*: Dr John Nguyen, University of California, San Diego.

blasts of all lineages. CD1a is a marker of immaturity specific to T-cells as it relates to the cortical thymocyte stage of T-cell maturation. Markers of T-cells include CD2, CD3, CD4, CD5, CD7, and CD8. The coexpression of T-cell markers with an immature phenotype (expression of CD34 and/or TdT) confirms the presence of T-lymphoblasts (Figure 3-8). Of these T-cell markers, only CD3 (cytoplasmic stain) appears to be the most reliable marker specific for T-cell lineage.[17,22] The expression intensity of CD3 is important because rare AMLs have been reported to be CD3 positive, although with weak expression in comparison to the bright CD3 characteristic of T-ALL.[21] Coexpression pattern of CD4 and CD8 particularly with phenotypes CD4+/CD8+ (double positive) or "CD4-/CD8-" (double negative) may also correspond to an immature T-cell of the cortical thymocyte stage and, therefore,

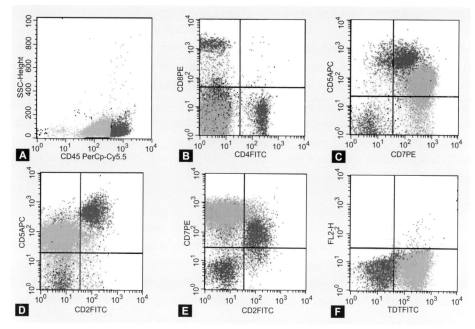

Figure 3-8 T-lymphoblastic leukemia/lymphoma. Flow cytometric studies demonstrate a population of immature T-lymphoid cells that are: **A,** dim CD45 positive (green population); **B,** that are CD4 and CD8 negative; **C,** CD5 dim positive and CD7 positive; **D,** CD5 positive and CD2 negative; **E,** CD7 positive and CD2 negative; and **F,** TdT positive.

represent T-lymphoblasts (Figure 3-8). However, the overall immunophenotype must be taken into consideration as the CD4/CD8 coexpression pattern is not unique to T-ALLs and have been reported in adult T-cell leukemia/lymphoma and T-prolymphocytic leukemia.[25] In certain situations, it might be difficult to distinguish T-ALL from thymocytes within a normal thymus or thymoma. The detection of immunophenotypic aberrancies, best performed through flow cytometry, is critical in such situations. Observing the loss of a pan T-cell marker or the abnormal expression of B-cell or myeloid antigens on the T-cell will support the diagnosis of T-ALL.

Genetics and Molecular Characteristics

Detection of T-cell receptor gene rearrangement by PCR can be performed on T-ALLs. Gene rearrangement studies are often not necessary for initial diagnosis and have greater utility in monitoring minimal residual disease (see Chapter 9). Since T-ALL represents a clonal proliferation of immature T-cells recapitulating various stages of normal T-cell development, molecular studies for TCR gene rearrangement can also show variable TCR loci rearrangement or germline confirmation of TCR.[26] In normal T-cell development, the most immature cells show germline configuration of TCR followed by rearrangements of the TCR loci from delta, gamma, beta, and then alpha. Unless the T-lymphoblasts phenotypically represent the later part of this maturation spectrum, most will have germline configuration of the alpha locus.[21] TCR rearrangements at the gamma locus can be detected in ~96% of T-ALL and may be useful in minimal disease monitoring.[26] However, it is important to keep in mind that T- or B-cell gene rearrangements do not confer lineage assignment as T-lymphoblasts can have rearranged B-cell Ig heavy chain infrequently and conversely B-ALL can have rearranged TCR genes.[26]

Cytogenetics

Unlike AMLs and B-lymphoblastic leukemias, there are no unique cytogenetic abnormalities associated with T-ALL and as such there is no cytogenetically defined T-ALL in the most current edition of the WHO 2008. It was recently recognized that T-ALL associated with eosinophilia are associated with abnormalities of FGFR-1 located on 8p11.[17] This rare and unique entity is currently classified as myeloid and lymphoid neoplasms with eosinophilia and abnormalities of FGFR. Unlike the other hematolymphoid disorders with eosinophilia, T-ALL associated with this abnormality do not respond to tyrosine kinase inhibitors.[27] Cytogenetics of T-ALL is discussed in detail in chapter 5.

DIFFERENTIAL DIAGNOSIS

Numerous non-neoplastic processes may manifest clinical or morphologic features that can show resemblance to ALL. These include lymphocytosis, increased BM hematogones (normal B-cell precursors), metastatic small cell tumors, Burkitt lymphoma, thymomas, and other chronic lymphoproliferative disorders. A few of these common categories are described in detail below.

Hematogones (Normal Bone Marrow B-Lymphocyte Precursors)

Hematogones are normally found in most BM specimens from infants and young children.[28] They are also increased in any condition leading to BM insult including severe infections, malignancies including lymphomas and metastatic tumors, and recovering BM following chemotherapy or hematopoietic stem cell transplantation where they may constitute up to half of nucleated marrow cells. On BM aspirate smears, hematogones are small to medium sized with a nucleus that is usually round to oval with condensed/homogenous chromatin and inconspicuous nucleoli with very scanty cytoplasm that is devoid of inclusions, granules, or vacuoles.[28,29] On BM biopsy sections, hematogones resemble lymphocytes and occur as single cells or tiny clusters. They are often confused for lymphoblasts on morphology, however, the nuclear contours which is usually smooth, with condensed chromatin, and lack of nucleoli would help to tell them apart. Hematogones may circulate in newborns and in umbilical cord blood but do not circulate in adults.[29]

It can be challenging to distinguish between residual B-ALL versus hematogones in post-chemotherapy BM specimens where there can be reactive increase in hemtogones. As hematogones are normally present in the BM of infants and small children, distinguishing increased hematogones from an occult B-ALL presenting without blood cytopenias or organomegaly may represent another potential diagnostic challenge.

Hematogones share a similar immunophenotypic profile with B-lymphoblasts in that both are positive for CD10, CD19, and TdT. However, hematogones can be dependably differentiated from neoplastic lymphoblasts in practically all cases by 3- or 4-color flow cytometry. Hematogones express B-lineage antigens that mimic the normal maturational pattern; this contrast from neoplastic lymphoblasts which demonstrate immunophenotypic asynchrony/aberrancy deviating from the normal B-cell antigen expression pattern.[29,30] In addition, immunohistochemical staining on BM biopsy sections can be helpful by highlighting the distribution of these cells. Hematogones are typically distributed as single cells with minimal small clustering while lymphoblasts typically form dense aggregates. Furthermore, DNA ploidy is normal in hematogones and clonality is not demonstrable by either cytogenetic or molecular analysis. Awareness of the conditions showing hematogone hyperplasia along with a thorough clinical history is important to avoid misinterpretation.

Reactive Lymphocytosis

Some infections can present with a reactive lymphocytosis in young children and may be confused with ALL. These reactive lymphocytes can mimic ALL due to their atypical morphology and may clinically be accompanied by blood cytopenias. This is particularly true in viral infections, such as infectious mononucleosis and *Bordetella pertussis* where children present with a profound lymphocytosis. However, clinical history and careful morphologic evaluation and immunophenotyping by flow cytometry will aid in making the right diagnosis.

Leukemic Phase of Burkitt Lymphoma

The leukemia phase of Burkitt lymphoma can clinically and morphologically mimic ALL presenting with prominent blood and BM involvement. While both these entities express pan B-cell antigens and CD10, Burkitt lymphoma is a mature B-cell lymphoma and, therefore, it expresses surface immunoglobulin and lacks TdT. In addition, detection of the characteristic t(8;14)(p24;q32.3) (MYC/IGH) or variant rearrangements, t(2;8) and t(8;22) by cytogenetics in Burkitt lymphoma aids in establishing the diagnosis as well.

Metastatic Small Cell Tumors

Metastatic small cell tumors may present with extensive BM involvement and may morphologically be indistinguishable from lymphoblasts. In children, these neoplasms include neuroblastoma, Ewing's sarcoma, primitive neuroectodermal tumors, retinoblastoma, medulloblastoma, and embryonal rhabdomyosarcoma. The diagnostic dilemma arises especially when these neoplasms present primarily with BM involvement without obvious extramedullary disease. Immunophenotyping will aid in the distinction of a nonhematolymphoid tumor metastatic to the BM from acute leukemia.

Normal Thymic Tissue and Thymoma

The major differential diagnoses of T-ALL presenting as a mediastinal mass are normal thymic tissue and thymoma. Since both thymic tissue and T-ALL are thymocyte derived, they share a similar immunophenotype. Comprehensive flow cytometry will aid in the detection of phenotypic abnormalities including cross-lineage aberrancy and abnormal maturational coexpression patterns that is not present in normal thymus or thymoma.[31] Cytokeratin staining for thymic epithelial cells is useful for highlighting the epithelial components of thymoma and normal thymus which are absent in T-ALLs.

SUMMARY

Acute lymphoblastic leukemia is an aggressive neoplasm and the diagnosis and treatment decisions have to be made with urgency. Accurate pathologic diagnosis is, therefore, critical for early initiation of appropriate therapy. The diagnosis of ALL requires the integration of clinical history and application of various diagnostic modalities, such as morphologic analysis, detailed immunophenotypic characterization, cytogenetics, and molecular studies. Accurate phenotypic, cyto-genetic, and molecular characterization of the neoplastic cells at diagnosis is critical in determining prognosis as well as monitoring minimal residual disease, a useful tool for tailoring therapy.

REFERENCES

1. Howlader N, Noone AM, Krapcho M, et al. (2011) SEER cancer statistics review, 1975–2008, National Cancer Institute. Bethesda, MD. [online] Available from: seer.cancer.gov/csr/1975_2008/. [Accessed August, 2013].
2. Smith MA, Seibel NL, Altekruse SF, et al. Outcomes for children and adolescents with cancer: challenges for the twenty-first century. *J Clin Oncol*. 2010;28:2625-34.
3. Hann IM, Richards SM, Eden OB, et al. Analysis of the immunophenotype of children treated on the Medical Research Council United Kingdom Acute Lymphoblastic Leukemia Trial XI (MRC UKALLXI). *Leukemia*. 1998;12:1249-55.
4. Fasching K, Panzer S, Haas OA, et al. Presence of clone-specific antigen receptor gene rearrangements at birth indicates an in utero origin of diverse types of early childhood acute lymphoblastic leukemia. *Blood*. 2000;95:2722-4.

5. Mc Neil DE, Cote TR, Clegg L, et al. SEER update of incidence and trends in pediatric malignancies acute lymphoblastic leukemia. *Med Pediatr Oncol.* 2002;39:554-7.
6. Pullarkat ST, Danley K, Bernstein L, et al. High lifetime incidence of adult acute lymphoblastic leukemia among Hispanics in California. *Cancer Epidemiol Biomarkers Prev.* 2009;18:611-5.
7. Borowitz MJ, Croker BP, Metzgar RS. Lymphoblastic lymphoma with the phenotype of common acute lymphoblastic leukemia. *Am J Clin Pathol.* 1983;79:387-91.
8. Ford AM, Bennett CA, Price CM, et al. Fetal origins of the TEL-AML1 fusion gene in identical twins with leukemia. *Proc Natl Acad Sci U S A.* 1998;95:4584-8.
9. Cavani S, Perfumo C, Argusti A, et al. Cytogenetic and molecular study of 32 Down syndrome families: potential leukemia predisposing role of the most proximal segment of chromosome 21q. *Br J Haematol.* 1998;103:213-6.
10. Krajinovic M, Labuda D, Richer C, et al. Susceptibility to childhood acute lymphoblastic leukemia: influence of CYP1A1, CYP2D6, GSTM1, and GSTT1 genetic polymorphisms. *Blood.* 1999;93:1496-501.
11. Klopfenstein KJ, Sommer A, Ruymann FB. Neurofibromatosis-Noonan syndrome and acute lymphoblastic leukemia: a report of two cases. *J Pediatr Hematol Oncol.* 1999;21:158-60.
12. Andersen MK, Christiansen DH, Jensen BA, et al. Therapy-related acute lymphoblastic leukaemia with MLL rearrangements following DNA topoisomerase II inhibitors, an increasing problem: report on two new cases and review of the literature since 1992. *Br J Haematol.* 2001;114:539-43.
13. Boue DR, LeBien TW. Expression and structure of CD22 in acute leukemia. *Blood.* 1988; 71:1480-6.
14. Tiacci E, Pileri S, Orleth A, et al. PAX5 expression in acute leukemias: higher B-lineage specificity than CD79a and selective association with t(8;21)-acute myelogenous leukemia. *Cancer Res.* 2004;64:7399-404.
15. Dabbs D. Diagnostic Immunohistochemistry, 2nd edition. Philadelphia: Elsevier; 2006.
16. Guglielmi C, Cordone I, Boecklin F, et al. Immunophenotype of adult and childhood acute lymphoblastic leukemia: changes at first relapse and clinic-prognostic implications. *Leukemia.* 1997;11:1501-7.
17. Swerdlow S, Campo E, Harris N, et al. WHO Classification of Tumours of Haematopoietic and Lymphoid Tissues, 4th edition. Lyon: IARC; 2008.
18. Reddy KS, Perkins SL. Advances in the diagnostic approach to childhood lymphoblastic malignant neoplasms. *Am J Clin Pathol.* 2004;122:S3-S18.
19. Cairo M, Raetz E, Perkins S. Non-Hodgkin Lymphoma in Children, Cancer Medicine. London: BC Decker Inc; 2006.
20. Racke F, Borowitz M. Precursor B- and T-cell Neoplasms. In: Jaffe E, Harris N, Vardiman J, Campo E, Arber DA, editors. Hematopathology. 1st ed. Philadelphia, PA: Elsevier; 2011. p. 629.
21. Jonsson OG, Sartain P, Ducore JM, et al. Bone pain as an initial symptom to childhood acute lymphoblastic leukemia: association with nearly normal hematologic indexes. *J Pediatr.* 1990;117:233-7.
22. Cortelazzo S, Ponzoni M, Ferreri AJ, et al. Lymphoblastic lymphoma. *Crit Rev Oncol Hematol.* 2011;79:330-43.
23. Dowell BL, Borowitz MJ, Boyett JM, et al. Immunologic and clinicopathologic features of common acute lymphoblastic leukemia antigen-positive childhood T-cell leukemia. A pediatric oncology group study. *Cancer.* 1987;59:2020-6.
24. Crist WM, Shuster JJ, Falletta J, et al. Clinical features and outcome in childhood T-cell leukemia-lymphoma according to stage of thymocyte differentiation: A Pediatric Oncology Group Study. *Blood.* 1988;72:1891-7.

25. Tkachuk D, Hirschmann J. Wintrobe's Atlas of Clinical Hematology, 1st edition. Philadelphia: Lippincott Williams & Wilkins; 2006.

26. Szezepanski T, Langerak AW, Willemse MJ, et al. T cell receptor gamma (*TCRG*) gene rearrangements in T cell acute lymphoblastic leukemia reflect 'end-stage' recombinations: implications for minimal residual disease monitoring. *Leukemia*. 2000;14:1208-14.

27. Chen J, De Angelo DJ, Kutok JL, et al. PKC412 inhibits the zinc finger 198 fibroblast growth factor receptor 1 fusion tyrosine kinase and is active in treatment of stem cell myeloproliferative disorder. *Proc Natl Acad Sci U S A*. 2004;101:14479-84.

28. Longacre TA, Foucar K, Crago S, et al. Hematogones: a multiparameter analysis of bone marrow precursor cells. *Blood*. 1989;73:543-52.

29. Rimsza LM, Larson RS, Winter SS, et al. Benign hematogone-rich lymphoid proliferations can be distinguished from B-lineage acute lymphoblastic leukemia by integration of morphology, immunophenotype, adhesion molecule expression, and architectural features. *Am J Clin Pathol*. 2000;114:66-75.

30. McKenna RW, Washington LT, Aquino DB, et al. Immunophenotypic analysis of hematogones (B-lymphocyte precursors) in 662 consecutive bone marrow specimens by 4-color flow cytometry. *Blood*. 2001;98:2498-507.

31. Tunkel DE, Erozan YS, Weir EG. Ectopic cervical thymic tissue: diagnosis by fine needle aspiration. *Arch Pathol Lab Med*. 2001;125:278-81.

Molecular Pathogenesis of Acute Lymphoblastic Leukemia

Enzi Jiang, Cynthia Hinh, Sajad Khazal, Yong-Mi Kim

INTRODUCTION

Despite much progress in cancer therapy over the last few decades, the overall survival of patients with acute lymphoblastic leukemia (ALL) is about 40% for adults and about 80% for children.[1,2] Although cure rates in children are high, long-term side effects of therapy remain a problem[3,4] and mortality in relapsed ALL is as high as 50–95%,[5] thereby warranting new treatment modalities. Improved therapy can only derive from an advanced understanding of the root causes of ALL. It remains unclear how and why ALL develops. ALL has been well characterized genetically as a heterogenous disease with various recurrent chromosomal translocations described for about 70% of childhood and adult ALL cases leading to deregulation of gene expression, fusion genes, mutations, or changes in chromosome copy number.[6] These chromosomal aberrations are commonly used to divide ALL into subgroups and have critical implications for diagnosis, risk stratification, therapy, and prognosis.[7,8] In B-cell precursor (BCP) ALL, favorable prognosis has been attributed to cytogenetic aberrations, such as hyperdiploidy (HD) (more than 50 chromosomes per leukemia cell) and the TEL-AML1 fusion gene, which occurs in about 50% of childhood cases but only 10% of adult cases. Childhood cases with E2A-rearranged ALL (often E2A-PBX1-positive; ~ 5% of cases) or trisomies 4, 10, and 17 may also be associated with favorable prognosis.[9-12] In contrast, poor prognosis has been described for hypodiploidy (fewer than 45 chromosomes per leukemia cell), found in less than 2% of pediatric or adult cases.[13,14] In addition, unfavorable prognosis has been linked to mixed-lineage leukemia gene *(*MLL*)*-rearrangements, which occurs in approximately 50% of cases in infants, 2% of cases in children, and 5–6% of cases in adults, and the BCR-ABL fusion gene, found in less than 5% of childhood ALL cases and over 20% of adult cases.[15-17] However, fusion proteins resulting from chromosomal translocations on their own are often not sufficient for leukemogenesis indicating that there are cooperating mutations required for overt leukemia. Of note, about 25% of ALL cases lack cytogenetic aberrations but constitute a large number of relapse cases.[18] Recently, mostly through genome-wide analyses, novel genomic alterations have been identified.[19-23] If they are validated in further studies, these novel alterations may require new risk stratification of ALL cases and an adjustment of current therapeutic interventions or the development of new ones.[24] Since pre-B ALL constitutes 85% of ALL cases, we will mostly focus on summarizing the molecular etiology of pre-B ALL. Details of specific cytogenetic alterations and their detection are discussed in detail in chapter 5.

TEL-AML1 (ETV6-RUNX1)

Balanced chromosomal translocations often affect genes that encode transcription factors, which play critical roles in normal hematopoiesis and are associated with hematopoietic malignancies. These chromosomal translocations give rise to fusion genes that act as oncoproteins as they contribute to leukemogenesis and serve as molecular markers for subtypes in ALL. The t(12;21)(p13;q22) chromosomal translocation generates the ETV6-RUNX1 fusion gene, the most common fusion gene in childhood ALLs occurring in about 25% of pediatric ALL cases[25] and in less than 4.4% of adult ALL cases.[26-29] The rearrangement results in the in-frame fusion of the 52 end of the ETS family gene, TEL (ETV6), to almost the entire AML1 (RUNX1) gene at the 32 end that encodes a deoxyribonucleic acid (DNA)-binding subunit of the transcription factor core-binding factor (CBF).[25,30,31] It has been shown that this fusion gene transforms a pre-B ALL cell during fetal hematopoiesis[32-34] into a preleukemic CD34+CD38$^{-/low}$CD19+ cell.[35,36] ETV6-RUNX1+ ALL involves multiple copy number alterations including deletions in genes regulating B-cell differentiation or cell cycling.[37] In addition, TEL-AML1 corrupts hematopoietic stem cells (HSCs) prone to transformation induced by ENU (N-ethyl-N-nitrosourea), a potent but nonspecific mutagen.[38] Although the frequency of children carrying the ETV6-RUNX1 fusion gene is high at birth as determined by the analysis of cord blood spots on Guthrie cards at birth (~1 in 100 newborns), only 1% of these children develop leukemia in their lifetime.[33] This implies that a fusion gene is necessary for leukemogenesis, but is not sufficient to trigger clinical disease, thereby generating the term "second or multiple hits", which are additional postnatal genetic mutation events that are required for overt leukemia.[39] The idea of "second or multiple hits" has been modeled experimentally in both mice and zebrafish suggesting that expression of the ETV6-RUNX1 fusion alone is insufficient for leukemogenesis, which may occur only after acquisition of cooperating mutations.[38,40-46]

The function of the TEL-AML1 fusion gene has recently been investigated using RNA interference (RNAi)[47] or shRNA (short hairpin RNA) to knock down the fusion gene *in vitro*.[48] Such studies have demonstrated that this mutation interferes with the differentiation, apoptosis, and self-renewal of the B-cell lineage during hematopoiesis.[42,49] Silencing the TEL-AML1 gene decreases levels of heat-shock proteins (HSP), such as HSP90 as well as survivin, an inhibitor of apoptosis protein (IAP), and inactivates the phosphoinositide 3-kinase (PI3K)/Akt/mammalian target of rapamycin (mTOR) pathway. On the other hand, ectopic expression of TEL-AML1 in Ba/F3 cells upregulates HSP90 and survivin, indicating the antiapoptotic effect of TEL-AML1[47] pointing to the potential usefulness of targeted therapy in TEL-AML1[+] ALL.[50,51]

HYPERDIPLOIDY

Hyperdiploidy is a form of aneuploidy where the number of chromosomes exceeds 50 (51–67 chromosomes)[52-55] and constitutes about 25–30% of pediatric ALL cases and 9% of adult ALL cases.[56,57] HD is associated with favorable prognosis[8,58,59] and occurs during a single abnormal nondisjunction event. HD may also develop by duplication of an initial near-haploid chromosome set or by the sequential gain of chromosomes during several cell divisions and the consecutive loss of chromosomes after a tetraploidization step.[53] HD may occur *in utero* and is not associated with recurrent structural abnormalities other than nonrandom tri- and tetrasomies of specific chromosomes.[39,60] However, the etiology of HD is unclear. Taketani et al.[61] have identified the receptor tyrosine-kinase FLT3-D835/I836 mutations as one of the second genetic events in infant ALL with MLL rearrangements or pediatric ALL with HD. It has also been demonstrated that FLT3 mutations found in HD patients[62] can be targeted[63] suggesting the benefit of possibly changing current therapies for the subtype of ALL using small-molecule tyrosine-kinase inhibitors.

MIXED-LINEAGE LEUKEMIA

Mixed-lineage leukemia rearrangements occurring in leukemia include MLL fusion genes, partial tandem duplications of MLL and MLL amplification. The MLL gene is located at chromosome 11q23 and about 104 MLL rearrangements have been characterized. About 64 translocation partner genes have been identified that may function as transcriptional factors.[64] The most common fusion partner genes of MLL are AF4, AF9, ENL, AF10, AF6, ELL, and AF1P, in order of frequency. The chromosomal translocation occurring between band 21 of the long arm of chromosome 4 and band 23 of the long arm of chromosome 11 [t(4;11)(q21;q23)], resulting in MLL-AF4, is detected in both pediatric and adult patients diagnosed with pro-B ALL, while fusion with AF9, AF6, or AF10 are commonly found in myelomonocytic or monoblastic acute myeloid leukemia (AML) subtypes.[65] This incidence in ALL has a characteristic bimodal age distribution with a major peak in early infancy, occurring in over 50% of ALL cases in infants aged less than 6 months, in 10–20% of older infants and in about 2% of children. In adults, t(4;11) (q21;q23) occurs in almost 10% of newly diagnosed B-cell ALL patients,[9,66,67] and in about 30–40% of pro-B ALL patients.[68-73]

The underlying mechanism by which the chromosomal translocation t(4;11) (q21;q23) leads to ALL is not clear yet. Epidemiologic associations and molecular analysis of breakpoints suggest an *in utero* origin of the translocations, with reactive metabolites of genotoxic chemicals playing a potential key role.[74-78] Exposure to topoisomerase II inhibitors etoposide, doxorubicin or dietary bioflavonoids can induce cleavage of the MLL gene and result in MLL rearrangement with partner genes, which are speculated to be involved in etiology of infant leukemia.[74,75] The MLL-associated leukemias, along with the hyperdiploid subtype, have been associated with alterations of genes encoding functional metabolic enzymes, indicating a risk of leukemia due to enzymes' substrates or products.[79-81] The development of mouse models with MLL fusion-mediated ALL remains difficult, as the first mouse models resulted in myelodysplasia or mature B-cell lymphomas.[82-84] Krivtsov et al.[85] have suggested a role for MLL partners in leukemogenesis by dysregulating gene expression in leukemic cells using a conditional MLL-AF4 knock-in mouse model. It was shown that the expression of MLL-AF4 in lymphoid cells leads to *in vitro* leukemic transformation, which was associated with an overexpression of HOXA9 and MEIS1 and caused by high H3K4 methyltransferase activity. Since the methyltransferase domain of MLL is invariably lost in MLL-fusion proteins, including MLL-AF4, it was found that MLL-AF4 recruits DOT1L to MLL target genes, and promotes methylation, stimulating transcriptional elongation of genes that are normally primed but not fully transcribed.[85]

Using a murine retroviral model, Faber et al.[86] demonstrated that HOXA9 is required for the survival of leukemic cells in the case of human MLL-rearranged acute leukemia, since it was shown that the suppression of HOXA9 causes apoptosis in cells expressing an MLL-fusion. Hsieh JJ et al.[87] have demonstrated that MLL may regulate HOX gene expression through direct promoter-binding and histone modification. MLL localization and stabilization depend on a proteolytic post-translational process activated by taspase1, a specialized protease that cleaves the MLL protein into N-terminal 320 kD (MLL^n) and C-terminal 180kD (MLL^c) fragments. These fragments are responsible for the transcriptional regulation of specific target genes, including many of the HOX genes regulating normal and malignant hematopoiesis.

Mixed-lineage leukemia fusion partners may interact with several proteins including positive transcription elongation factor b (P-TEFb) and DOT1L, which stimulate the activity of RNA polymerase II to induce leukemogenesis.[88,89] P-TEFb phosphorylates the C-terminal domain of RNA polymerase II (CTD) to cause transcriptional elongation.[90] Yokohama et al.[91] demonstrated that P-TEFb is a part of a core complex termed AF4 family/ENL family/P-TEFb that is physically distinct from the DOT1L complex. It was shown that fusing the P-TEFb-interacting domain of AF4 family members to MLL is necessary and sufficient for leukemic transformation, while DOT1L is not sufficient. Other studies suggest that DOT1L methyltransferase activity is crucial for homeobox (HOX) gene deregulation and transformation seen in leukemias with MLL rearrangements.[92] MLL fusions and amplification upregulate

HOX expression and may, therefore, block hematopoietic differentiation. Thus, development of new therapies for MLL-associated leukemia may target HOX gene upregulation.[93,94]

E2A-PBX1

The second most common translocation in pediatric ALL is t(1;19), which fuses the 5' end of E2A to most of PBX1, yielding a chimeric protein that has cell transformation capability in both *in vitro* and *in vivo* models.[95] E2A-PBX1 represents 5% of childhood and adult ALL and occurs in about 25% of the pre-B cell (CD10$^+$, CD19$^+$, CD34$^-$, cIgµ$^+$, and sIgµ$^-$) leukemia.[96]

However, the underlying mechanism by which this genetic rearrangement results in leukemia is unclear. E2A-PBX1 leukemias have germline-rearranged immunoglobulin (Ig) heavy chain (IGH) rearrangements like most leukemias of B-cell origin.[97] The characteristics of the leukemic IGH CDR3 region distinguish early (prenatal) from later (postnatal) development of normal lymphocytes as well as various ALL subtypes.[98-100] Wiemels et al.[101] have demonstrated that the presence of extensive N-nucleotides at the point of fusion in the E2A-PBX1 translocation as well as specific characteristics of the IGH/T-cell receptor (TCR) rearrangements pointing to a postnatal, pre-B cell origin.

BCR-ABL1/BCR-ABL1-LIKE

The t(9;22) translocation, or the Philadelphia (Ph) chromosome, is the result of the reciprocal translocation between chromosomes 9 (region q34) and 22 (region q11). The resulting fusion of the BCR (breakpoint cluster region) signaling protein to the ABL1 (Abelson) nonreceptor tyrosine kinase leads to constitutive tyrosine-kinase activity that is essential for BCR-ABL leukemogenesis and interaction with other signaling pathways involved in cell differentiation, proliferation, and survival [e.g., RAS, SHP2 (Src homology protein tyrosine phosphatase 2), Jun N-terminal protein kinase (JNK), SRC, and PI3K-AKT pathway].[102,103] The Ph chromosome is found in more than 95% of patients with chronic myelogenous leukemia (CML),[104] in 20–40% of adult and 2–10% of pediatric patients with ALL,[105,106] and in 1–2% of patients with AML.[107,108] The product of the BCR-ABL oncogene, exists in three isoforms (P190, P210, and P230 BCR-ABL) that are found in distinct types of Ph-positive (Ph$^+$) leukemia, suggesting that the three oncoproteins have different leukemogenic activity. P190 BCR-ABL is characterized by higher transforming activity, inducing mainly ALL with shorter latency than P210, which is generally associated with CML, or P230, which is associated with chronic neutrophilic leukemia. The more aggressive acute lymphoid leukemias—with a particularly more unfavorable prognosis than CML[109]—have provirus integration patterns that are limited to malignant cells, suggesting a B lineage-restricted target cell with a requirement for gene lesions in addition to BCR-ABL transduction for full malignant transformation and progression.[103,110,111]

A frequently occurring cooperating lesion with BCR-ABL1 is the deletion of the IKZF1 locus on 7p12, encoding the nuclear zinc-finger transcription factor IKAROS required for early B-cell differentiation.[112,113] IKZF1 deletion results in haploinsufficiency, homozygous loss, or expression of dominant-negative IKAROS isoforms, which interferes with the activity of functional isoforms that bind to DNA.[114,115] IZKF1 alteration is a hallmark of Ph⁺ ALL with BCR-ABL1 fusion, but it is also expressed in Ph⁻ ALL.[113,116,117] In a study done by Cazzaniga et al.[118] on two pairs of monozygotic twins bearing the same clonotype of BCR-ABL1 fusion gene, one pair was concordant, the other disconcordant for childhood Ph⁺ ALL, it was suggested that fetal origin of BCR-ABL1 and postnatal genetic mutation events are required for the onset of ALL (e.g., IKZF1). One twin with ALL and an IKZF1 deletion died of isolated BM relapse after transplantation, while the other twin with HD but no IKZF1 deletion is still in remission 8 years after transplantation, suggesting that IKZF1 deletion is secondary to BCR-ABL1 and accelerates BCR-ABL1-driven leukemogenesis.[118] A genome-wide analysis of leukemia samples taken at diagnosis from 304 patients with ALL, including 43 BCR-ABL1 B-progenitor ALLs and 23 CML cases,[116] showed that IKZF1 was deleted in 83.7% of BCR-ABL1 ALL, but not in chronic-phase CML. However, similar deletion of IKZF1 was also identified as an acquired lesion during lymphoid blast crisis at the time of conversion of CML to ALL.[116] Sequencing of IKZF1 deletion breakpoints suggested that aberrant RAG (recombination-activating gene)-mediated V(D)J recombination is related to the deletions.[113,119] These findings suggest that the loss of IKAROS function by IKZF1 gene deletion is a crucial event in the development of BCR-ABL1 ALL.

Interestingly, *BCR-ABL1*-negative cases commonly exhibit a gene expression profile similar to BCR-ABL1-positive ALL, and are thus referred to as "BCR-ABL1/Ph-like ALL".[120,121] Den Boer et al.[120] showed that these BCR-ABL-like cases represent 15–20% of ALL cases and have a highly unfavorable outcome compared to other precursor B-ALL cases, similar to the poor prognosis of *BCR-ABL*-positive ALL. BCR-ABL1-like leukemic cells were found to be more resistant to selected chemotherapeutic agents, such as L-asparaginase and daunorubicin compared to other precursor B-ALL cases, although less resistant to prednisolone and vincristine.[120] Several studies have identified, using genome-wide analyses and single nucleotide polymorphism (SNP) array analysis, genetic alterations targeting transcriptional regulators of lymphoid development including PAX5, EBF1 and IKZF1 in over 60% of B-ALL patients.[20,120-123]

Similar to BCR-ABL1-positive ALL, IZKF1 alteration is also associated with poor outcome in BCR-ABL1-negative ALL.[120,121,124] The fact that IKZF1-mutated, BCR-ABL1-negative cases have a similar gene expression profile to BCR-ABL1-positive

ALL[120,121] may have critical therapeutic consequences, as Ph-like ALL patients if identified at diagnosis may benefit from the addition of tyrosine-kinase inhibitor treatment to current chemotherapeutic regimens. Approximately 50% of Ph-like patients harbor rearrangements of CRLF2 (CRLF2r),[125] with concomitant Janus kinase (JAK) mutations detected in approximately 50% of *CRLF2*r cases.[121,126-128] However, the underlying mechanism and specific genetic alterations responsible for activated kinase signaling in the remaining Ph-like cases are unknown. Using transcriptome and whole genome sequencing on 15 cases of Ph-like ALL, Roberts et al.[23] identified rearrangements involving ABL1, JAK2, PDGFRB, CRLF2 and EPOR, activating mutations of IL7R and FLT3, as well as deletion of SH2B3, which encodes the JAK2-negative regulator LNK. Importantly, some of these rearrangements induce transformation that is attenuated with tyrosine-kinase inhibitors, suggesting that such patients may benefit from kinase inhibitor therapy.

CREB-BINDING PROTEIN

The Wnt pathway has been implicated in the self-renewal and differentiation of normal hematopoietic stem/progenitor cells.[129-131] Aberrant Wnt/β-catenin signaling has been shown to play critical roles in AML cells[132] and CML cells,[133,134] and leukemic drug-resistant clones are associated with increased nuclear β-catenin levels.[135] However, less is known about the role of Wnt/β-catenin signaling in ALL. Wnt/β-catenin-signaling has been described as dispensable for BCR-ABL1 B-cell lineage leukemia.[136] In one ALL subtype, endogenous Wnt16b expression is upregulated by the E2A-PBX1 leukemogenic fusion gene.[137] siRNA knockdown of Wnt16b, which decreases canonical Wnt/β-catenin signaling, has been shown to initiate apoptosis and reduce the expression of the Wnt-regulated inhibitor of apoptosis protein family member, survivin (BIRC5),[138] implicated in both the survival and drug resistance of leukemia cells.[138,139] In addition, it has been noted that Wnt-3a mediates the proliferation of precursor B-ALL.[140] The Wnt pathway is classically mediated through the central signaling effector molecule β-catenin.[141] Recently, novel sequence or deletion mutations of CBP (CREB-binding protein), a transcriptional coactivator recruited by β-catenin, have been identified at diagnosis and relapse of ALL.[142-144] Interestingly, of the hundreds of sequenced samples, most occurred within the HAT domain while only one of these mutations was found in the extreme N-terminus of CBP.[144]

A variety of ways to inhibit Wnt signaling are under investigation for other hematological malignancies,[145-147] β-catenin has been targeted using nonsteroidal anti-inflammatory drugs (NSAIDs),[148] PKF115-584 in multiple myeloma,[149,150] or AV65 in CML cells.[151] However, ICG-001 and its second generation clinical compound PRI-724 are the only well-characterized small molecule-inhibitors that bind specifically to a small region in the N-terminal of the CBP cofactor (region 1–110) thereby blocking its interaction with the C-terminal β-catenin coactivation domain (region 647–781) and leaving the rest of the large CBP protein (300 kDa) functionally active.[152] In addition, and of critical importance to its therapeutic utility, despite the close homology of CBP and p300, the specificity of ICG-001 avoids interference with p300/catenin-dependent signaling,[152] thereby allowing for normal cellular differentiation and maintenance of normal stem cell populations.[153]

PAX5

The highly conserved paired-box (PAX) domain family of transcription factors is involved in cell differentiation. Among them, PAX5 on chromosome 9p13, a master regulator of B-cell development, is the only PAX family member expressed in the hematopoietic system and its expression occurs during pro-B to pre-B cell transition and persists until B-cells differentiate into plasma cells.[154-157] PAX5 has a dual function in both fetal and adult B lymphopoiesis, through which it represses lineage-inappropriate genes (e.g., NOTCH1) while activating B-lymphoid-specific genes (e.g., SLP-65).[157-159]

Interestingly, in a genome-wide analysis of 242 pediatric ALL cases, PAX5 was found to be altered in 31.7% of cases such that the mutant PAX5 encoded proteins lacked the DNA-binding domain and/or transcriptional domains, resulting in a loss of function.[20] The analysis of PAX5 in 117 adult BCP (B-cell progenitor)-ALL patients in the protocol Group for Research on Adult Acute Lymphoblastic Leukemia (GRAALL)-2003/GRAAPH-2003 revealed mutations in 34% of adult pre-B-ALL cases that involved partial or complete deletion, partial or complete amplification, point mutation, or fusion genes.[160] PAX5 alterations occur heterogeneously, consisting of complete loss in 17%, focal deletions in 10%, point mutations in 7% and translocations in 1% of the cases.[160] In a study of 89 adults with BCR-ABL1-positive ALL, Iacobucci I et al.[161] detected PAX5 genomic deletions in 29 patients (33%) with the extent of deletions ranging from a complete loss of chromosome 9 to the loss of a subset of exons. It was suggested that deletions are the main mechanism of inactivation of PAX5 in BCR-ABL1-positive ALL since in contrast to BCR-ABL1-negative ALL, no PAX5 point mutations were found.[161] Genomic analysis of 40 childhood ALL cases identified the most frequently affected genes as those controlling G1/S cell cycle progression (e.g., CDKN2A, CDKN1B and RB1), followed by genes associated with B-cell development, including microdeletions of the B-lineage transcription factor genes PAX5, EBF, E2-2, and IKZF1.[122]

In addition to PAX5 loss-of-function mutations, PAX5 rearrangements are present in 2.6% of BCP ALL.[162] PAX5-TEL was the first reported translocation, resulting in a novel chimeric transcription factor by the fusion of the N-terminal of the DNA-binding domain (DBD) of PAX5 to almost the entire TEL transcription factor encompassing the helix-loop-helix and DBDs.[163] To date, 17 different PAX5 fusion partners have been identified, indicating variability of rearrangements. Among them, the most frequently observed rearrangements include PAX5-ETV6[164] and PAX5-C20orf112,[165] followed by PAX5-ELN, PAX5-FOXP1, and PAX5-JAK2.[162,166-168] All these fusion proteins contain the N-terminal DBD domain (paired domain) but lack the C-terminal transactivation domain (TAD) of PAX5.[165,169] They are thus associated with leukemogenesis as potent dominant-negative inhibitors of wild-type PAX5 by blocking PAX5-dependent B-cell differentiation.[167,170] Some PAX5 fusion partners are indeed transcriptional repressors (e.g., ETV6) and resulting fusion proteins may function as constitutive repressors during B-cell development.[20,167] Notably, it was found that abnormalities of PAX5 copy number or detection of PAX5 fusion failed to act as a predictor of poor outcome in children with high-risk B-cell-progenitor ALL.[121,171]

PRENATAL ORIGIN OF LEUKEMIA

There is compelling evidence that some common chromosome translocations that are seen in pediatric leukemia often originate prenatally *in utero* during fetal hematopoiesis.[39] Screening of neonatal cord-blood samples has revealed a putative leukemic clone with the TEL-AML1 (ETV6-RUNX1) fusion gene in 1% of newborn babies, a frequency 100 times higher than the prevalence of ALL defined by this fusion gene later in childhood.[52] Infant ALL is a biologically and clinically distinct disease from childhood ALL. It would be more appropriate to consider concordance rates separately for infant versus childhood ALL. In twins with infant leukemia, the concordance rate seems to be close to 100% for those with a shared placenta. For acute leukemia in older children, the twin concordance rate is approximately 10%.[172] TEL-AML1 fusion gene is an acquired or nonconstitutive leukemia clone-specific genetic abnormality thought to be critically involved in the pathogenesis of childhood common ALL. The presence of this gene at birth is direct evidence that this disease can originate *in utero*. This conclusion applies to the subset of patients with common ALL who have TEL-AML1 fusion gene, but it may also be true for ALLs that are of the same cell type (B-cell precursor) and age distribution, but that have other molecular abnormalities, including HD.[32] Evidence for an *in utero* initiation of this important genetic event in ALL is available from blood spots but remains limited.[60] Maia et al. described a pair of 2-year-old monozygotic twins with concordant BCP ALL and hyperdiploid karyotypes based on sharing of chromosomal gains and identical TCRD and IGH genomic sequences.[60] Evidence to support the "intraplacental metastasis" idea has been provided by an international study of concordant twin cases of leukemia. This used the unique genomic breakpoints in chromosome translocations for MLL fusions and TEL-AML1 and IGH and TCR clonotypic rearrangements. In each twin pair investigated, their leukemic cells were found to share the same fusion gene sequence or IGH/TCR sequences. These acquired, nonconstitutive clonal events are shared by each pair of twins pointing to the possibility of a single-cell origin followed by metastasis.[39]

NOTCH SIGNALING IN T-LINEAGE ALL

T-ALL occurs in 10–15% of pediatric and in 25% of adult ALL cases current therapies achieve 5-year relapse-free survival rates of about 75% in pediatric and 50% in adult patients.[173,174] Drug resistance remains a main problem for T-ALL, as the outcome for patients with relapse of the disease is poor.[175,176] Over 50% of T-ALLs harbor activating mutations in the NOTCH signaling pathway making NOTCH1 the most prominent T-ALL specific oncogene and defining T-ALL as a disease primarily characterized by aberrant NOTCH1 activation.[177] Over 70% of T-ALL patients have deletions of cyclin-dependent kinase inhibitor 2A (CDKN2A),[178,179] which is located in the short arm of chromosome 9 encompassing tumor suppressor genes p16INK4A and p14ARF. Therefore, oncogenic T-cell transformation is associated with constitutive activation of NOTCH signaling and loss of p16INK4A and p14AR.

Four NOTCH genes (NOTCH 1–4) have been described in mammals, which encode unusual type I transmembrane receptors composed of a characteristic series of iterated structural motifs.[180] Newly synthesized NOTCH receptors are proteolytically cleaved in the Golgi apparatus during their transport to the cell surface by a furin-like protease. This cleavage generates a heterodimeric receptor consisting of an extracellular subunit (N^{EC}) that is non-covalently linked to a second subunit containing the extracellular heterodimerization domain and the trans-membrane domain followed by cytoplasmic region of the NOTCH receptor (N^{TM}). The extracellular part of the receptors contains 29–36 epidermal growth factor-like repeats involved in ligand binding, followed by three cysteine-rich LIN12 repeats that prevent ligand-independent activation and hydrophobic stretch of amino acids mediating heterodimerization between N^{EC} and N^{TM} [2]. The cytoplasmic tail of the receptor harbors multiple conserved elements including nuclear localization signals, as well as protein-protein interaction and transactivation domains including the C-terminal PEST (rich in proline, glutamic acid E, serine, and threonine domain that regulates the intracellular portion of NOTCH1). Activation of NOTCH signaling is ligand mediated (delta like 1, 3 and 4 and jagged 1 and 2). When NOTCH ligand binds to N^{EC} receptor on an adjacent cell, conformational changes will occur within the NOTCH receptors to express the S2 cleavage site for proteolysis mediated by ADAM10 metalloprotease. After shedding of the extracellular domain, a second cleavage within the transmembrane domain (at site S3) is mediated by the γ-secretase activity of a multiprotein complex.[181] A series of proteolytic cleavages occurs resulting in release of the NOTCH intracellular domain that subsequently translocates into the nucleus and binds to CBF1 and with cofactors of the mastermind-like (MAML) family that result in the formation of tertiary complex that functions as transcriptional activator which increases the expression of various NOTCH target genes including those belonging to the HES, MYC, and HRT (HEY) families.[182] Termination of NOTCH1 signaling occurs following phosphorylation of the C-terminal PEST domain of the receptor, which leads to the recruitment of the FBXW7/SCF ubiquitin ligase to the transcriptional complex and triggers the polyubiquitination and proteasomal degradation of intracellular NOTCH1 (ICN1).[180]

NOTCH signaling appears to play diverse roles in different malignancies, effecting differentiation, metastasis, cancer "stem cells", and angiogenesis.[183] Analysis of patient samples with T-ALL has revealed a chromosomal translocation, t(7;9)(q34:q34.3), that juxtapose the coding region of the C-terminal domain of epidermal growth factor (EGF) repeat 34 of the human NOTCH1 gene adjacent to the TCR-β locus enhancer. This translocation results in the expression of a truncated constitutively active NOTCH1 protein referred to as translocation-associated NOTCH1 (TAN1). Less than 1% of human T-ALLs exhibit the t(7;9) translocation. The proof that TAN1 is indeed causative for T-cell ALL development was shown by murine bone marrow (BM) reconstitution experiments. Mice transplanted with BM progenitors expressing TAN1 developed T cell neoplasms as early as 2 weeks after BM transplantation.[184] Aster and colleagues analyzed 96 pediatric primary T-ALL tumors and found that 55% of the samples had at least one mutation in the HD (heterodimerization) or the PEST domain within the NOTCH1 gene, with approximately 20% of the tumors having a mutation in both domains.[185] Mutations within the HD domain render NOTCH1 susceptible to ligand-independent S2 cleavage.[186] Mutations and/or deletions of the PEST domain stabilize the ICN1 protein.[187] Additionally, mutations in FBXW7 are present in 8.6% of primary T-ALL cases, and similar to NOTCH1 PEST domain mutations, impair the proteasomal degradation of ICN1.[188,189]

The high frequency of NOTCH mutations in T-ALL led to the growing field of anti-NOTCH1-targeted therapies for the treatment of T-ALL. Gamma-secretase inhibitors (GSI), which block the proteolytic cleavage of the NOTCH receptors and preclude the release of ICN1 from the membrane, have been proposed as a potential targeted therapy in T-ALL. GSIs are nonspecific and block the function of all four NOTCH family members, however, may result in gastrointestinal toxicity.[190] Another strategy for inhibiting NOTCH signaling explored by Bradner and colleagues aims at inhibiting the NOTCH transcription complex with small alpha helical peptides, and thereby blocks the intracellular protein-protein interaction. Treatment of leukemic cells with such a peptide resulted in the suppression of the NOTCH-activated transcriptome. The peptide inhibited the proliferation of leukemic cells *in vitro* as well as in a NOTCH1 driven T-ALL mouse model without causing gut toxicity (which is the major side effect of GSI).[191]

SUMMARY

Although the full etiology of ALL remains unclear, chromosomal aberrations can be analyzed and used to divide ALL into subtypes. These ALL subtypes dictate additional diagnostic evaluation, treatment choice, and prognostic stratification. However, 25% of cases still have no described cytogenetic aberrations and constitute a large number of relapsed cases. Chromosomal aberrations alone are often not sufficient to cause leukemogenesis as described for some leukemia subtypes including TEL-AML1. Only a better understanding of the molecular pathogenesis through mutational analysis of genes along with an improved knowledge of their biological functions will allow us to develop truly novel and improved therapies. Novel therapies specifically tailored to target key molecular alterations are on the way and should improve the outcome of ALL therapy.

REFERENCES

1. Larson S, Stock W. Progress in the treatment of adults with acute lymphoblastic leukemia. *Curr Opin Hematol.* 2008;15(4):400-7.
2. Faderl S, O'Brien S, Pui CH, et al. Adult acute lymphoblastic leukemia: concepts and strategies. *Cancer.* 2010;116(5):1165-76.
3. Pui CH, Evans WE. Treatment of acute lymphoblastic leukemia. *N Engl J Med.* 2006;354(2): 166-78.
4. Robison LL, Bhatia S. Late-effects among survivors of leukaemia and lymphoma during childhood and adolescence. *Br J Haematol.* 2003;122(3):345-59.
5. Gaynon PS, Trigg ME, Heerema NA, et al. Children's Cancer Group trials in childhood acute lymphoblastic leukemia: 1983-1995. *Leukemia.* 2000;14(12):2223-33.
6. Teitell MA, Pandolfi PP. Molecular genetics of acute lymphoblastic leukemia. *Annu Rev Pathol.* 2009;4:175-98.
7. Gilliland DG. Molecular genetics of human leukemias: new insights into therapy. *Semin Hematol.* 2002;39(4 Suppl 3):6-11.
8. Armstrong SA, Look AT. Molecular genetics of acute lymphoblastic leukemia. *J Clin Oncol.* 2005;23(26):6306-15.
9. Pui CH, Relling MV, Downing JR. Acute lymphoblastic leukemia. *N Engl J Med.* 2004; 350(15):1535-48.
10. Pieters R, Carroll WL. Biology and treatment of acute lymphoblastic leukemia. *Pediatr Clin North Am.* 2008;55(1):1-20.
11. Pui CH, Raimondi SC, Hancock ML, et al. Immunologic, cytogenetic, and clinical characterization of childhood acute lymphoblastic leukemia with the t(1;19) (q23; p13) or its derivative. *J Clin Oncol.* 1994;12(12):2601-6.
12. Pieters R, Schrappe M, De Lorenzo P, et al. A treatment protocol for infants younger than 1 year with acute lymphoblastic leukaemia (Interfant-99): an observational study and a multicentre randomised trial. *Lancet.* 2007;370(9583):240-50.
13. Ramos ML, Palacios JJ, Fournier BG, et al. Prognostic value of tumoral ploidy in a series of spanish patients with acute lymphoblastic leukemia. *Cancer Genet Cytogenet.* 2000;122(2):124-30.
14. Nachman JB, Heerema NA, Sather H, et al. Outcome of treatment in children with hypodiploid acute lymphoblastic leukemia. *Blood.* 2007;110(4):1112-5.
15. Dombret H, Gabert J, Boiron JM, et al. Outcome of treatment in adults with Philadelphia chromosome-positive acute lymphoblastic leukemia—results of the prospective multicenter LALA-94 trial. *Blood.* 2002;100(7):2357-66.

16. Gao C, Zhao XX, Li WJ, et al. Clinical features, early treatment responses, and outcomes of pediatric acute lymphoblastic leukemia in China with or without specific fusion transcripts: a single institutional study of 1,004 patients. *Am J Hematol.* 2012;87(11):1022-7.

17. Abdulwahab A, Sykes J, Kamel-Reid S, et al. Therapy-related acute lymphoblastic leukemia is more frequent than previously recognized and has a poor prognosis. *Cancer.* 2012;118(16): 3962-7.

18. Möricke A, Reiter A, Zimmermann M, et al. Risk-adjusted therapy of acute lymphoblastic leukemia can decrease treatment burden and improve survival: treatment results of 2169 unselected pediatric and adolescent patients enrolled in the trial ALL-BFM 95. *Blood.* 2008; 111(9):4477-89.

19. Pui CH, Mulligan CG, Evans WE, et al. Pediatric acute lymphoblastic leukemia: where are we going and how do we get there? *Blood.* 2012;120(6):1165-74.

20. Mulligan CG, Goorha S, Radtke I, et al. Genome-wide analysis of genetic alterations in acute lymphoblastic leukaemia. *Nature.* 2007;446(7137):758-64.

21. Mulligan CG. New strategies in acute lymphoblastic leukaemia: translating advances in genomics into clinical practice. *Clin Cancer Res.* 2011;17(3):396-400.

22. Mulligan CG, Zhang J, Kasper LH, et al. CREBBP mutations in relapsed acute lymphoblastic leukaemia. *Nature.* 2011;471(7337):235-9.

23. Roberts KG, Morin RD, Zhang J, et al. Genetic alterations activating kinase and cytokine receptor signaling in high-risk acute lymphoblastic leukemia. *Cancer Cell.* 2012;22(2):153-66.

24. Pui CH, Carroll WL, Meshinchi S, et al. Biology, risk stratification, and therapy of pediatric acute leukemias: an update. *J Clin Oncol.* 2011;29(5):551-65.

25. Shurtleff SA, Buijs A, Behm FG, et al. TEL/AML1 fusion resulting from a cryptic t(12;21) is the most common genetic lesion in pediatric ALL and defines a subgroup of patients with an excellent prognosis. *Leukemia.* 1995;9(12):1985-9.

26. Aguiar RC, Sohal J, van Rhee F, et al. TEL-AML1 fusion in acute lymphoblastic leukaemia of adults. M.R.C Adult Leukaemia Working Party. *Br J Haematol.* 1996;95(4):673-7.

27. Burmeister T, Gökbuget N, Schwartz S, et al. Clinical features and prognostic implications of TCF3-PBX1 and ETV6-RUNX1 in adult acute lymphoblastic leukemia. *Haematologica.* 2010;95(2):241-6.

28. Lee DS, Kim YR, Cho HK, et al. The presence of TEL/AML1 rearrangement and cryptic deletion of the TEL gene in adult acute lymphoblastic leukemia (ALL). *Cancer Genet Cytogenet.* 2005;162(2):176-8.

29. Jabber Al-Obaidi MS, Martineau M, Bennett CF, et al. ETV6/AML1 fusion by FISH in adult acute lymphoblastic leukemia. *Leukemia.* 2002;16(4):669-74.

30. Romana SP, Mauchauffé M, Le Coniat M, et al. The t(12;21) of acute lymphoblastic leukemia results in a tel-AML1 gene fusion. *Blood.* 1995;85(12):3662-70.

31. Wiemels JL, Greaves M. Structure and possible mechanisms of TEL-AML1 gene fusions in childhood acute lymphoblastic leukemia. *Cancer Res.* 1999;59(16):4075-82.

32. Wiemels JL, Cazzaniga G, Daniotti M, et al. Prenatal origin of acute lymphoblastic leukaemia in children. *Lancet.* 1999;354(9189):1499-503.

33. Mori H, Colman SM, Xiao Z, et al. Chromosome translocations and covert leukemic clones are generated during normal fetal development. *Proc Natl Acad Sci U S A.* 2002;99(12):8242-7.

34. Ford AM, Bennett CA, Price CM, et al. Fetal origins of the TEL-AML1 fusion gene in identical twins with leukemia. *Proc Natl Acad Sci U S A.* 1998;95(8):4584-8.

35. Hong D, Gupta R, Ancliff P, et al. Initiating and cancer-propagating cells in TEL-AML1-associated childhood leukemia. *Science.* 2008;319(5861):336-9.

36. Ford AM, Palmi C, Bueno C, et al. The TEL-AML1 leukemia fusion gene dysregulates the TGF-beta pathway in early B lineage progenitor cells. *J Clin Invest.* 2009;119(4):826-36.

37. Bateman CM, Colman SM, Chaplin T, et al. Acquisition of genome-wide copy number alterations in monozygotic twins with acute lymphoblastic leukemia. *Blood.* 2010;115(17):3553-8.

38. Schindler JW, Van Buren D, Foudi A, et al. TEL-AML1 corrupts hematopoietic stem cells to persist in the bone marrow and initiate leukemia. *Cell Stem Cell.* 2009;5(1):43-53.

39. Greaves MF, Wiemels J. Origins of chromosome translocations in childhood leukaemia. *Nat Rev Cancer.* 2003;3(9):639-49.

40. Higuchi M, O'Brien D, Kumaravelu P, et al. Expression of a conditional AML1-ETO oncogene bypasses embryonic lethality and establishes a murine model of human t(8;21) acute myeloid leukemia. *Cancer Cell.* 2002;1(1):63-74.

41. Bernardin F, Yang Y, Cleaves R, et al. TEL-AML1, expressed from t(12;21) in human acute lymphocytic leukemia, induces acute leukemia in mice. *Cancer Res.* 2002;62(14):3904-8.

42. Tsuzuki S, Seto M, Greaves M, et al. Modeling first-hit functions of the t(12;21) TEL-AML1 translocation in mice. *Proc Natl Acad Sci U S A.* 2004;101(22):8443-8.

43. Fischer M, Schwieger M, Horn S, et al. Defining the oncogenic function of the TEL/AML1 (ETV6/RUNX1) fusion protein in a mouse model. *Oncogene.* 2005;24(51):7579-91.

44. Sabaawy HE, Azuma M, Embree LJ, et al. TEL-AML1 transgenic zebrafish model of precursor B cell acute lymphoblastic leukemia. *Proc Natl Acad Sci U S A.* 2006;103(41):15166-71.

45. van der Weyden L, Giotopoulos G, Rust AG, et al. Modeling the evolution of ETV6-RUNX1-induced B-cell precursor acute lymphoblastic leukemia in mice. *Blood.* 2011;118(4):1041-51.

46. Zelent A, Greaves M, Enver T. Role of the TEL-AML1 fusion gene in the molecular pathogenesis of childhood acute lymphoblastic leukaemia. *Oncogene.* 2004;23(24):4275-83.

47. Diakos C, Krapf G, Gerner C, et al. RNAi-mediated silencing of TEL/AML1 reveals a heat-shock protein- and survivin-dependent mechanism for survival. *Blood.* 2007;109(6):2607-10.

48. Fuka G, Kantner HP, Grausenburger R, et al. Silencing of ETV6/RUNX1 abrogates PI3K/AKT/mTOR signaling and impairs reconstitution of leukemia in xenografts. *Leukemia.* 2012; 26(5):927-33.

49. Morrow M, Horton S, Kioussis D, et al. TEL-AML1 promotes development of specific hematopoietic lineages consistent with preleukemic activity. *Blood.* 2004;103(10):3890-6.

50. Mosad E, Hamed HB, Bakry RM, et al. Persistence of TEL-AML1 fusion gene as minimal residual disease has no additive prognostic value in CD 10 positive B-acute lymphoblastic leukemia: a FISH study. *J Hematol Oncol.* 2008;1:17.

51. Fuka G, Kauer M, Kofler R, et al. The leukemia-specific fusion gene ETV6/RUNX1 perturbs distinct key biological functions primarily by gene repression. *PLoS One.* 2011;6(10):e26348.

52. Pui CH, Robison LL, Look AT. Acute lymphoblastic leukaemia. *Lancet.* 2008;371(9617): 1030-43.

53. Paulsson K, Johansson B. High hyperdiploid childhood acute lymphoblastic leukemia. *Genes Chromosomes Cancer.* 2009;48(8):637-60.

54. Ito C, Kumagai M, Manabe A, et al. Hyperdiploid acute lymphoblastic leukemia with 51 to 65 chromosomes: a distinct biological entity with a marked propensity to undergo apoptosis. *Blood.* 1999;93(1):315-20.

55. Heerema NA, Raimondi SC, Anderson JR, et al. Specific extra chromosomes occur in a modal number dependent pattern in pediatric acute lymphoblastic leukemia. *Genes Chromosomes Cancer.* 2007;46(7):684-93.

56. Liang DC, Shih LY, Yang CP, et al. Frequencies of ETV6-RUNX1 fusion and hyperdiploidy in pediatric acute lymphoblastic leukemia are lower in far east than west. *Pediatr Blood Cancer.* 2010;55(3):430-3.

57. Gómez-Seguí I, Cervera J, Such E, et al. Prognostic value of cytogenetics in adult patients with Philadelphia-negative acute lymphoblastic leukemia. *Ann Hematol.* 2012;91(1):19-25.

58. Sutcliffe MJ, Shuster JJ, Sather HN, et al. High concordance from independent studies by the Children's Cancer Group (CCG) and Pediatric Oncology Group (POG) associating favorable prognosis with combined trisomies 4, 10, and 17 in children with NCI Standard-Risk B-precursor Acute Lymphoblastic Leukemia: a Children's Oncology Group (COG) initiative. *Leukemia.* 2005;19(5):734-40.

59. Harrison CJ, Foroni L. Cytogenetics and molecular genetics of acute lymphoblastic leukemia. *Rev Clin Exp Hematol.* 2002;6(2):91-113.

60. Maia AT, van der Velden VH, Harrison CJ, et al. Prenatal origin of hyperdiploid acute lymphoblastic leukemia in identical twins. *Leukemia.* 2003;17(11):2202-6.

61. Taketani T, Taki T, Sugita K, et al. FLT3 mutations in the activation loop of tyrosine kinase domain are frequently found in infant ALL with MLL rearrangements and pediatric ALL with hyperdiploidy. *Blood.* 2004;103(3):1085-8.

62. Stam RW, den Boer ML, Schneider P, et al. D-HPLC analysis of the entire FLT3 gene in MLL rearranged and hyperdiploid acute lymphoblastic leukemia. *Haematologica.* 2007; 92(11):1565-8.

63. Brown P, Levis M, Shurtleff S, et al. FLT3 inhibition selectively kills childhood acute lymphoblastic leukemia cells with high levels of FLT3 expression. *Blood.* 2005;105(2):812-20.

64. Meyer C, Kowarz E, Hofmann J, et al. New insights to the MLL recombinome of acute leukemias. *Leukemia.* 2009;23(8):1490-9.

65. Kohlmann A, Schoch C, Dugas M, et al. New insights into MLL gene rearranged acute leukemias using gene expression profiling: shared pathways, lineage commitment, and partner genes. *Leukemia.* 2005;19(6):953-64.

66. Pui CH, Frankel LS, Carroll AJ, et al. Clinical characteristics and treatment outcome of childhood acute lymphoblastic leukemia with the t(4;11)(q21;q23): a collaborative study of 40 cases. *Blood.* 1991;77(3):440-7.

67. Pui CH, Kane JR, Crist WM. Biology and treatment of infant leukemias. *Leukemia.* 1995; 9(5):762-9.

68. Moorman AV, Harrison CJ, Buck GA, et al. Karyotype is an independent prognostic factor in adult acute lymphoblastic leukemia (ALL): analysis of cytogenetic data from patients treated on the Medical Research Council (MRC) UKALLXII/Eastern Cooperative Oncology Group (ECOG) 2993 trial. *Blood.* 2007;109(8):3189-97.

69. Mancini M, Scappaticci D, Cimino G, et al. A comprehensive genetic classification of adult acute lymphoblastic leukemia (ALL): analysis of the GIMEMA 0496 protocol. *Blood.* 2005;105(9):3434-41.

70. Cimino G, Elia L, Mancini M, et al. Clinico-biologic features and treatment outcome of adult pro-B-ALL patients enrolled in the GIMEMA 0496 study: absence of the ALL1/AF4 and of the BCR/ABL fusion genes correlates with a significantly better clinical outcome. *Blood.* 2003;102(6):2014-20.

71. Ludwig WD, Rieder H, Bartram CR, et al. Immunophenotypic and genotypic features, clinical characteristics, and treatment outcome of adult pro-B acute lymphoblastic leukemia: results of the German multicenter trials GMALL 03/87 and 04/89. *Blood.* 1998;92(6):1898-909.

72. Huguet F, Leguay T, Raffoux E, et al. Pediatric-inspired therapy in adults with Philadelphia chromosome-negative acute lymphoblastic leukemia: the GRAALL-2003 study. *J Clin Oncol.* 2009;27(6):911-8.

73. Bassan R, Spinelli O, Oldani E, et al. Improved risk classification for risk-specific therapy based on the molecular study of minimal residual disease (MRD) in adult acute lymphoblastic leukemia (ALL). *Blood.* 2009;113(18):4153-62.

74. Strick R, Strissel PL, Borgers S, et al. Dietary bioflavonoids induce cleavage in the MLL gene and may contribute to infant leukemia. *Proc Natl Acad Sci U S A.* 2000;97(9):4790-5.

75. Alexander FE, Patheal SL, Biondi A, et al. Transplacental chemical exposure and risk of infant leukemia with MLL gene fusion. *Cancer Res.* 2001;61(6):2542-6.

76. Ford AM, Ridge SA, Cabrera ME, et al. In utero rearrangements in the trithorax-related oncogene in infant leukaemias. *Nature.* 1993;363(6427):358-60.

77. Gale KB, Ford AM, Repp R, et al. Backtracking leukemia to birth: identification of clonotypic gene fusion sequences in neonatal blood spots. *Proc Natl Acad Sci U S A.* 1997; 94(25):13950-4.

78. Ross JA, Potter JD, Reaman GH, et al. Maternal exposure to potential inhibitors of DNA topoisomerase II and infant leukemia (United States): a report from the Children's Cancer Group. *Cancer Causes Control.* 1996;7(6):581-90.

79. Wiemels JL, Pagnamenta A, Taylor GM, et al. A lack of a functional NAD(P)H:quinone oxidoreductase allele is selectively associated with pediatric leukemias that have MLL fusions. United Kingdom Childhood Cancer Study Investigators. *Cancer Res.* 1999;59(16):4095-9.

80. Wiemels JL, Smith RN, Taylor GM, et al. Methylenetetrahydrofolate reductase (MTHFR) polymorphisms and risk of molecularly defined subtypes of childhood acute leukemia. *Proc Natl Acad Sci U S A.* 2001;98(7):4004-9.

81. Smith MT, Wang Y, Skibola CF, et al. Low NAD(P)H:quinone oxidoreductase activity is associated with increased risk of leukemia with MLL translocations in infants and children. *Blood.* 2002;100(13):4590-3.

82. Dobson CL, Warren AJ, Pannell R, et al. Tumorigenesis in mice with a fusion of the leukaemia oncogene Mll and the bacterial lacZ gene. *EMBO J.* 2000;19(5):843-51.

83. Chen W, Li Q, Hudson WA, et al. A murine Mll-AF4 knock-in model results in lymphoid and myeloid deregulation and hematologic malignancy. *Blood.* 2006;108(2):669-77.

84. Lobato MN, Metzler M, Drynan L, et al. Modeling chromosomal translocations using conditional alleles to recapitulate initiating events in human leukemias. *J Natl Cancer Inst Monogr.* 2008;(39):58-63.

85. Krivtsov AV, Feng Z, Lemieux ME, et al. H3K79 methylation profiles define murine and human MLL-AF4 leukemias. *Cancer Cell.* 2008;14(5):355-68.

86. Faber J, Krivtsov AV, Stubbs MC, et al. HOXA9 is required for survival in human MLL-rearranged acute leukemias. *Blood.* 2009;113(11):2375-85.

87. Hsieh JJ, Ernst P, Erdjument-Bromage H, et al. Proteolytic cleavage of MLL generates a complex of N- and C-terminal fragments that confers protein stability and subnuclear localization. *Mol Cell Biol.* 2003;23(1):186-94.

88. Bitoun E, Oliver PL, Davies KE. The mixed-lineage leukemia fusion partner AF4 stimulates RNA polymerase II transcriptional elongation and mediates coordinated chromatin remodeling. *Hum Mol Genet.* 2007;16(1):92-106.

89. Monroe SC, Jo SY, Sanders DS, et al. MLL-AF9 and MLL-ENL alter the dynamic association of transcriptional regulators with genes critical for leukemia. *Exp Hematol.* 2011;39(1):77-86.e1-5.

90. Estable MC, Naghavi MH, Kato H, et al. MCEF, the newest member of the AF4 family of transcription factors involved in leukemia, is a positive transcription elongation factor-b-associated protein. *J Biomed Sci.* 2002;9(3):234-45.

91. Yokoyama A, Lin M, Naresh A, et al. A higher-order complex containing AF4 and ENL family proteins with P-TEFb facilitates oncogenic and physiologic MLL-dependent transcription. *Cancer Cell.* 2010;17(2):198-212.

92. Benedikt A, Baltruschat S, Scholz B, et al. The leukemogenic AF4-MLL fusion protein causes P-TEFb kinase activation and altered epigenetic signatures. *Leukemia.* 2011;25(1):135-44.

93. Marchesi F, Girardi K, Avvisati G. Pathogenetic, Clinical, and Prognostic Features of Adult t(4;11)(q21;q23)/MLL-AF4 Positive B-Cell Acute Lymphoblastic Leukemia. *Adv Hematol.* 2011;2011:621627.

94. Milne TA, Briggs SD, Brock HW, et al. MLL targets SET domain methyltransferase activity to Hox gene promoters. *Mol Cell.* 2002;10(5):1107-17.

95. Aspland SE, Bendall HH, Murre C. The role of E2A-PBX1 in leukemogenesis. *Oncogene.* 2001;20(40):5708-17.

96. Borowitz MJ, Hunger SP, Carroll AJ, et al. Predictability of the t(1;19)(q23;p13) from surface antigen phenotype: implications for screening cases of childhood acute lymphoblastic leukemia for molecular analysis: a Pediatric Oncology Group study. *Blood.* 1993;82(4):1086-91.

97. Brumpt C, Delabesse E, Beldjord K, et al. The incidence of clonal T-cell receptor rearrangements in B-cell precursor acute lymphoblastic leukemia varies with age and genotype. *Blood*. 2000;96(6):2254-61.

98. Wasserman R, Galili N, Ito Y, et al. Predominance of fetal type DJH joining in young children with B precursor lymphoblastic leukemia as evidence for an in utero transforming event. *J Exp Med*. 1992;176(6):1577-81.

99. Steenbergen EJ, Verhagen OJ, van Leeuwen EF, et al. B precursor acute lymphoblastic leukemia third complementarity-determining regions predominantly represent an unbiased recombination repertoire: leukemic transformation frequently occurs in fetal life. *Eur J Immunol*. 1994;24(4):900-8.

100. Fasching K, Panzer S, Haas OA, et al. Presence of N regions in the clonotypic DJ rearrangements of the immunoglobulin heavy-chain genes indicates an exquisitely short latency in t(4;11)-positive infant acute lymphoblastic leukemia. *Blood*. 2001;98(7):2272-4.

101. Wiemels JL, Leonard BC, Wang Y, et al. Site-specific translocation and evidence of postnatal origin of the t(1;19) E2A-PBX1 fusion in childhood acute lymphoblastic leukemia. *Proc Natl Acad Sci U S A*. 2002;99(23):15101-6.

102. McLaughlin J, Chianese E, Witte ON. In vitro transformation of immature hematopoietic cells by the P210 BCR/ABL oncogene product of the Philadelphia chromosome. *Proc Natl Acad Sci U S A*. 1987;84(18):6558-62.

103. Ren R. Mechanisms of BCR-ABL in the pathogenesis of chronic myelogenous leukaemia. *Nat Rev Cancer*. 2005;5(3):172-83.

104. Sawyers CL. Chronic myeloid leukemia. *N Engl J Med*. 1999;340(17):1330-40.

105. Gleissner B, Gökbuget N, Bartram CR, et al. Leading prognostic relevance of the BCR-ABL translocation in adult acute B-lineage lymphoblastic leukemia: a prospective study of the German Multicenter Trial Group and confirmed polymerase chain reaction analysis. *Blood*. 2002;99(5):1536-43.

106. Schrappe M, Hunger SP, Pui CH, et al. Outcomes after induction failure in childhood acute lymphoblastic leukemia. *N Engl J Med*. 2012;366(15):1371-81.

107. Paietta E, Racevskis J, Bennett JM, et al. Biologic heterogeneity in Philadelphia chromosome-positive acute leukemia with myeloid morphology: the Eastern Cooperative Oncology Group experience. *Leukemia*. 1998;12(12):1881-5.

108. Cuneo A, Ferrant A, Michaux JL, et al. Philadelphia chromosome-positive acute myeloid leukemia: cytoimmunologic and cytogenetic features. *Haematologica*. 1996;81(5):423-7.

109. Faderl S, Jeha S, Kantarjian HM. The biology and therapy of adult acute lymphoblastic leukemia. *Cancer*. 2003;98(7):1337-54.

110. Li S, Ilaria RL, Million RP, et al. The P190, P210, and P230 forms of the BCR/ABL oncogene induce a similar chronic myeloid leukemia-like syndrome in mice but have different lymphoid leukemogenic activity. *J Exp Med*. 1999;189(9):1399-412.

111. Ribeiro RC, Abromowitch M, Raimondi SC, et al. Clinical and biologic hallmarks of the Philadelphia chromosome in childhood acute lymphoblastic leukemia. *Blood*. 1987;70(4): 948-53.

112. Molnár A, Georgopoulos K. The Ikaros gene encodes a family of functionally diverse zinc finger DNA-binding proteins. *Mol Cell Biol*. 1994;14(12):8292-303.

113. Iacobucci I, Storlazzi CT, Cilloni D, et al. Identification and molecular characterization of recurrent genomic deletions on 7p12 in the IKZF1 gene in a large cohort of BCR-ABL1-positive acute lymphoblastic leukemia patients: on behalf of Gruppo Italiano Malattie Ematologiche dell'Adulto Acute Leukemia Working Party (GIMEMA AL WP). *Blood*. 2009; 114(10):2159-67.

114. Sun L, Heerema N, Crotty L, et al. Expression of dominant-negative and mutant isoforms of the antileukemic transcription factor Ikaros in infant acute lymphoblastic leukemia. *Proc Natl Acad Sci U S A*. 1999;96(2):680-5.

115. Liu P, Lin Z, Qian S, et al. Expression of dominant-negative Ikaros isoforms and associated genetic alterations in Chinese adult patients with leukemia. *Ann Hematol.* 2012;91(7): 1039-49.

116. Mullighan CG, Miller CB, Radtke I, et al. BCR-ABL1 lymphoblastic leukaemia is characterized by the deletion of Ikaros. *Nature.* 2008;453(7191):110-4.

117. Iacobucci I, Iraci N, Messina M, et al. IKAROS deletions dictate a unique gene expression signature in patients with adult B-cell acute lymphoblastic leukemia. *PLoS One.* 2012; 7(7):e40934.

118. Cazzaniga G, van Delft FW, Lo Nigro L, et al. Developmental origins and impact of BCR-ABL1 fusion and IKZF1 deletions in monozygotic twins with Ph+ acute lymphoblastic leukemia. *Blood.* 2011;118(20):5559-64.

119. Kirstetter P, Thomas M, Dierich A, et al. Ikaros is critical for B cell differentiation and function. *Eur J Immunol.* 2002;32(3):720-30.

120. Den Boer ML, van Slegtenhorst M, De Menezes RX, et al. A subtype of childhood acute lymphoblastic leukaemia with poor treatment outcome: a genome-wide classification study. *Lancet Oncol.* 2009;10(2):125-34.

121. Mullighan CG, Su X, Zhang J, et al. Deletion of IKZF1 and prognosis in acute lymphoblastic leukemia. *N Engl J Med.* 2009;360(5):470-80.

122. Kuiper RP, Schoenmakers EF, van Reijmersdal SV, et al. High-resolution genomic profiling of childhood ALL reveals novel recurrent genetic lesions affecting pathways involved in lymphocyte differentiation and cell cycle progression. *Leukemia.* 2007;21(6):1258-66.

123. Paulsson K, Cazier JB, Macdougall F, et al. Microdeletions are a general feature of adult and adolescent acute lymphoblastic leukemia: Unexpected similarities with pediatric disease. *Proc Natl Acad Sci U S A.* 2008;105(18):6708-13.

124. Martinelli G, Iacobucci I, Papayannidis C, et al. New targets for Ph+ leukaemia therapy. *Best Pract Res Clin Haematol.* 2009;22(3):445-54.

125. Harvey RC, Mullighan CG, Wang X, et al. Identification of novel cluster groups in pediatric high-risk B-precursor acute lymphoblastic leukemia with gene expression profiling: correlation with genome-wide DNA copy number alterations, clinical characteristics, and outcome. *Blood.* 2010;116(23):4874-84.

126. Russell LJ, Capasso M, Vater I, et al. Deregulated expression of cytokine receptor gene, CRLF2, is involved in lymphoid transformation in B-cell precursor acute lymphoblastic leukemia. *Blood.* 2009;114(13):2688-98.

127. Harvey RC, Mullighan CG, Chen IM, et al. Rearrangement of CRLF2 is associated with mutation of JAK kinases, alteration of IKZF1, Hispanic/Latino ethnicity, and a poor outcome in pediatric B-progenitor acute lymphoblastic leukemia. *Blood.* 2010;115(26):5312-21.

128. Yoda A, Yoda Y, Chiaretti S, et al. Functional screening identifies CRLF2 in precursor B-cell acute lymphoblastic leukemia. *Proc Natl Acad Sci U S A.* 2010;107(1):252-7.

129. Reya T, Duncan AW, Ailles L, et al. A role for Wnt signalling in self-renewal of haematopoietic stem cells. *Nature.* 2003;423(6938):409-14.

130. Luis TC, Naber BA, Roozen PP, et al. Canonical wnt signaling regulates hematopoiesis in a dosage-dependent fashion. *Cell Stem Cell.* 2011;9(4):345-56.

131. Chan WI, Hannah RL, Dawson MA, et al. The transcriptional coactivator Cbp regulates self-renewal and differentiation in adult hematopoietic stem cells. *Mol Cell Biol.* 2011; 31(24):5046-60.

132. Wang Y, Krivtsov AV, Sinha AU, et al. The Wnt/beta-catenin pathway is required for the development of leukemia stem cells in AML. *Science.* 2010;327(5973):1650-3.

133. Zhao C, Blum J, Chen A, et al. Loss of beta-catenin impairs the renewal of normal and CML stem cells in vivo. *Cancer Cell.* 2007;12(6):528-41.

134. Hu Y, Chen Y, Douglas L, et al. beta-Catenin is essential for survival of leukemic stem cells insensitive to kinase inhibition in mice with BCR-ABL-induced chronic myeloid leukemia. *Leukemia.* 2009;23(1):109-16.

135. Jamieson CH, Ailles LE, Dylla SJ, et al. Granulocyte-macrophage progenitors as candidate leukemic stem cells in blast-crisis CML. *N Engl J Med.* 2004;351(7):657-67.

136. Zhao C, Blum J, Chen A, et al. Loss of beta-catenin impairs the renewal of normal and CML stem cells in vivo. *Cancer Cell.* 2007;12(6):528-41.

137. Mazieres J, You L, He B, et al. Inhibition of Wnt16 in human acute lymphoblastoid leukemia cells containing the t(1;19) translocation induces apoptosis. *Oncogene.* 2005;24(34):5396-400.

138. Altieri DC. Survivin, cancer networks and pathway-directed drug discovery. *Nat Rev Cancer.* 2008;8(1):61-70.

139. Park E, Gang EJ, Hsieh YT, et al. Targeting survivin overcomes drug resistance in acute lymphoblastic leukemia. *Blood.* 2011;118(8):2191-9.

140. Khan NI, Bradstock KF, Bendall LJ. Activation of Wnt/beta-catenin pathway mediates growth and survival in B-cell progenitor acute lymphoblastic leukaemia. *Br J Haematol.* 2007;138(3):338-48.

141. Reya T, Clevers H. Wnt signalling in stem cells and cancer. *Nature.* 2005;434(7035):843-50.

142. Mullighan CG, Zhang J, Kasper LH, et al. CREBBP mutations in relapsed acute lymphoblastic leukaemia. *Nature.* 2011;471(7337):235-9.

143. Zhang J, Mullighan CG, Harvey RC, et al. Key pathways are frequently mutated in high-risk childhood acute lymphoblastic leukemia: a report from the Children's Oncology Group. *Blood.* 2011;118(11):3080-7.

144. Inthal A, Zeitlhofer P, Zeginigg M, et al. CREBBP HAT domain mutations prevail in relapse cases of high hyperdiploid childhood acute lymphoblastic leukemia. *Leukemia.* 2012; 26(8):1797-803.

145. Takahashi-Yanaga F, Kahn M. Targeting Wnt signaling: can we safely eradicate cancer stem cells? *Clin Cancer Res.* 2010;16(12):3153-62.

146. Takebe N, Harris PJ, Warren RQ, et al. Targeting cancer stem cells by inhibiting Wnt, Notch, and Hedgehog pathways. *Nat Rev Clin Oncol.* 2011;8(2):97-106.

147. Verkaar F, van der Stelt M, Blankesteijn WM, et al. Discovery of novel small molecule activators of β-catenin signaling. *PLoS One.* 2011;6(4):e19185.

148. Maier TJ, Janssen A, Schmidt R, et al. Targeting the beta-catenin/APC pathway: a novel mechanism to explain the cyclooxygenase-2-independent anticarcinogenic effects of celecoxib in human colon carcinoma cells. *FASEB J.* 2005;19(10):1353-5.

149. Sukhdeo K, Mani M, Zhang Y, et al. Targeting the beta-catenin/TCF transcriptional complex in the treatment of multiple myeloma. *Proc Natl Acad Sci U S A.* 2007;104(18):7516-21.

150. Doghman M, Cazareth J, Lalli E. The T cell factor/beta-catenin antagonist PKF115-584 inhibits proliferation of adrenocortical carcinoma cells. *J Clin Endocrinol Metab.* 2008;93(8):3222-5.

151. Nagao R, Ashihara E, Kimura S, et al. Growth inhibition of imatinib-resistant CML cells with the T315I mutation and hypoxia-adaptation by AV65—a novel Wnt/β-catenin signaling inhibitor. *Cancer Lett.* 2011;312(1):91-100.

152. Emami KH, Nguyen C, Ma H, et al. A small molecule inhibitor of beta-catenin/CREB-binding protein transcription [corrected]. *Proc Natl Acad Sci U S A.* 2004;101(34):12682-7.

153. Kahn M. Symmetric division versus asymmetric division: a tale of two coactivators. *Future Med Chem.* 2011;3(14):1745-63.

154. Nutt SL, Heavey B, Rolink AG, et al. Commitment to the B-lymphoid lineage depends on the transcription factor Pax5. *Nature.* 1999;401(6753):556-62.

155. Nutt SL, Eberhard D, Horcher M, et al. Pax5 determines the identity of B cells from the beginning to the end of B-lymphopoiesis. *Int Rev Immunol.* 2001;20(1):65-82.

156. Fuxa M, Skok JA. Transcriptional regulation in early B cell development. *Curr Opin Immunol.* 2007;19(2):129-36.

157. Cobaleda C, Schebesta A, Delogu A, et al. Pax5: the guardian of B cell identity and function. *Nat Immunol.* 2007;8(5):463-70.

158. Souabni A, Cobaleda C, Schebesta M, et al. Pax5 promotes B lymphopoiesis and blocks T cell development by repressing Notch1. *Immunity*. 2002;17(6):781-93.

159. Medvedovic J, Ebert A, Tagoh H, et al. Pax5: a master regulator of B cell development and leukemogenesis. *Adv Immunol*. 2011;111:179-206.

160. Familiades J, Bousquet M, Lafage-Pochitaloff M, et al. PAX5 mutations occur frequently in adult B-cell progenitor acute lymphoblastic leukemia and PAX5 haploinsufficiency is associated with BCR-ABL1 and TCF3-PBX1 fusion genes: a GRAALL study. *Leukemia*. 2009;23(11):1989-98.

161. Iacobucci I, Lonetti A, Paoloni F, et al. The PAX5 gene is frequently rearranged in BCR-ABL1-positive acute lymphoblastic leukemia but is not associated with outcome. A report on behalf of the GIMEMA Acute Leukemia Working Party. *Haematologica*. 2010;95(10):1683-90.

162. Nebral K, Denk D, Attarbaschi A, et al. Incidence and diversity of PAX5 fusion genes in childhood acute lymphoblastic leukemia. *Leukemia*. 2009;23(1):134-43.

163. Cazzaniga G, Daniotti M, Tosi S, et al. The paired box domain gene PAX5 is fused to ETV6/TEL in an acute lymphoblastic leukemia case. *Cancer Res*. 2001;61(12):4666-70.

164. Strehl S, König M, Dworzak MN, et al. PAX5/ETV6 fusion defines cytogenetic entity dic(9;12)(p13;p13). *Leukemia*. 2003;17(6):1121-3.

165. Kawamata N, Pennella MA, Woo JL, et al. Dominant-negative mechanism of leukemogenic PAX5 fusions. *Oncogene*. 2012;31(8):966-77.

166. Put N, Deeren D, Michaux L, et al. FOXP1 and PAX5 are rare but recurrent translocations partners in acute lymphoblastic leukemia. *Cancer Genet*. 2011;204(8):462-4.

167. Bousquet M, Broccardo C, Quelen C, et al. A novel PAX5-ELN fusion protein identified in B-cell acute lymphoblastic leukemia acts as a dominant negative on wild-type PAX5. *Blood*. 2007;109(8):3417-23.

168. Kearney L, Gonzalez De Castro D, Yeung J, et al. Specific JAK2 mutation (JAK2R683) and multiple gene deletions in Down syndrome acute lymphoblastic leukemia. *Blood*. 2009;113(3):646-8.

169. Coyaud E, Struski S, Prade N, et al. Wide diversity of PAX5 alterations in B-ALL: a Groupe Francophone de Cytogenetique Hematologique study. *Blood*. 2010;115(15):3089-97.

170. Kurahashi S, Hayakawa F, Miyata Y, et al. PAX5-PML acts as a dual dominant-negative form of both PAX5 and PML. *Oncogene*. 2011;30(15):1822-30.

171. Krentz S, Hof J, Mendioroz A, et al. Prognostic value of genetic alterations in children with first bone marrow relapse of childhood B-cell precursor acute lymphoblastic leukemia. *Leukemia*. 2013;27(2):295-304.

172. Greaves MF, Maia AT, Wiemels JL, et al. Leukemia in twins: lessons in natural history. *Blood*. 2003;102(7):2321-33.

173. Marks DI, Paietta EM, Moorman AV, et al. T-cell acute lymphoblastic leukemia in adults: clinical features, immunophenotype, cytogenetics, and outcome from the large randomized prospective trial (UKALL XII/ECOG 2993). *Blood*. 2009;114(25):5136-45.

174. Pui CH, Pei D, Sandlund JT, et al. Long-term results of St Jude Total Therapy Studies 11, 12, 13A, 13B, and 14 for childhood acute lymphoblastic leukemia. *Leukemia*. 2010;24(2):371-82.

175. Goldberg JM, Silverman LB, Levy DE, et al. Childhood T-cell acute lymphoblastic leukemia: the Dana-Farber Cancer Institute acute lymphoblastic leukemia consortium experience. *J Clin Oncol*. 2003;21(19):3616-22.

176. Oudot C, Auclerc MF, Levy V, et al. Prognostic factors for leukemic induction failure in children with acute lymphoblastic leukemia and outcome after salvage therapy: the FRALLE 93 study. *J Clin Oncol*. 2008;26(9):1496-503.

177. Paganin M, Ferrando A. Molecular pathogenesis and targeted therapies for NOTCH1-induced T-cell acute lymphoblastic leukemia. *Blood Rev*. 2011;25(2):83-90.

178. Hebert J, Cayuela JM, Berkeley J, et al. Candidate tumor-suppressor genes MTS1 (p16INK4A) and MTS2 (p15INK4B) display frequent homozygous deletions in primary cells from T- but not from B-cell lineage acute lymphoblastic leukemias. *Blood.* 1994;84(12):4038-44.

179. Ferrando AA, Neuberg DS, Staunton J, et al. Gene expression signatures define novel oncogenic pathways in T cell acute lymphoblastic leukemia. *Cancer Cell.* 2002;1(1):75-87.

180. Aster JC, Pear WS, Blacklow SC. Notch signaling in leukemia. *Annu Rev Pathol.* 2008;3: 587-613.

181. Radtke F, Fasnacht N, Macdonald HR. Notch signaling in the immune system. *Immunity.* 2010;32(1):14-27.

182. Leong KG, Karsan A. Recent insights into the role of Notch signaling in tumorigenesis. *Blood.* 2006;107(6):2223-33.

183. Zweidler-McKay PA. Notch signaling in pediatric malignancies. *Curr Oncol Rep.* 2008; 10(6):459-68.

184. Pear WS, Aster JC, Scott ML, et al. Exclusive development of T cell neoplasms in mice transplanted with bone marrow expressing activated Notch alleles. *J Exp Med.* 1996; 183(5):2283-91.

185. Weng AP, Ferrando AA, Lee W, et al. Activating mutations of NOTCH1 in human T cell acute lymphoblastic leukemia. *Science.* 2004;306(5694):269-71.

186. Malecki MJ, Sanchez-Irizarry C, Mitchell JL, et al. Leukemia-associated mutations within the NOTCH1 heterodimerization domain fall into at least two distinct mechanistic classes. *Mol Cell Biol.* 2006;26(12):4642-51.

187. Chiang MY, Xu ML, Histen G, et al. Identification of a conserved negative regulatory sequence that influences the leukemogenic activity of NOTCH1. *Mol Cell Biol.* 2006;26(16):6261-71.

188. O'Neil J, Grim J, Strack P, et al. FBW7 mutations in leukemic cells mediate NOTCH pathway activation and resistance to gamma-secretase inhibitors. *J Exp Med.* 2007;204(8):1813-24.

189. Thompson BJ, Buonamici S, Sulis ML, et al. The SCFFBW7 ubiquitin ligase complex as a tumor suppressor in T cell leukemia. *J Exp Med.* 2007;204(8):1825-35.

190. Van Vlietrberghe P, Ferrando A. The molecular basis of T cell acute lymphoblastic leukemia. *J Clin Invest.* 2012;122(10):3398-406.

191. Moellering RE, Cornejo M, Davis TN, et al. Direct inhibition of the NOTCH transcription factor complex. *Nature.* 2009;462(7270):182-8.

Cytogenetics of Acute Lymphoblastic Leukemia

Marilyn L Slovak

INTRODUCTION

Acute lymphoblastic leukemia (ALL) is a malignant disorder of the lymphoid progenitor cells. With a worldwide incidence of 1–4.75 cases per 100,000 individuals, ALL represents 12% of all cases of leukemia.[1] In the United States alone, ALL accounts for ~6,000 cancer diagnoses and 1,400 deaths annually.[2] Data from the 2012 Surveillance, Epidemiology and End Results (SEER) program indicate that 30% of acute leukemia cases in the United States are ALL. The age distribution is bimodal, with a predominant childhood peak between the ages of 1 years and 5 years and a minor peak in adults over age 50 years.[3]

Acute lymphoblastic leukemia arises from recurrent genetic insults that block B- and T-cell differentiation and drive aberrant cell proliferation and survival. These genetic insults include chromosomal translocations, aneuploidy, and gene-specific alterations that define specific cytogenetic subgroups in ALL with differing clinical courses and distinct responses to therapy.[4-6] In 2008, the World Health Organization (WHO) refined the pathological classification of B-cell acute lymphoblastic leukemia (B-ALL) and T-cell acute lymphoblastic leukemia/lymphoma (T-ALL) to include cell lineage, morphology, immunophenotyping, and genetic factors.[7]

B-cell acute lymphoblastic leukemia, a malignancy of the lymphoblasts or precursor cells committed to the B-cell lineage, represents 85% of ALL. Most cases (~75%) are reported in children less than 6 years of age. The WHO defines seven cytogenetic B-ALL subtypes based on the presence or absence of specific recurring cytogenetic aberrations.[7] These aberrations are present in both pediatric and adult B-ALL but show clear differences in their frequency and prognosis, supporting the supposition of different disease etiology/pathogenesis (Figure 5-1). Mature B-ALL, or Burkitt leukemia, is characterized by one of the 8q24.1/MYC-translocations. It is not grouped within the B-ALL WHO classification, because patients with Burkitt leukemia are treated using Burkitt lymphoma protocols. T-ALL, which accounts for ~15% of childhood and 25% of adult ALL, is an aggressive neoplastic disorder characterized by the proliferation of malignant thymocytes at various stages of T-cell development.[7,8]

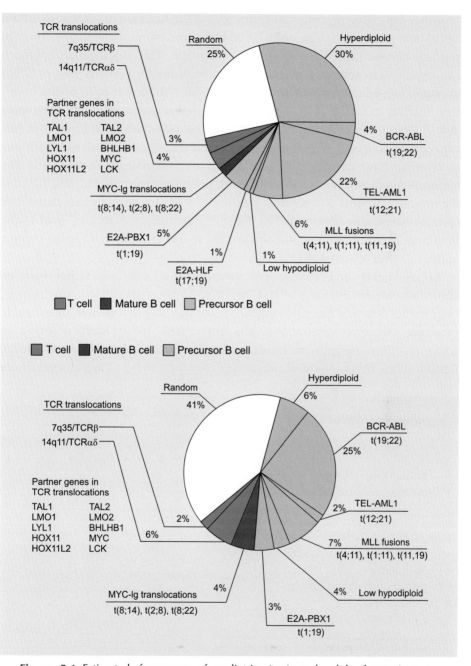

Figure 5-1 Estimated frequency of pediatric (top) and adult (bottom) acute lymphoblastic leukemia (ALL) by cytogenetics. The frequencies of the most common B-ALL and T-ALL cytogenetic subgroups are listed. Exclusive T-ALL aberrations are noted in purple. *From* Pui CH, Relling MV, Downing JR. Acute lymphoblastic leukemia. *N Engl J Med.* 2004;350(15):1535-48, *with permission.*

Risk-adapted therapeutic categories relevant to ALL take into account several key parameters, such as age, white blood cell count, immunophenotype, minimal residual disease (MRD) detection, and karyotype. This stratification approach has improved treatment, survival, and quality of life for patients with ALL. For example, risk-adapted treatments for childhood ALL have lead to 5-year event-free survival rates of ~80% and 5-year overall survival rates approximating 90%.[4,9] Despite these recent treatment advances, ~15–20% of children with ALL experience a relapse.[10-12] Features associated with a high risk of relapse or adverse outcome in patients with B-ALL or T-ALL are summarized in table 5-1. The strongest prognostic factor associated with poor outcome in B-ALL and T-ALL is the presence of MRD or molecular failure,[13-15] a finding strongly associated with specific cytogenetic aberrations in B-ALL.[16] Accordingly, a focused goal in the treatment of ALL is to determine the specific role of genetics in directing therapy in patients with relapsed ALL.

Secker-Walker and colleagues[17] described the first association between chromosomal aberrations and ALL in 1978. Today, conventional (metaphase) cytogenetics remains the gold standard screening method used to detect these recurring karyotypic aberrations. The aberrations are typically observed as whole chromosome gains or losses, leukemic-specific balanced or unbalanced translocations, inversions, and deletions (Tables 5-2 and 5-3). Fluorescence *in situ*

Table 5-1	Features Associated with Relapse or Adverse Outcomes in B-ALL and T-ALL/Lymphoma	
B-ALL		**T-ALL**
Specific cytogenetic subgroups[1]		High WBC ($>$ 50,000/mm^3)
• t(9;22)(q34.1;q11.2)		
• Intrachromosomal amplification of chromosome 21 or iAMP21		
• MLL translocations		
• Abnormal 17p/TP53		
• Deletion 13q (secondary aberration)		
• Near-haploidy		
• Low hypodiploidy/near triploidy		
• t(17;19)(q22;p13.3)		
Age $<$ 12 months or $>$ 10 years		Multiple lymphadenopathies
High WBC ($>$ 50,000/mm^3)		Mediastinal enlargement
Slow response to induction therapy		Central nervous system involvement
MRD		MRD

ALL, acute lymphoblastic leukemia; WBC, white cell count; MLL, mixed lineage leukemia; MRD, minimal residual disease; near-haploidy, less than 30 chromosomes; low hypodiploidy, ~30–39 chromosomes.

[1]See table 2 for the most common cytogenetic subgroups and their characteristic features. See reference 16 for risk of relapse details. Deletion 13q is usually a secondary aberration reported in just 3% of ALL patients.

Table 5-2   Recurrent Cytogenetic and Molecular Abreviations in B-ALL

Genetic grouping	Abnormality	Chromosome number, site or genes involved	Estimated frequency (%)			Comments/associations
			Pediatric	Both	Adults	
Numerical aberrations						
	Near haploidy	~ 23–29 chromosomes	< 1.0%			Restricted to children (<15 years old); Gains of X/Y, 14, 18, and 21; often with duplication of near-haploid clone; FISH needed to detect both clones; usually no apparent structural abnormalities
	Low hypodiploidy	~ 30–39/~ 60–78 chromosomes	< 1.0%		1.0%	Low hypodiploid seen often with a near-triploid duplicated clone. Consistent loss of chr 7 and 17 and gain of chr 1, 11, 19, 10, and 22
	High hypodiploidy	~ 42–45 chromosomes	1.0%	~ 5.0%	2.0%	Heterogeneous group. Prognosis should be deferred to specific primary structural aberration, if known; otherwise intermediate observed in children and adults. Usually complex karyotypes. Losses due to monosomy or unbalanced/dicentric chromosomes
	Low hyperdiploidy	~ 47–50 chromosomes	~ 1.0%		~ 10%	Includes acquired + 21, +X
	High hyperdiploidy	~ 51–65 chromosomes	~ 25–30%		~ 2–10%	Common gains of chr X, 4, 6, 10, 14, 17, 18, 21, and 1q. CD19+,CD10+, TdT+, often CD34+,CD45. Frequent microdeletions of ETV6, CKDN2A, PAX5, PAN3, and CN-LOH of chr 9 and 11. Only 10% in DS-B-ALL. Not seen in infant ALL. Favorable prognosis

Continued

Continued

Genetic grouping	Abnormality	Chromosome number, site or genes involved	Estimated frequency (%)			Comments/associations
			Pediatric	Both	Adults	
Structural aberrations						
MLL trans-locations	t(4;11)(q21;q23)	MLL, AFF1	~6.0%		~10%	ALL and AML; CD10−, CD19+, CD24, CD15+; 60% in infant ALL
	t(6;11)(q27;q23)	MLLT4, MLL	~2.0%	~2.0%		Most common translocation in infant ALL (~50%); overexpression of FLT3
	t(9;11)(p21;q23)	MLLT3, MLL				Mainly infants in pediatric cases ~10% of infant ALL
	t(11;19)(q23;p13.3)	MLLT1, MLL	1%			~10% of infant ALL (poor prognosis); also seen pediatric B-ALL (1–9 years and T-ALL (good prognosis in T-ALL)
Philadelphia translocation	t(9;22)(q34.1;q11.2)	BCR, ABL1	~2–4%		~25–30%	CD10+, CD19+, TdT+, CD13+, CD33+, CD117−; historically poor OS, however, clinical trials with TKIs show increased DFS. Associated with -7, CDKN2A and IKZF1 deletions, t(8;14)(q11;q32); IGH-CEBPE without DS
BCR-ABL1 like	del(5)(q31q33)	EBF1;PDGFRB		8%		Activates various kinase genes such as ABL1, PDGFRB, and JAK2. May respond to targeted kinase inhibitors*
ETV6-RUNX1	t(12;21)(p13;q22)	ETV6, RUNX1	~20–25%		2.0%	CD19+, CD34+, TdT+, CD10+, CD24+, CD13+; CDKN2A deletions occur in 15%. Favorable prognosis. Only seen ~10% of DS-ALL
IGH/14q32 aberrations	t(X;14)(p22;q32) or t(Y;14)(p11;q32)	CRLF2; IGH		5.0%		Older children (median age, 13 years) and young adults. Frequent +X and del(9p). Risk elevates with IKZF1 deletions. High frequency in DS and Hispanic ethnicity
	t(5;14)(q31;q32)	IL3; IGH		<1.0%		CD19+, CD10+ with variable (reactive) eosinophilia

Continued

Continued

Genetic grouping	Abnormality	Chromosome number, site or genes involved	Estimated frequency (%)			Comments/associations
			Pediatric	Both	Adults	
	Other 14q32/iGH aberrations	CEBPA,B,D,EID4/6p22EPO4/19p13	~1.0%		~5.0%	Common in AYA; associated with CDKN2A and PAX5 deletions; also reported in CML-BC, T-ALL and NHL. CEBPA/19q13, CEBPB/20q13, CEBPD/8q11 and CEBPE/14q11. t(8;14) associated with DS-ALL
Amplification	iAMP21 amp21q22.11q22.12	Possibly RUNX1	~3–5%		<1.0%	Often observed as a structural abnormal chromosome 21. Older children (age range 7–14 years) with lower WBC
TCF3 translocations	t(1;19)(q23;p13.3)	TCF3, PBX1	~2–6%		3.0%	CD19+, CD10+, cytoplasmic μ heavy chain +, CD9+, CD20 variable and CD34 +/−. With antimetabolite therapy considered favorable to intermediate in children; less favorable in adults
	t(17;19)(q22;p13.3)	TCF3, HLF	<1%			Adverse prognosis, unlike t(1;19)
MYC translocations	t(8;14)(q24.2;q32.3) t(2;8)(p11.2;q24.2) t(8;22)(q24.2;q11.2)	MYC; IGH IGK; MYC MYC; IGL	~2.0%			Associated with mature B-cell ALL or Burkitt leukemia; treated on Burkitt lymphoma protocols
PAX5				~35%		PAX5 alterations (deletion, mutations, and translocations)
PAX5 - balanced translocations	t(7;9)(p12.1;p13.2) t(9;12)(p13.2;p12) t(9;20)(p13.2;q11.1) t(3;9)(p13;p13.2)	LOC392027 SLCO1B3 ASXL1/KIF3B or C20orf112 FOXP1		2.0%		Over 17 partner chromosomes. Balanced PAX5 translocations in simple karyotypes (suggests primary change). Other partners reported include HIPK1, POM121, ELN, JAK2, ETV6, DACH1, IGH, PML; ZNF521, BRD1 and AUTS2. ELN-PAX5 may be more common in adults. CDKN2A deletions are common

Continued

Continued

Genetic grouping	Abnormality	Chromosome number, site or genes involved	Estimated frequency (%)			Comments/associations
			Pediatric	Both	Adults	
PAX5 – unbalanced translocations	dic(7;9)(p11.2;p13)	PAX5; LOC392027			<1.0%	3% of childhood ALL with 9p aberrations, Usually seen in age <6 years. At times, seen with t(9;22)
	dic(9;12)(p13;p13)	PAX5, ETV6 or SLCO1B3	~4.0%		<1.0%	Predominantly seen in B-progenitor ALL of childhood and young adults. May be seen with t(12;21). Trisomy 8 common secondary change
	dic(9;20)(p13.2;q11.2)	PAX5; ASXL1/ KIF3B or C20orf112	~1–2%			Frequency may be ~5.0% if FISH is used routinely for detection; additional changes including loss of CDKN2A and +X, +21
Deletions	deletion 7p12.2	IKZF1		30%		Cryptic. Associated with JAK2 mutations, deletion CDKN2A/B, DS-ALL and t(9;22) and "BCR-ABL1-like" GEP
	Deletion 9p21.3	CDKN2A	~20%			Secondary aberration seen commonly in t(9;22) or t(1;19) ALL. 60% have PAX5 alteration
	Deletion 12q22	BTG1	~7.0%			~30% cryptic deletions in DS-ALL
	del(X)(p22.33p22.33) del(Y)(p11.32p11.32)	P2RY8-CRLF2		7.0%	Unknown	Small cryptic fusion in PAR1 region of the sex chromosomes; Frequent IKZF1 deletions. Seen in ~60% of DS-ALL usually with +X and del(9p)
Mutations		JAK2	<20%		N/A	Predominant in high risk B-ALL; found in 20% of DS-ALL

*Weston BW, Hayden MA, Roberts KG, Bowyer S, Hsu J, Fedoriw G, Rao KW, Mullighan CG. Tyrosine kinase inhibitor therapy induces remission in a patient with refractory EBF1-PDGFRB-positive acute lymphoblastic leukemia. *J Clin Oncol.* 2013;31(25):e413-6.

ALL, acute lymphoblastic leukemia; FISH, fluorescence *in situ* hybridization; DS, Down syndrome; AYA, adolescences and young adults; OS, overall survival; CML-BC, chronic myeloid leukemia in blast crisis; GEP, gene expression profiling; NHL, non-Hodgkin lymphoma; N/A, not available; TKI, tyrosine kinase inhibitors; PAR1, pseudoautosomal.

Table 5-3 Recurrent Cytogenetic and Molecular Aberrations in T-ALL

Risk/type category	Abnormality	Genes involved	Frequency (%)			Comments/associations
			Pediatric	Both	Adults	
TLX3	t(5;14)(q35.1;q32.2)	TLX3; BCL11B;	~15%		~25%	
	t(5;7)(q35.1;q21)	TLX3; CDK6	~20%		~5.0%	Cryptic; detected by FISH and microarrays; frequently seen with NOTCH1/FBXW7 mutations. Poorer prognosis than TLX1 aberrations
	t(5;14)(q35.1;q11.2) del(5)(q35.1)	TLX3; TRD				
T-cell receptor aberrations			~35%			
	t(1;7)(p34;q34)	LCK; TRB		<1%		Results in overexpression of the LCK SRC kinase
	t(1;14)(p32;q11.2) t(1;7)(p32;q34)	TAL1; TRA/D TAL1;TRB	~3%		11%	Median survival >5 years in children; TAL1 is more often fused with STIL (by interstitial cryptic deletion)
	t(6;7)(q23;q34)	MYB; TRB	~7%			Seen in pediatric T-ALL (median age 2.2 year)
	inv(7)(p15q34) or t(7;7)(p15q34) t(7;14) (p15;q11.2) t(7;14) (p15;q32)	HOXA; TRB HOXA; TRB HOXA; TRD HOXA; BCL11B		5%		inv(7) associated with CD2-, CD4+,CD8- lymphoblasts and deletion CDKN2A and NOTCH1 mutations. Elevated expression of HOXA genes
	t(7;9)(q34;q32)	TAL2; TRB		<1%		Often cryptic
	t(7;9)(q34;q34.3)	NOTCH1; TRB		<1%		Often cryptic
	t(7;11)(q34;p15) and t(11;14)(p15;q11.2)	LMO2; TRB orTRA/TRD		3%		Activates LMO2
	t(7;11)(q34;p13) and t(11;14)(p13;q11.2)	LMO1; TRB orTRA/TRD		2%		Activates LMO1
	t(7;12)(q34;p13.3) t(12;14)(p13.3;q11.2)	CCND2; TRB CCND2; TRA		<1%		Activates CCND2

Continued

Continued

Risk/type category	Abnormality	Genes involved	Frequency (%)			Comments/associations
			Pediatric	Both	Adults	
	t(7;10)(q34;q24)	TLX1; TRB	7%	~10%	30%	Shows early cortical phenotype, CD1 positivity, Favorable outcome. TLX1 also known as HOX11
	t(10;14)(q24.32;q11.2)	TLX1; TRA				
	t(7;19)(q34;p13)	LYL1; TRB	<2.0%		3.0%	Rare. Thought to have a poor prognosis
	t(14;21)(q11.2;q22)	OLIG2; TRA	<1%			Seen with del(6q); Cryptic translocations may exist
Fusion genes	t(11;19)(q23;p13.3)	MLL; MLLT1		<1%		Rare in T-ALL; confers a favorable prognosis. Elevated expression of HOXA genes
	ABL1 fusion genes	NUP214; ABL1 EML1; ABL1 BCR; ABL1ETV6; ABL1		6.0%		NUP214-ABL1 is the most common; Cryptic fusions results in gain of ABL1 (duplication, episomal amplification or rare hsr); ABL1 fusion is a late event associated with NOTCH1 activating mutation, CDKN2A deletion, and ectopic expression of TLX1 or TLX3. Rare cases of BCR-ABL1 and ETV6-ABL1 T-ALL reported. May benefit from TKI
	Deletion 9q34 resulting in fusion	SET; NUP214		N/A		Only detected by microarrays so frequency is not known. Elevated expression of HOXA genes
	t(10;11)(p12;q14)	PICALM; MLLT10		~10%		Poor prognosis; specific for early stages development of the TCRγδ lineage; No CDKN2A deletions. Elevated expression of HOXA genes
	Deletion 1p32 resulting in fusion	TAL1; STIL	~20%		~13%	Often submicroscopic deletion (detected best by microarray); frequently seen with deletion 6q and less often (~3.0%) with TCR translocations
Deletion	Deletion 6q	CASP8AP2		25%		Reports focus on 6q15q16.1 and CASP8AP (aka FLASH) downregulation. Associated with inferior prognosis; determinant in glucocorticoid signaling

Continued

Continued

Risk/type category	Abnormality	Genes involved	Frequency (%)			Comments/associations
			Pediatric	Both	Adults	
	Deletion 9p21	CDKN2A	~50–65%	70%	45%	Often cryptic. FISH detection suggested. Monoallelic or biallelic deletions. Acquired isodisomy or CN-LOH in 8% of pediatric ALL
	Deletion 11p12p13	LMO2	~4.0%			Cryptic deletion detected in pediatric T-ALL results in upregulation of LMO2
	Deletion 18p11.21	PTPN2		~6%		Associated with aberrant expression of the TLX1 and NUP214-ABL1 fusion
Gains	MYB duplication	MYB/6q23.3	~8.0%			Small duplication; may represent therapeutic target
	ABL1 gain/amplification	ABL1/9q34		~6%		See ABL1 fusion gene comments in this table
Common Mutations	9q34.3	NOTCH1	~50%		~60%	Prognosis first reported as favorable but recent reports are conflicting. May response to NOTCH inhibitors. Cooperates with loss of EZH2 and SUZ12; may be seen with or without FBXW7 mutations
	4q31.3	FBXW7	~11–31%	~15%	~18%	Prognostic value uncertain
	Xq26.2	PHF6	~16%		~38%	X-linked TSG almost exclusively in males

ALL, acute lymphoblastic leukemia; FISH, fluorescence *in situ* hybridization; TCR, T-cell receptor; aka, also known as; N/A, not available; TKI, tyrosine kinase inhibitors; CN-LOH, copy neutral loss of heterozygosity.

hybridization (FISH), a molecular cytogenetic technique that typically uses ~150–300 kb DNA probes to target specific areas of the genome, is used routinely to detect "cryptic" (not visible by conventional cytogenetics) aberrations that have prognostic significance in ALL [e.g., t(12;21)(p13;q22), t(9;9)(q34;q34), and t(5;14)(q35;q32)]. A combination of conventional cytogenetics and FISH has been reported to enable detection of recurring chromosome abnormalities in ~80% of ALL cases.[5,6,18,19] These well-established tumor markers play a pivotal role in the emergence of the neoplastic phenotype, resulting in their use as strong prognostic indicators of outcome. Recently, high-resolution oligonucleotide/single nucleotide polymorphism (SNP) (oligo/SNP) microarrays, gene expression profiling (GEP), and deep sequencing studies have identified novel submicroscopic alterations that disrupt genes that encode regulators of lymphocyte development and proliferation.[20-22] These efforts are helping to distinguish alterations that "drive" ALL leukemogenesis from so-called "passenger" aberrations that have little or pathogenetic role in ALL. Furthermore, recurrent somatic alterations that affects key signaling pathways—such as B-cell development/differentiation, the TP53/RB tumor suppressor, Janus kinase, and RAS signaling pathways—provides the rationale for future targeted or personalized therapeutic approaches.[23-25]

The etiology and pathogenetic events leading to the development of ALL remain largely unknown.[26] A small percentage of ALL cases (<5%) have been associated with predisposing genetic syndromes, such as trisomy 21 (Down) syndrome, Bloom syndrome, ataxia-telangiectasia, and Nijmegen syndrome, or with exposure to cytotoxic agents and ionizing radiation. Moreover, emerging data from genome-wide association studies (GWAS) suggest that germline SNPs at loci involved in lymphoid regulation and differentiation directly influence susceptibility to pediatric ALL; these loci include IKZF1 at 7p12.2, CDKN2A at 9p21.3, ARID5B at 10q21.1, and CEBPE at 14q11.2.[27-31]

In this chapter, I reviewed the diagnostic and prognostic criteria associated with the most commonly acquired cytogenetic abnormalities in B-ALL and T-ALL and the cytogenetic methodologies used for their detection. As you read through this chapter, it is important to keep in mind that the prognostic impact of any given genetic abnormality is also dependent upon the treatment protocol used and other risk factors, such as age, cooperating genetic abnormalities, treatment response, and MRD.

CYTOGENETIC METHODS

A cytogenetic screening strategy in ALL should take into account clinical indication, age, and the clinical trial requirements. In the United States, the National Comprehensive Cancer Network ALL guidelines provide a consensus of the laboratory tests recommended to confirm a diagnosis and detect the clinically relevant aberrations for determining appropriate patient management.[32] Europeans follow a similar approach.[33]

Conventional or Metaphase Cytogenetics

Chromosome analysis should be performed on diagnostic bone marrow (preferred) or peripheral blood samples. It is very important that the samples are collected before any treatment including steroid treatment. Due to the fragility and poor growth of lymphoblasts *in vitro*, extreme care must be taken when seeding, harvesting, and the slide preparation of short-term ALL cultures. Two unstimulated short-term cultures (direct preparations, overnight, or 24 hours) should be evaluated using standard procedures. When possible, a minimum of 20 cells should be analyzed to define all clonal populations, and the abnormal karyotype should be described according to International System of Human Cytogenetic Nomenclature.[34] Periodic follow-up cytogenetic studies are recommended to confirm remission or relapse, detect clonal evolution of disease, and the possibility of an evolving therapy-related neoplasm.

Poor chromosome morphology and low mitotic indexes hinder detailed karyotyping in ALL. It is not uncommon to find only a few karyotypically-aberrant cells in ALL samples with high lymphoblasts counts. Typically, many slides are analyzed to detect the clonal ALL populations. As a result, conventional cytogenetics is supplemented with additional tests, such as FISH, reverse transcription-polymerase chain reaction (RT-PCR), multiplex ligation-dependent probe amplification (MLPA), and oligo/SNP microarrays to detect or confirm cytogenetically hidden, cryptic, or submicroscopic abnormalities within a suboptimal, complex or incomplete karyotypic study.

Fluorescence *In Situ* Hybridization

Two significant limitations of conventional cytogenetics preclude the detection of subtle structural aberrations (<~5-10 Mb in size): the requirement for actively dividing (metaphase) cells to visualize the chromosomes; and the poor morphological appearance of lymphoblasts in metaphase. Thus, FISH screening for the prognostically significant aberrations is often performed on all patients registered on clinical trials.

Fluorescence *in situ* hybridization is a molecular cytogenetic technology that can reliably detect specific cytogenetic abnormalities in interphase (non-dividing) and metaphase cells. For ALL, FISH assays are used to detect known prognostic recurrent gains or losses (numerical abnormalities) of specific chromosomes and structural aberrations (translocations, deletions, amplification). FISH studies should be performed for all newly-diagnosed B-ALL to rule out the high risk translocations (BCR-ABL1 and MLL), the favorable risk "cryptic" 12;21 (ETV6-RUNX1) translocation, and favorable risk high hyperdiploidy by screening for trisomy 4 and trisomy 10. The ETV6-RUNX1 probe set will also detect iAMP21, deletion 12p, and trisomy/tetrasomy chromosome 21. Together, these FISH probes will also confirm the presence of near haploidy and its endoduplicated hyperdiploid subclone (discussed in detail below). In T-ALL, the BCR-ABL1 probe set is routinely used to rule out ABL1 gene amplification. FISH may be performed on the fixed cell suspensions used for chromosome analysis, touch preparations, or destained G-banded slides using standard procedures. Interphase or I-FISH detects its intended target only and provides no information about additional abnormalities that are present or may signal disease progression. Metaphase FISH is an excellent tool to define and refine suspected aberrations in poor quality metaphase spreads or define the partner translocation chromosome. Most FISH probes are between 150 kb to 300 kb in size; however, break-apart probe sets using two probes on either side of a targeted sequence can be as large as 1 Mb. Prior to implementation of any FISH assay for clinical use, cytogenetic laboratories must verify the performance characteristics of the assay (e.g., accuracy, precision, sensitivity and specificity, reference ranges, and reproducibility).

Multiplex Ligation-dependent Probe Amplification

When targeting small (50–70 nucleotides) sequences for single gene aberrations that are too small to be detected by FISH, a technique known as MLPA may be used.[35] Using purified DNA, MLPA is a rapid, high-throughput multiplex PCR method for detecting abnormal copy numbers of up to 50 different genomic DNA sequences. This technology can distinguish sequences differing by only one nucleotide. MLPA is not suitable for genome-wide screening, but commercially-available or customized disease-specific kits allow for selective genes to be interrogated in a limited sample following the manufacturers' instructions. MLPA results should be reported in accordance with International Sustainable Campus Network (ISCN) guidelines.[34] Quantitative MRD assessments by RT-PCR and other molecular assays are described in chapters 4 and 9.

Genome-wide Microarray Approaches

Genome-wide information on copy number alterations in bone marrow samples can be obtained with array comparative genomic hybridization (aCGH) or high resolution oligo/SNP arrays. These DNA-based arrays are highly effective in determining the chromosomal site, size, and genetic content of copy number alterations and defining the minimal region of gain or loss. Together with GEP, mutation analysis, and methylation studies, these genomic tools have the potential to identify candidate genes important in the pathogenesis of ALL and to establish a new molecular risk stratification models.

B-ALL

Cytogenetic analysis and FISH reveal recurring chromosome abnormalities in ~85% of B-ALL. Seven well-characterized WHO B-ALL subgroups associated with aneuploidy (numerical) and specific translocations characteristic of B-ALL are described (Table 5-2). The distribution of chromosomal changes in B-ALL varies according to age, with adolescents and young adults (AYAs; usually defined between the ages of 13–24 years) having the highest incidence of ill-defined abnormalities[16] (Figure 5-2). The incidences of individual chromosomal abnormalities are well-established in childhood B-ALL, with high hyperdiploidy and the translocation, t(12;21)(p13;q22) being the most common. The Philadelphia translocation or t(9;22)(q34.1;q11.2) and the MLL/11q23 translocations are more common in adult ALL (Figures 5-1 and 5-2). Importantly, five chromosomal abnormalities are strong independent indicators of risk of relapse in B-ALL.[16] These aberrations include intrachromosomal amplification of chromosome 21 (iAMP21), t(9;22), MLL translocations, abnormal 17p, and deletion 13q, and are described in greater detail below along with the other common B-cell ALL cytogenetic subgroups. Several versions of B-ALL cytogenetic risk groups have been reported.[4,5,16] Table 5-2 lists the consensus of the most common cytogenetic risk groups for B-ALL.

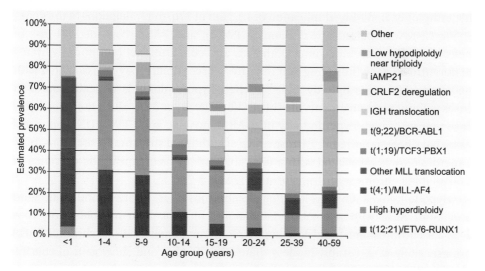

Figure 5-2 Age-specific frequency of the common ALL cytogenetic aberrations. The estimated prevalence is based on the number of samples tested by conventional cytogenetics, fluorescence *in situ* hybridization, or multiplex ligation-dependent probe amplification for the abnormality listed. A minimum of 80 cases per age group was tested with the exception of infant cohort (defined as < 12 months of age). Total study cohort was composed of 7,113 patients. *From* Moorman AV. The clinical relevance of chromosomal and genomic abnormalities in B-cell precursor acute lymphoblastic leukaemia. *Blood Rev.* 2012;26(3):123-35, *with permission.*

Numerical Chromosomal B-ALL Subgroups

Distinct B-ALL hyperdiploid and hypodiploid cytogenetic subgroups are well-established (Table 5-2). High hyperdiploidy is readily detected by flow cytometry because a DNA index between 1.16 and 1.6 corresponds to the 51–65 chromosome range, which defines this subgroup. High hyperdiploidy is the most common pediatric B-ALL subtype, accounting for ~25–30% of childhood B-ALL.[36] High hyperdiploidy occurs in an estimated ~2–10% among AYA and adults with B-ALL but is not observed in infants.[5,19]

High hyperdiploidy shows frequent gain (trisomy or tetrasomy) of chromosomes X, 4, 6, 10, 14, 17, 18, and 21. The simultaneous presence of trisomy 4 and 10 has been associated with a favorable prognosis.[37] By the WHO criteria, this favorable childhood ALL subgroup is associated with a typical B-cell immunophenotype (CD19+, CD10+, TdT+, often CD34+, CD45–), low white blood cell count, and median age of 4 years (most cases presenting between ages 3–5 years), with cures rate greater than 90% of children. At the typical 300–400 band level of karyotype resolution in ALL, recurring structural aberrations have not been detected in high hyperdiploidy. This suggests that chromosome or gene dosage underlies the pathological consequences of this subgroup. However, high-resolution microarray studies have detected many additional abnormalities in 80% of high hyperdiploidy, including duplication of 1q, gain of 17q, microdeletions of the genes ETV6, CDKN2A, paired-box domain 5 (PAX5), and PAN3, copy-neutral loss of heterozygosity of chromosomes 9 and 11, and constitutional (germline) variants of the *ARID5B* gene indicating that inherited susceptibility may be associated with pediatric high hyperdiploidy ALL.[22,38] High hyperdiploidy is typically found in cases without rearrangements of MLL, ETV6-RUNX1, or BCR-ABL1; however, a few case reports of high hyperdiploidy BCR-ABL1-positive and ETV6-RUNX1-positive cases have been reported.[39,40] Irrespective of additional structural aberrations, high hyperdiploidy is associated with a favorable prognosis except in the presence of Philadelphia chromosome translocation (Table 5-2).

Hypodiploidy, defined as less than 46 chromosomes, is rare in both childhood and adult ALL, with a combined incidence of ~5%. Near-haploid karyotypes (~23–29 chromosomes) and low hypodiploid karyotypes (~30–39 chromosomes) are especially rare, comprising less than 1% of B-ALL, and show gain of specific chromosomes onto the haploid chromosome set. Most patients in this subgroup show a related doubling product (hyperdiploidy) of the near-haploid clone.[41] FISH studies are required to confirm the presence of near haploidy and its endoduplicated hyperdiploid subclone.

In the near haploid group, the most common chromosome gains to the haploid set are chromosomes 21, 14, 18, and the sex chromosomes. Similarly, the pattern of chromosome gains in the low hypodiploid subgroup shows gains of chromosomes 1,

11, 19, 10, and 22 to the near haploid clone, with loss (monosomy) of chromosomes 7 and 17. Age restrictions separate these adverse risk hypodiploid groups with less than 40 chromosomes. Near haploidy is restricted to children (median age of 7 years, age range 2–15 years), whereas low hypodiploidy includes adults and children (range 9–54 years), with most reported cases in the AYA age group.[18,41]

Structural Chromosomal B-ALL Subgroups

Structural abnormalities with an associated prognostic risk group used in treatment stratification are discussed individually below. Translocations may be detected by conventional cytogenetics, FISH, or RT-PCR. The translocations t(12;21), t(9;22), t(1;19), and t(4;11) have unique gene expression signatures and associated responses to treatment.[42-45] These gene expression observations are currently being further validated in independent prospective and unselected clinical trial-based studies.

B-ALL with t(9;22)(q34.1;q11.2); BCR-ABL1

The t(9;22)(q34.1;q11.2), or the Philadelphia chromosome translocation, is the most common primary karyotypic aberration in adult ALL and conveys a poor prognosis in both children and adults. The incidence of t(9;22) increases with age. This translocation is found in ~30% of adult ALL but only ~3% of childhood ALL.[8,23,46] The translocation results in the fusion of breakpoint cluster region (BCR) at 22q11.2 with the cytoplasmic tyrosine kinase gene ABL1 at 9q34.1. Because of heterogeneity in the BCR breakpoint, this translocation can result in one of three different molecular weight fusion products that upregulates tyrosine kinase activity: p190 (minor BCR breakpoint found in pediatric and most adult BCR-ABL ALL), p210 (major BCR breakpoint found in some adult ALL), or the very rare p230 (micro-BCR breakpoint). B-ALL with t(9;22) is frequently CD10+, CD19+, TdT+, with frequent expression of the myeloid markers CD13 and CD33.[47] Secondary aberrations are frequently observed, but the primary 9;22 translocation determines treatment. Monosomy 7 is the most common numeric loss in this ALL subgroup and implies loss of the IKZF1/7p12.2 gene, which encodes the lymphoid transcription factor IKAROS.[48] Deletion of CDKN2A/9p21 is also common (~30%) in newly diagnosed BCR-ABL1-positive adult ALL, with a higher incidence (~50%) detected at relapse.[49] Submicroscopic deletions/alterations IKZF1 and CKDN2A deletions are easily detected by SNPs/oligo microarrays (Figures 5-3). In addition, t(8;14)(q11;q32), an IGH gene rearrangement with the CCAAT/enhancer binding protein delta or CEBPD, has been associated with "cryptic" BCR-ABL1-positive ALL.[50] Twin studies provide compelling evidence that the BCR-ABL1 fusion detected in prenatal samples is an initiating genetic event, which in the absence of additional, secondary changes remains clinically silent. IKZF1 deletions represent secondary cooperating postnatal events that trigger fulminant BCR-ABL1-positive childhood B-ALL.

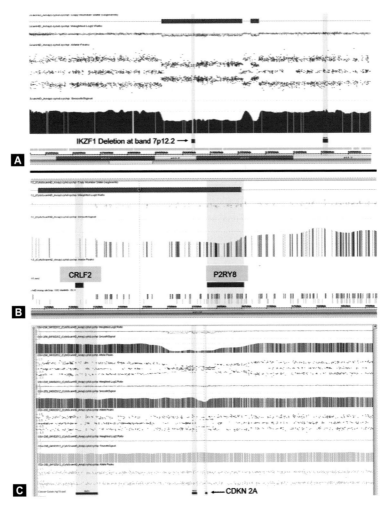

Figure 5-3 Microdeletions detected by oligo/single nucleotide polymorphism microarrays. **A,** IKZF1 deletion within band 7p12.2 in a patient with B-ALL. The larger red bar marks the area with the IKZF1 deletion. The weighted log2 ratio shows a small dip and the SNP allele peak tract is pinched in indicating loss of one allele. The smooth signal tract clearly shows the loss of one copy of IKZF1. Blue block and gray vertical line, gene position of IKZF1 on chromosome 7; **B,** The red bar marks the ~320 kb deleted segment which leads to fusion of P2RY8-CRLF2, resulting in CRLF2 overexpression. The smooth signal tract shows the deletion in relation to the normal two allele ratio seen to the right of the deletion; **C,** Examples of three different CDKN2A aberrations. The first example (purple) shows biallelic CDKN2A deletions with a very clear pinched in SNP allele peak. The middle example (pink) shows a monoallelic CDKN2A deletion. The third example shows copy-number neutral loss of homozygosity for the entire short arm of chromosome 9. Note, the allele peak showed two instead of three SNP tracts and the smooth signaling tract indicates a normal two copy number pattern.

Historically, the presence of the 9;22 translocation has been associated with an adverse outcome. The addition of tyrosine kinase inhibitors (TKIs), as an integral part of frontline therapy for BCR/ABL1-positive ALL, results in high remission rates (>90%) and encouraging event-free survival rates of 60% in adults and ~80% in children.[51-53] Unfortunately, acquired resistance on TKI treatment occurs in ~30% of patients, meaning that many patients receive only short-lived clinical benefit. Thus, allogeneic stem cell transplantation (SCT) in first complete remission (CR) remains the standard strategy and best curative option for BCR-ABL1 positive ALL[53]

B-ALL with t(v;11q23); MLL Rearranged

The MLL gene on band 11q23 is known as the most promiscuous gene in the genome because it has fused with over 100 partner genes in the acute leukemias. MLL rearrangements occur in ~6-10% of children and adults ALL. The most common MLL translocation in ALL is t(4;11)(q21;q23) (Figure 5-4A), which results in an MLL-AFF1 fusion and accounts for ~50% of ALL cases in infants younger than 6 months (*see* Infant Leukemia). The frequency decreases by two- to three-fold in children 6-11 months of age.[54] In older children and adults, MLL-AFF1 accounts for only less than 5% of ALL cases.[18,47] The age-associated incidence is thought to be related with environmental factors. In particular, DNA topoisomerase II is highly expressed in developing fetuses and exposure to DNA topoisomerase II inhibitors, possibly by diet, could induce MLL rearrangements *in utero*.[55,56]

B-cell acute lymphoblastic leukemia with t(4;11)(q21;q23); MLL-AFF1 is frequently associated with a high WBC (>100,000/μL) at diagnosis and CNS involvement.[54] MLL-rearranged lymphoblasts are typically positive for CD19, CD34, and terminal deoxynucleotidyl transferase (TdT) and negative or weakly positive for CD10, CD24, and CD20, and frequently express the myeloid-associated antigens CD15 and/or CD65.[46] Two other common MLL fusion partners in B-ALL are MLLT1/19p13.3 (previously known as ENL), occurring in approximately 1% of childhood ALL,[57] and MLLT3/9p21 (previously known as AF9). In general, the prognosis of MLL-rearranged B-ALL is poor. Cooperative efforts are now in progress to determine if specific MLL translocations convey a better or worse prognosis, particularly among infants.

B-ALL with t(12;21)(p13;q22); ETV6-RUNX1

The "cryptic" t(12;21)(p13;q22) was not discovered until the mid-1990s, because this rearrangement results in the exchange of two G-negative bands of equal size[58-60] but is easily detected by FISH.[60] The 12;21 translocation results in an ETV6-RUNX1 fusion, previously known as TEL-AML1, and is thought to represent an initiating event in the most common genetically aberrant subgroup of childhood ALL.[61] The ETV6-RUNX1 fusion occurs in approximately 25% of younger B-ALL

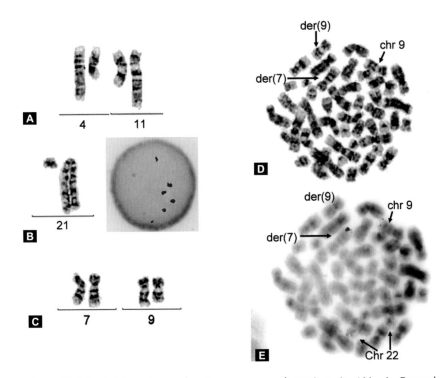

Figure 5-4 Partial karyotypes showing common aberrations in ALL. **A,** Example of t(4;11)(q21;q23) in B-ALL; **B,** Example of intrachromosomal amplification of chromosome 21 or iAMP21 in B-ALL (left) and interphase ETV6-RUNX1 fluorescence in situ hybridization (FISH) shows six (red) RUNX1 signals; **C,** Chromosome 7 and 9 pairs showing the t(7;9)(q34;q32) found in T-ALL. This subtle translocation is difficult to see by conventional cytogenetics. The normal chromosome 7 and 9 are on the left; the derivative chromosome 7 and 9 are on the right. FISH was performed on the G-banded metaphase cell to confirm chromosome 9 material had translocated to chromosome 7; **D,** The derivative chromosomes 7 and 9 are labeled in the G-banded cell; **E,** The same cell is destained and hybridized using the BCR-ABL1 probe set. The ABL1/9q34 probe (red) hybridizes to the normal chromosome 9 and the derivative chromosome 7. The BCR probe (green) hybridizes to the normal chromosomes 22.

patients (mostly between the ages of 1 year and 9 years), whereas only a few adult cases have been described.[58,59,62,63] ETV6-RUNX1 positive ALL is positive for CD19, CD34, TdT, and CD10, often positive for CD33 and/or CD13, and negative for CD20 and CD66.[46] Because the 12;21 translocation is not visible by conventional karyotyping, all newly diagnosed ALL patients between the ages of 1 year and 9 years are routinely tested for this fusion using either RT-PCR and FISH. This FISH-based approach is important in revealing complex (three-way) or hidden ETV6-RUNX1 translocations (Figure 5-5).

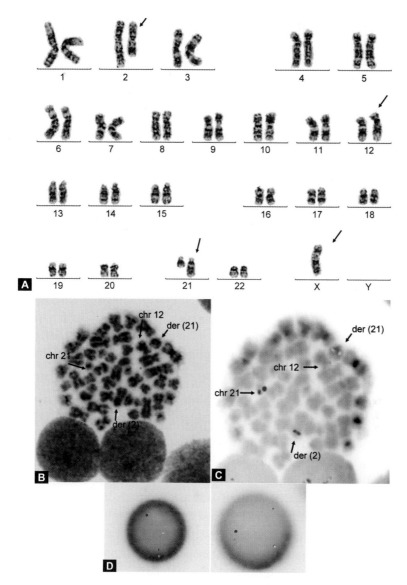

Figure 5-5 Karyotype showing a hidden ETV6-RUNX1 translocation. **A,** Karyotype with a 4-break chromosome rearrangement. In this case, the 12;21 occurred followed by second translocation involving chromosome 2 with the derivative chromosome 21; **B,** A G-banded metaphase cell was destained and hybridized with the ETV6-RUNX1 probe set; **C,** The fused (red-green) ETV-RUNX1 signal is on the derivative chromosome 21. The smaller (extra) red signal which would normally hybridize to the derivative chromosome 12 is on the derivative chromosome 2. The non-translocated chromosome 21 (red signal) and chromosome 12 (green signal) are also shown; **D,** Two interphase cells showing the typical ETV6-RUN1 positive pattern of one fusion, one red, one green and one small (extra) red signal. Only metaphase FISH allow for the detection of the small red (extra) signal to chromosome 2 and not chromosome 12.

ETV6-RUNX1 karyotypes frequently show additional (secondary) aberrations, including deletion of ETV6 on the non-translocated chromosome 12, +21, +der(21)t(12;21), +16, and CDKN2A/9p21 deletions.[64] These frequent secondary aberrations have been confirmed by oligo/SNP arrays, which detected an average of 3.5 copy number aberrations (CNAs) per ETV6-RUNX1 positive case (range, 0–13 CNAs/case).[65,66]

Acute lymphoblastic leukemia patients with ETV6-RUNX1 fusions have a favorable prognosis,[4] especially when using MRD-guided treatment protocols with intensive asparaginase and high-dose methotrexate.[67] Unfortunately, ~20% of ETV6-RUNX1 positive ALL patients relapse. To gain insight into the relapse mechanisms of this subgroup, Kuster et al.[68] analyzed 18 paired diagnostic and relapsed ALL samples by SNP arrays. SNP analysis detected on average five more CNAs at relapse (12.5) than at diagnosis (7.5). Patterns of recurring deletions also suggested that glucocorticoid-associated drug resistance may be linked to relapse of ETV6-RUNX1-positive B-ALL: in particular, the deletions housed genes associated with glucocorticoid-mediated apoptosis targeting the BMF (BCL2 modifying factor) gene, glucocorticoid receptor NR3C1 gene, and components of the mismatch repair pathways. Continued detection of these potentially clinically relevant submicroscopic deletions may guide future therapies in relapsed ETV6-RUNX1 positive ALL.

B-ALL with t(1;19)(q23;p13.3); TCF3-PBX1 (Previously known as E2A-PBX1)

Translocation (1;19)(q23;p13) occurs in ~5% of children and adults with ALL, usually resulting in a TCF3-PBX1 fusion.[69,70] The functional fusion gene resides on the derivative chromosome 19, thus either a balanced or unbalanced form with loss of the derivative chromosome 1 may occur. TCF3-PBX1 positive lymphoblasts are typically positive for CD19, CD10, cytoplasmic μ Ig heavy chain, CD9+, CD20 variable and CD34+/−.[46] Using antimetabolite-based therapy, this subgroup was regarded as high risk; however, with the more recent use of intensive multiagent regimens, this subgroup is now considered standard risk.[8,71] CNS relapse has been associated with this subgroup.[4] Rare cases of t(1;19) positive ALL have hyperdiploid DNA content and do not involve TCF3-PBX1 and should be classified as hyperdiploid ALL.[72]

A rare variant of the t(1;19) is the t(17;19)(q22;p13), which results in the TCF3-HLF fusion.[73] This translocation, found in less than 1% of children (age range, 5–18 years) with B-ALL, has an adverse prognosis and thus must be identified and distinguished from other TCF3-positive B-ALL.[4]

Intrachromosomal Amplification of Chromosome 21 or iAMP21

First described in 2001 by Busson-Le Coniat and colleagues[74] as multiple copies of the RUNX1 gene on a derivative chromosome 21, iAMP21 now defines a small

(~3–5%) but distinct subgroup of childhood B-ALL.[13,75,76] The cytogenetic clue of this subgroup is the presence of a structurally abnormal chromosome 21 with uneven repetitions of the chromosomal material (Figure 5-4B).[74,75] Because iAMP is not associated with any other known recurrent aberration in ALL, FISH using a targeted *RUNX1* probe is the only reliable detection method for this abnormality. iAMP is defined as ~3–4 or more copies of *RUNX1* observed as multiple signals in interphase cells (Figure 5-4B) or in tandem repetition along the length of the derivative chromosome 21 by metaphase FISH.[77] The common region of amplification on chromosome 21 has been narrowed down to a 5.1 Mb region, 21q22.11 to 21q22.12 which includes RUNX1, microRNA802, or *miR802*, and genes within the Down syndrome (DS) critical region, thus it is not known if RUNX1 is a driver or passenger target of this distinct subgroup. Recurrent secondary abnormalities observed in iAMP ALL are IKZF1 (22%), CDKN2A/B (17%), PAX5 (8%), ETV6 (19%), and RB1 (37%).[78] In addition, a deletion of the pseudoautosomal region 1 of a sex chromosome resulting in fusion of P2RY8-CRLF2 and overexpression of the type 1 cytokine receptor CRLF2 gene has been detected in ~40% of iAMP21 patients.[79]

Intrachromosomal amplification of chromosome 21 usually presents in older children or young adolescents (median age 9.4 years, range 5–20 years) with low WBC and a common/pre-B immunophenotype. In comparison with other pediatric ALL patients, iAMP21 patients show an increased risk of both early and late relapses and a uniformly poor outcome with standard ALL regimens;[16,76] however, intensive therapeutic approaches, including allogeneic SCT look promising and are clearly warranted for this ALL subgroup.[13]

IGH Gene Rearrangements in B-ALL

Translocations involving the immunoglobulin heavy chain or IGH gene within band 14q32 are emerging as a significant subgroup in B-ALL (Table 5-2), especially in the AYA subgroup. The overall incidence is thought to be ~2–3% in B-ALL,[80,81] with a slightly higher incidence of ~8% in childhood B-ALL.[82] However, this frequency could be underestimated because of the prevalence of "cryptic" IGH gene rearrangements that are not detected by conventional cytogenetics. These rearrangements are surprisingly first detected by interphase FISH, followed by metaphase FISH to determine the partner chromosome.

B-ALL with t(5;14)(q13;q32); IL3-IGH

The WHO classification system recognizes B-ALL with t(5;14)(q13;q32); IL3-IGH as a rare but distinct ALL subgroup based on immunophenotypic (CD19+ and CD10+) and cytogenetic findings, regardless of the blast count.[7] The 5;14 translocation results in breaks in the promoter region of IL3 and in the JH region of IGH, leading to overexpression of IL3.[83] A unique feature of this ALL subgroup is a reactive hypereosinophilia. Surprisingly, the eosinophils do not show the t(5;14) and they are not part of the leukemic clone. This rare ALL subgroup is not associated with a specific prognosis; however, the trend appears to be intermediate to poor.

CRLF2 and Other IGH Rearrangements in B-ALL

Fluorescence *in situ* hybridization and high-resolution microarray studies have identified several recurring IGH translocations in B-ALL that are more commonly seen in the AYA age group (Table 5-2). The most frequent IGH translocations juxtapose the IGH enhancer to a cytokine receptor-like factor 2 gene (CRLF2) in the pseudoautosomal region (PAR1) of the X and Y chromosomes: t(X;14) (p22;q32) and t(Y;14)(p11;q32). Other IGH rearrangements in B-ALL involve inhibitor of DNA binding 4 (ID4), the collective CCAAT enhancer-binding protein (CEBPA, B, D, and E) translocations, and the cytokine receptor for erythropoietin (EPO4).[18,79,84-87] The CRLF2-IGH translocation leads to overexpression of CRLF2 at both the transcript and protein levels. Similarly, a 320 kb microdeletion within PAR1, giving rise to an intrachromosomal P2RY8-CRLF2 fusion also results in overexpression of CRLF2 (Figure 5-3B). The PAR1 deletion variant has been reported in ~60% of DS-ALL, usually in association with +X and del(9p)/CDKN2A.[87] CRLF2 alterations, including activating mutations of the CRLF2 receptor (e.g., CRLF2-F232C), are associated with activating mutations of JAK kinases, which together result in constitutive activation of the JAK-STAT signaling pathway.[87-89] Importantly, CRLF2 alterations have also been associated with IKZF1 alterations and Hispanic/Latino ethnicity.[89] Reports on the prognostic relevance of CRLF2 alterations are conflicting, with an associated poor prognosis in adults and children in some clinical trials[89,90] but an intermediate outcome in the UK ALL97 trial.[91] Nevertheless, clinical trials of JAK inhibitors in high-risk B-ALL are currently under investigation.

Several other recurrent IGH translocations have been reported (Table 5-2; reviewed in reference 18). IGH translocations are known to deregulate the expression of their partner gene by juxtaposition with IGH transcriptional enhancers. The diversity of the targeted genes, including cytokine receptors, transcription factors, signaling adapter molecules, and miRNAs reflects the heterogeneity of pathogenic mechanisms that underlie B-ALL. Many genes targeted by IGH translocations are also deregulated in B-ALL by other genetic or epigenetic mechanisms. The clinical importance of infrequent IGH translocations in B-ALL remains to be determined from prospective studies.

9p/PAX5 Balanced and Unbalanced Translocations

The PAX5 gene plays an essential role in B-cell lymphocyte development,[92] underscoring its significance as a critical mutation target in adult and childhood B-ALL.[93-96] FISH studies have confirmed that dicentric and apparently balanced chromosome rearrangements involving the short arm of chromosome 9 frequently hit PAX5, resulting in partial or complete deletion of PAX5 at 9p13.2.[93,95,96] B-lymphoblasts carrying PAX5 balanced translocations usually displayed a simple karyotype.[95,96] Over 17 partner genes are known to fuse with PAX5, including FOXP1/3p13, LOC392027/7p12.1, SLCO1B3/12p12, ASXL1/20q11.1, KIF3B/20q11.21, and C20orf112/20q11.1 (Table 5-2).[96,97] These fusion genes result in underexpressed PAX5 with concomitant differential expression of the corresponding PAX5 target genes EBF1, ALDH1A1, ATP9A, and FLT3. Deletion and mutation of the homologous PAX5 allele on the non-translocated chromosome 9 provides further support for a critical role of PAX5 in B-ALL.[96]

In 153 adult and childhood, B-ALL patients with deletion 9p detected by conventional cytogenetics, Coyaud and colleagues[95] detected PAX5 internal rearrangements in 21% of the cases. Recurrent and new PAX5 translocations, involving NCOR1, DACH2, GOLGA6, and TAOK1 genes gave rise to truncated PAX5 proteins in simple karyotypes, suggesting that PAX5 translocations are a primary aberration in some B-ALL cases. In contrast, deletions of PAX5 in association with other 9p alterations and complex karyotypes support the contention for a late or secondary event in a larger subset of B-ALL. Finally, using deep exon sequencing, Familiades et al.[94] detected PAX5 mutations in approximately one-third of adult B-ALL. It appears that PAX5 alterations are very heterogeneous, consisting of complete, partial or focal deletions, point mutations, and less frequently (~2%) translocations. Complete loss of PAX5 is thought to represent a secondary event in BCR-ABL1 and TCF3-PBX1 fusion-positive ALL, whereas PAX5 point mutations and the balanced translocations are most consistent with a primary or causal B-ALL event.

dic(9;20)(p13.2;q11.2)

Dicentric (9;20)(p13.2;q11.2) is a characteristic abnormality reported in ~1–2% of childhood B-ALL, resulting in loss of 9p and 20q. The 9p breakpoints cluster within a 1.5 Mb segment of band 9p13.2.[98] The true frequency of this unbalanced translocation may be higher because fusion of the short arm of chromosome 20 with the long arm of chromosome 9 often masks the chromosome 9 alteration. It is, therefore, essential to rule out a dic(9;20) aberration by metaphase FISH or microarray analysis when a karyotype shows an apparent loss of one copy of chromosome 20. In a Nordic study, the dic(9;20) cohort showed a modal chromosome distribution of ~45–50 chromosomes with frequent homozygous loss of CDKN2A, gain of chromosomes 21 and X, and less frequently gain of the derivative chromosome 20.[98]

The median patient age of this ALL subgroup is 3 years, with a female predominance and a median WBC of 24×10^9/L. Nearly 11% of reported patients have CNS involvement, and 5% present with a mediastinal mass. Consistent immunophenotypic features include positivity for HLA-DR, CD10, CD19, CD20, and CD22. Twenty-nine dic(9;20)-positive cases were treated according to the NOPHO ALL 2000 protocol.[99] Relapses occurred in 24% (7/29), resulting in a 5-year event-free survival of 0.69, which was significantly worse than for t(12;21) and high hyperdiploidy.[99] Although relapses, especially in the CNS, are common, post-relapse treatment of many dic(9;20) patients is successful.[99] In addition, dic(9;20) patients treated on a four drug induction and subsequent consolidation acute lymphoblastic leukemia-Berlin-Frankfurt-Münster (ALL-BFM) protocol were all good responders to prednisone and in CR after induction therapy.[100] In conclusion, with aggressive multiagent ALL therapy, dic(9;20)-positive B-ALL appears to have a favorable prognosis.

dic(9;12)(p13;p13) ALL

The dicentric (9;12) is most common in B-progenitor ALL in children and young adults, but is rarely detected in infants. It is easily identified by conventional cytogenetics and usually results in a PAX5-ETV6 gene rearrangement; however, PAX5-SLCO1B3 has also been reported.[96] Although most patients have at least one adverse prognostic indicator, most notably age greater than 10 years or WBC greater than 100×10^9/L, this ALL subgroup is associated with an excellent prognosis overall.[93,101] Trisomy 8 and additional structural chromosomal changes are commonly seen as secondary aberrations. Dicentric (9;12) has also been reported in rare cases of chronic myeloid leukemia in lymphoid blast crisis, T-cell lymphoblastic lymphoma, and T-cell non-Hodgkin lymphoma.

Down Syndrome and ALL

Children with DS have an increased risk of developing ALL, yet DS-ALL accounts for a surprisingly low frequency (20% vs. 66%) of the well-established childhood B-ALL cytogenetic aberrations described above.[102-105] For example, high hyperdiploidy-positive DS-ALL accounts for only ~10% of childhood B-ALL, compared to ~25–30% for the non DS-ALL children. Given that high-hyperdiploidy DS-ALL and high-hyperdiploidy non-DS-ALL share the same chromosomal gains, these entities likely have a common etiology/pathogenesis mechanism.[102] Conversely, DS-ALL shows an over representation of cases with +X, t(8;14)(q11;q32) and del(9p).[50] Unlike, DS-acute myeloid leukemia (AML), which is characterized by the unique genetic event of acquired mutations of the globin transcription factor 1, or GATA1 gene, cytogenetic and gene expression studies have shown that DS-ALL is a highly heterogeneous disease.[88] Regardless, as discussed above, two cytogenetic aberrations that result in CRLF2 overexpression have been described in ~60% of DS-ALL: a CRLF2-IGH translocation and an interstitial deletion of *PAR1* within a sex chromosome, resulting in P2RY8-CRLF2 fusion (Figure 5-3B). Because CRLF2 alterations cooperate with activating mutations of JAK kinases, most DS-ALL patients may benefit from therapy blocking the CRLF2/JAK2 pathways.

Infant ALL

Infant ALL, defined as presentation of ALL within the first 12 months of life, is a rare but distinct acute leukemia subgroup with a particularly high risk of treatment failure [5-year overall survival (OS) rate of ~50%].[106] Within this poor prognosis acute leukemia subgroup, 60% of infants present with ALL and 40% with AML and show an MLL/11q23 gene rearrangement.[107-110] The biologic features of infant ALL differ from those seen in older children (> 1 year) with ALL. The presence or absence of an 11q23/*MLL* rearrangement is used to subdivide infant ALL. Characteristics of MLL-positive infant ALL include high WBC, CD10-negative lymphoblasts, and frequent CNS involvement. The most common translocation in infant ALL is t(4;11)(q21;q23) (~50%), followed by t(11;19)(q23;p13.3) and t(9;11)(p21;q23)(~10% each).[109] On the other hand, infants whose lymphoblasts show a germline *MLL* gene configuration (~20%) frequently present with CD10-positive B-ALL and have a significantly better outcome than infants with MLL-positive B-ALL.[107,108,110] Additionally, microarray studies show striking differences in gene expression profiles among infants with ALL based on the presence or absence of MLL status[111] and age of presentation (≤90 vs >90 days of age).[112] Statistical modeling of GEP data in infant ALL suggests that the expression pattern of just three genes (FLT3, TACC2, and IRX2) may be helpful in predicting event-free survival and possibly provide novel insights into the various mechanisms associated with infant leukemogenesis.[112]

Genomic Profiling Reveals Submicroscopic Co-operative Abnormalities in B-ALL

High-resolution oligo/SNP arrays have advanced our understanding of how the disruption of genes involved in B-cell development and differentiation contribute to B-ALL pathogenesis.[20] These heterogenous genetic abnormalities may present as submicroscopic deletions, duplications, amplification, point mutations, cryptic fusions, and copy-neutral loss of heterozygosity (CN-LOH) (i.e., acquired isodisomy or uniparental disomy) that target genes and their cellular pathways known to play a critical role in lymphocyte differentiation and cell cycle progression.[20,113,114] The B-cell developmental pathway genes frequently altered include PAX5, TCF3, TCF4, EBF1, LEF1, IKZF1, and IKZF3; the cell cycle regulator and tumor suppressor genes CDKN2A, CDKN1B, RB1, and PTEN; the lymphoid signaling genes CD200, BTLA, BTG1, and BLNK and the glucocorticoid receptor drug response gene NR3C1.[20,68,115] Some of these deletions are large enough to be detected by FISH, but high-resolution microarrays provide an overall comprehensive genomic analysis (Figures 5-3A–C). The association of submicroscopic gene alterations with cytogenetically-defined B-ALL subgroups, e.g., IKZF1 deletions and mutations of the JAK kinases with poor prognosis in BCR-ABL1 positive and CRLF2-rearranged B-ALL, has identified critical drug resistant genetic alterations with a high risk of treatment failure.[48,79,89,112,113,116-118] Expanding these studies using extensive deep-mutation sequencing, Zhang et al. defined four central signaling pathways in high-risk pediatric B-ALL, the B-cell development/differentiation, the TP53/RB tumor suppressor pathway, RAS signaling, and the Janus kinase pathway.[24] Such results portend the basis for new therapeutic strategies in high-risk childhood B-ALL.

T-ALL

T-cell acute lymphoblastic leukemia and T-cell lymphoblastic lymphoma are classified together by the WHO classification as "T-lymphoblastic leukemia/lymphoma," simply differing by the extent of bone marrow infiltration. T-ALL is a genetically heterogeneous disease that is more often seen in males and in AYA more frequently than in younger children. T-ALL is defined by expression of T-cell associated antigens (e.g., cytoplasmic CD3 with CD7 plus CD2 or CD5; see chapter 3 for further details) with TdT positivity.[46] Recurring cytogenetic aberrations are identified in ~50% of T-ALL patients using conventional cytogenetics (Table 5-3);[119] however, the WHO does not classify T-ALL by specific karyotypic aberrations. Unlike B-ALL, numerical changes in T-ALL are rare and have no prognostic significance. Because many of the T-ALL aberrations are "cryptic" (e.g., CDKN2A, NUP-ABL1, and the 5;14 translocation), FISH, MLPA, PCR, and high-resolution microarrays are the best assays for defining these aberrations.[120,121] High-resolution microarray studies estimate a case of T-ALL to have on average four CNAs (usually focal deletions).[20,122] T-ALL genetic aberrations may be grouped into five molecular pathways based on cooperating mutations that promote aberrant proliferation and survival that contribute to T-ALL leukemogenesis. These pathways involve cell cycle perturbations, blocked differentiation, uncontrolled proliferation, selective survival advantage, and unrestricted self-renewal capacity.[120,123-126]

T-Cell Receptor Gene Rearrangements

T-cell receptor (TCR) gene translocations have been described in ~35% of patients with T-ALL. These translocations juxtapose the regulatory region (promoter or enhancer) of TCR genes (the alpha, TRA, or delta, TRD, genes at 14q11.2 or the beta, TRB gene at 7q34) to various transcription factor genes, such as the basic helix-loop-helix genes (MYC, TAL1, TAL2, LYL1, and OLIG2) or the cysteine-rich LIM-domain-only genes (LMO1 or LMO2) involved in transcriptional regulation (Table 5-3).[119,127] TCR translocations also involve the cell cycle regulator cyclin D2 gene (CCND2),[128] the class II TLX1 and TLX3 homeobox genes, and the other class I genes of the HOXA gene cluster (Table 5-3).[129-133] The TLX1 (previously known as HOX11) homeobox gene at 10q24 is translocated to either TRB or TRA in t(7;10)(q34;q24) and t(10;14) (q24.32;q11.2), respectively. These αβ TCR translocations are more often seen in adults than children, show an early cortical phenotype, and are associated with a more favorable outcome compared to other types of T-ALL.[125]

TAL1 can fuse to many target genes. The TAL1-TCR translocations are observed in ~3% of childhood T-ALL; however, the majority of TAL1 rearrangements occur by a cryptic ~90 kb interstitial deletion resulting in a STIL-TAL1 fusion (Table 5-3). Likewise, TAL2 is juxtaposed to TRB in the t(7;9)(q34;q32) (Figures 5-4C, D, and F), suggesting that TAL1 and TAL2 have similar properties and promote T-ALL by a common mechanism.[134] These mutually exclusive TCR translocations are considered the driving or primary aberrations that result in oncogenetic activation of TAL1, LMO2, TLX1, TLX3, MYB, and HOXA. GEP has confirmed mutually exclusive aberrant expression patterns for TAL1/LMO, LYL1, TLX1, TLX3, HOXA, and the two T-ALL translocations involving PICALM and MLL, consistent with distinct genetically defined T-cell subgroups.[123,126,135] Currently, no recurring T-cell receptor gamma (TRG) locus maps to band 7p14) chromosomal translocations have been reported.

t(5;14)(q35;q32) T-ALL

Nearly 20% of pediatric and 5% of adult T-ALL cases are characterized by overexpression of TLX3 due to the cryptic t(5;14)(q35;q32) or its variant translocations (Table 5-3).[130-133] The 5;14 translocation results in the TLX3-BCL11B gene rearrangement, whereas the two variant rearrangements juxtapose TLX3 with NKX2-5 or CDK6/7q21.[132,136] Deletion 5q35 occurs in ~25% of TLX3 rearranged T-ALL cases, with frequent deletion of WT1 (a transcription factor that plays an important role in cell development and survival) and FBXW7 (a U3-ubiquitin ligase that mediates the degradation of NOTCH1). Other cooperating genetic events identified in TLX3-rearranged T-ALL patients include NOTCH1 mutations, CDKN2A/2B/9p deletions, NUP214-ABL1 aberrations, and deletions of 1p36, 5q35, 13q14.3, 16q22.1, and 19p13.2.[137] TLX3 aberrations in T-ALL patients are associated with γδ-lineage and immature T-cell development.[138]

Fusion Genes Associated with T-ALL

The fusion genes of MLL and ABL1 in T-ALL are characterized by arrest at an early stage of thymocyte differentiation with commitment to γδ-lineage.[119,124,139,140] MLL-rearranged T-ALL has a reported frequency of ~4–8%.[124,139] The most common translocation in T-ALL is t(11;19)(q23;p13.3), which results in an MLL-MLLT1 fusion (previously known as MLL-ENL). Unlike other MLL-rearranged forms of B-ALL, that are generally associated with an adverse prognosis, MLL-MLLT1 is associated with an excellent prognosis in pediatric T-ALL.[57] Similar to MLL-rearranged B-ALL, GEP in T-ALL shows increased expression of HOXA9, HOXA10, and HOXC6 genes and the HOX gene cofactor MEIS1, suggesting that dysregulation of the HOX gene family is the dominant leukemic transformation mechanism in MLL-rearranged T-ALL.[124]

The t(10;11)(p12;q14) was first reported in 1991 and results in a PICALM-MLLT10 fusion.[141,142] This translocation is also restricted to mature T-ALL expressing TCRγδ and their precursor, immature IMγδ T-ALL, with an immunophenotype positive for cCD3, CD5, CD7, and TdT but negative for CD2. The reported frequency is ~10% in pediatric and adult T-ALL, although this may be an underestimate because detection by conventional cytogenetics often fails in ALL. The best way to detect this translocation is to use a combination of FISH or PCR, immunophenotype, and TCR assays. GEP studies have characterized t(10;11)-positive T-ALL with exclusive overexpression of BMI1/10p12.3, a gene in close proximity to MLLT10 that is associated with self-renewal of leukemia stem cells and concurrent upregulation of HOXA5, HOXA9, and HOXA10 and their co-regulator MEIS1.[143,144] Unique overexpression of BMI1 apparently inhibits CDKN2A without deleting the gene, resulting in aberrant cell proliferation.[145] In general, the prognosis of this subgroup is thought to be poor.[142,146]

Various ABL1 fusions have been identified in roughly 8% of T-ALL cases. The most common of these, NUP214-ABL1, is found in 6% of T-ALL. In the AYA group (median age, 15 years), this fusion is associated with the usual high risk T-ALL features.[147] NUP214-ABL1 results from an intrachromosomal deletion within band 9q34 that is not visible by conventional cytogenetics. The chimeric NUP214-ABL1 fusion protein is a constitutively active tyrosine kinase with weak oncogenetic properties, which explains why this specific ABL1-fusion is always duplicated or amplified in T-ALL.[148] NUP214-ABL1 must be tested for by FISH, microarrays, or RT-PCR. Although NUP214-ABL1 is easily detected by FISH on amplified episomes (extrachromosomal elements not visible by G-band analyses), microarrays are best for detection of internal tandem duplications, insertions, and small homogenously staining region.[147,149,150] ABL1 fusions are considered secondary or late genetic events associated with NOTCH1 activating mutations, CDKN2A deletions, and TLX1 or TLX3 overexpression.[147-150] Rare ABL1-fusions detected in T-ALL include the EML1-ABL1 fusion due to a cryptic t(9;14)(q34;q32) and the BCR-ABL1 and ETV6-ABL1 chimeric genes.[148] TKIs in combination with chemotherapy may impart a therapeutic benefit in ABL1-fusion positive T-ALL;[148,151] however, microdeletions of the protein tyrosine phosphatase, non-receptor type 2 gene (PTPN2) appear to modulate the drug responsiveness.[152]

Common Gains and Deletions in T-ALL

Gains in T-ALL are infrequent and restricted to ABL1 (discussed above) or to MYB, which maps to band 6q23.[127,153] Clappier and colleagues[127] reported two types of MYB genomic alterations in T-ALL: the t(6;7)(q23;q34), which juxtaposes TRB and MYB; and small duplications usually detected by microarray studies. In contrast to the duplicated MYB alteration, the TRB-MYB gene rearrangement is found exclusively in very young children (median age 2.2 years) with an associated proliferation/ mitosis expression signature.

Deletions are frequent and often cryptic in T-ALL. Deletions of 9p are the most common. Chromosome band 9p21.3 houses the genes for CDKN2A and CDKN2B, which are inhibitors of cyclin/CDK-4/6 complexes and block cell division. Loss of CDKN2A and/or CDKN2B results in loss of cell proliferation control. Deletion CDKN2A/9p21 is detected in 70% of T-ALL, in sharp contrast to the ~20% deletion rate in B-ALL.[64] Monoallelic and biallelic deletions are observed by FISH using a probe that targets CNDN2A or by oligo/SNP arrays. Inactivation of this tumor suppressor gene may also occur by hypermethylation, mutation, and acquired isodisomy, the latter detected only by SNP arrays (Figure 5-3C).[64] In a pediatric T-ALL study, CDKN2A deletions detected by microarrays showed monoallelic and biallelic deletions ranging 23.3 Mb to 25 kb; most (~80–90%) were associated with TLX3 or TLX1 gene rearrangements.[64] Because CDKN2A deletions are considered secondary events, prognosis is deferred to the primary T-ALL aberration.

Variable 6q deletions detected by conventional cytogenetics are seen in ~25% of T-ALL cases.[119] Detailed molecular cytogenetic studies have focused on deletions involving region 6q15q16.1 and the CASP8AP2 gene. Deletion of CASP8AP2, which encodes a protein mediator of apoptosis and a determinant of glucocorticoid signaling, has been associated poor early treatment response.[154,155]

New T-ALL Cytogenetic Aberrations

A combination of GEP and detailed molecular-cytogenetic studies has recently uncovered two T-ALL entities, each in ~20% of T-ALL lacking other oncogenic hits: NKX2-1/NKX2-2 gene rearrangement and MEF2C-activing rearrangements.[138,156] NKX2-1 is known to rearrange with TRA, IGH, and TRB, whereas NKX2-2 rearranges with TRD. Lymphoblasts with this entity are arrested in the early corticoid stage of development and share a gene expression signature with T-ALL harboring TLX1 translocations (a related NKL homeobox gene). The second group is associated with immature T-cell development and rearrangements that upregulates expression of MEF2C, a key lymphoid development regulator that is activated by PU.1.[157] This entity includes aberrations disrupting band 5q14, such as del(5)(q14) or der(5)t(4;5) (q26;q14), and t(5;14)(q34;q32.2), the latter resulting in a BCL11B-NKX2-5 gene rearrangement. Because these genetic aberrations were found in two T-ALL gene expression clusters for which no known "driver" hits were previously identified, continued efforts using such a strategy may further classify and strengthen our understanding of novel entities in T-ALL.[138,156]

Early T-Cell Precursor-ALL

In 2009, a distinct subset of childhood early precursor T-cell ALL was identified by flow cytometry and microarray studies.[158] ETP-ALL comprises ~15% of T-ALL and is associated with a high risk of treatment failure using standard intensive chemotherapy.[158,159] Early T-cell precursor (ETP)-ALL is negative for CD1a and CD8 with weak or no expression of CD5 and hematopoietic stem-cell or myeloid markers; shows no distinct genetic aberration(s); has increased genomic instability; and does not demonstrate biallelic deletion of the TRG locus (a characteristic feature of early thymic-precursor cells).[158,159] These data indicate that ETP-ALL is an aggressive, poorly differentiated stem cell leukemia.[25] Zhang et al. sequenced the entire genome of 12 pediatric ETP-ALL cases to identify the recurring genetic aberrations in this newly-defined subgroup.[25] Overall, the mutational and transcriptional profile of ETP-ALL was similar to that of normal and myeloid leukemia hematopoietic stem cells. Two-thirds of samples showed activating mutations in the cytokine receptor and RAS signaling regulator genes (NRAS, KRAS, FLT3, IL7R, JAK3, JAK1, SH2B3, and BRAF), more than half had mutations targeting genes involved with hematopoietic development (GATA3, ETV6, RUNX1, IKZF1, and EP300), and almost half had mutations of genes involved in histone modification (EZH2, EED, SUZ12, SETD2, and EP300). In a related study, van Vlierberghe and colleagues[160] reported myeloid-specific mutations (IDH1, IDH2, DNMT3A, FLT3, and NRAS) and ETV6 aberrations in adult immature T-ALL. These data suggest the genetics of ETP-ALL could modify the diagnosis and treatment for patients with this disease and provide a basis for prospective clinical trials to determine if myeloid-directed therapies might improve the poor outcome of ETP-ALL.

Submicroscopic Deletions and Mutations Studies in T-ALL

High-resolution oligo/SNP array analyses have detected recurring CNAs in greater than 95% of the T-ALL samples tested.[20,122] In addition to focal CDKN2A deletions, small deletions within band 1p32 activate TAL1 by a TAL1-STIL fusion in ~20% of childhood T-ALL cases.[149,161] van Vlierberghe and colleagues[122] detected a cryptic deletion on the short arm of chromosome 11, or del(11)(p12p13), in ~4% of pediatric T-ALL patients. This deletion activates the LMO2 oncogene in the same manner as the LMO2-TCR translocations. These data indicate that LMO2 abnormalities represent ~9% of pediatric T-ALL cases. Lastly, 2.5 Mb deletions within band 9q34 may lead to a SET-NUP214 fusion and contribute leukemogenesis through HOXA activation.[121,149]

The NOTCH1 signaling pathway is essential for normal T-cell development, so it is not surprising that the activating NOTCH1 mutations are the most common mutations in T-ALL. Nearly 60% of patients with T-ALL harbor NOTCH1 mutations, and an additional 15% show deletions or mutations in FBXW7, a gene that impairs the degradation of activated NOTCH1 in the nucleus. Together, NOTCH1/FBXW7 mutations are found in ~75% of T-ALL. Conflicting results have been reported on whether these mutations carry a favorable prognosis[162,163] or are non-predictive;[164-166] however, the mutually exclusive T-ALL genetic aberrations discussed above may be more predictive of outcome. NOTCH1 and/or FBXW7 mutations are frequently associated with TLX3 rearrangements and less frequently identified in cases with TAL1 or LMO2 rearrangements.[166] Other genome-wide profiling and deep-sequencing approaches have revealed recurrent gene mutations affecting NRAS, FLT3, JAK1, PTPN2, PHF6, LEF1, PTEN, and WT1 in T-cell ALL.[122,152,167,168] Investigations of the prognostic significance, incidence, and mutational spectrum of these acquired T-cell alterations are in progress. A number of associations between these mutations and other acquired genetic alterations are beginning to reveal relationships between T-ALL cytogenetic subgroups and molecular pathways, which should provide a means to stratify patients and develop new therapeutic strategies in T-ALL.

SUMMARY

In summary, ALL is characterized by recurring numerical cytogenetic changes (high hyperdiploidy and hypodiploidy) and well-established structural karyotypic rearrangements (deletions, translocations, inversions, and amplification). These cytogenetic aberrations pinpoint the underlying molecular events that deregulate hematopoietic regulators, transcription factors, and tyrosine kinases, assisting practitioners in diagnosis, prognosis, and selection of therapeutic options. Multiple genetic subgroups defined by recurring chromosomal alterations are being used worldwide in the diagnosis and risk stratification of ALL. Recent discoveries arising from genome-wide DNA microarrays and GEP have uncovered multiple gene CNAs that define novel characteristics of ALL subgroups and cooperate with known cytogenetic alterations in leukemogenesis. Clinically, some of these genetic aberrations are being utilized as significant predictors of relapse risk, whereas others are potential targets for therapeutic intervention. Continued use of the advanced molecular technologies with next-generation and whole-genome sequencing as part of the pediatric cancer genome project[23] should enhance our understanding of the molecular interactions and biology of ALL, which should in turn lead to treatment strategies that may include molecular therapeutics or enhance the antileukemic effects of chemotherapy.

REFERENCES

1. Redaelli A, Laskin BL, Stephens JM, et al. A systematic literature review of the clinical and epidemiological burden of acute lymphoblastic leukaemia (ALL). *Eur J Cancer Care (Engl)*. 2005;14(1):53-62.
2. Siegel R, Naishadham D, Jemal A. Cancer statistics, 2012. *CA Cancer J Clin*. 2012;62(1):10-29.
3. Dores GM, Devesa SS, Curtis RE, et al. Acute leukemia incidence and patient survival among children and adults in the United States, 2001-2007. *Blood*. 2012;119(1):34-43.

4. Pui CH, Carroll WL, Meshinchi S, et al. Biology, risk stratification, and therapy of pediatric acute leukemias: an update. *J Clin Oncol.* 2011;29(5):551-65.

5. Pullarkat V, Slovak ML, Kopecky KJ, et al. Impact of cytogenetics on the outcome of adult acute lymphoblastic leukemia: results of Southwest Oncology Group 9400 study. *Blood.* 2008;111(5):2563-72.

6. Marks DI, Paietta EM, Moorman AV, et al. T-cell acute lymphoblastic leukemia in adults: clinical features, immunophenotype, cytogenetics, and outcome from the large randomized prospective trial (UKALL XII/ECOG 2993). *Blood.* 2009;114(25):5136-45.

7. Swerdlow S, Campo E, Harris N, et al. WHO classification of tumors of hematopoietic and lymphoid tissues. 4th edition. Lyon, France: International Agency for Research on Cancer; 2008.

8. Pui CH, Robison LL, Look AT. Acute lymphoblastic leukaemia. *Lancet.* 2008;371(9617): 1030-43.

9. Hunger SP, Lu X, Devidas M, et al. Improved survival for children and adolescents with acute lymphoblastic leukemia between 1990 and 2005: a report from the children's oncology group. *J Clin Oncol.* 2012;30(14):1663-9.

10. Moricke A, Zimmermann M, Reiter A, et al. Long-term results of five consecutive trials in childhood acute lymphoblastic leukemia performed by the ALL-BFM study group from 1981 to 2000. *Leukemia.* 2010;24(2):265-84.

11. Salzer WL, Devidas M, Carroll WL, et al. Long-term results of the pediatric oncology group studies for childhood acute lymphoblastic leukemia 1984-2001: a report from the children's oncology group. *Leukemia.* 2010;24(2):355-70.

12. Nguyen K, Devidas M, Cheng SC, et al. Factors influencing survival after relapse from acute lymphoblastic leukemia: a Children's Oncology Group study. *Leukemia.* 2008;22(12): 2142-50.

13. Attarbaschi A, Mann G, Panzer-Grumayer R, et al. Minimal residual disease values discriminate between low and high relapse risk in children with B-cell precursor acute lymphoblastic leukemia and an intrachromosomal amplification of chromosome 21: the Austrian and German acute lymphoblastic leukemia Berlin-Frankfurt-Munster (ALL-BFM) trials. *J Clin Oncol.* 2008;26(18):3046-50.

14. Silverman LB, Stevenson KE, O'Brien JE, et al. Long-term results of Dana-Farber Cancer Institute ALL Consortium protocols for children with newly diagnosed acute lymphoblastic leukemia (1985-2000). *Leukemia.* 2010;24(2):320-34.

15. Gokbuget N, Kneba M, Raff T, et al. Adults with acute lymphoblastic leukemia and molecular failure display a poor prognosis and are candidates for stem cell transplantation and targeted therapies. *Blood.* 2012;120(9):1868-76.

16. Moorman AV, Ensor HM, Richards SM, et al. Prognostic effect of chromosomal abnormalities in childhood B-cell precursor acute lymphoblastic leukaemia: results from the UK Medical Research Council ALL97/99 randomised trial. *Lancet Oncol.* 2010;11(5):429-38.

17. Secker-Walker LM, Lawler SD, Hardisty RM. Prognostic implications of chromosomal findings in acute lymphoblastic leukaemia at diagnosis. *Br Med J.* 1978;2(6151):1529-30.

18. Moorman AV. The clinical relevance of chromosomal and genomic abnormalities in B-cell precursor acute lymphoblastic leukaemia. *Blood Rev.* 2012;26(3):123-35.

19. Moorman AV, Harrison CJ, Buck GA, et al. Karyotype is an independent prognostic factor in adult acute lymphoblastic leukemia (ALL): analysis of cytogenetic data from patients treated on the Medical Research Council (MRC) UKALLXII/Eastern Cooperative Oncology Group (ECOG) 2993 trial. *Blood.* 2007;109(8):3189-97.

20. Mulligan CG, Goorha S, Radtke I, et al. Genome-wide analysis of genetic alterations in acute lymphoblastic leukaemia. *Nature.* 2007;446(7137):758-64.

21. Mulligan CG, Su X, Zhang J, et al. Deletion of IKZF1 and prognosis in acute lymphoblastic leukemia. *N Engl J Med.* 2009;360(5):470-80.

22. Paulsson K, Forestier E, Lilljebjorn H, et al. Genetic landscape of high hyperdiploid childhood acute lymphoblastic leukemia. *Proc Natl Acad Sci U S A.* 2010;107(50):21719-24.
23. Downing JR, Wilson RK, Zhang J, et al. The pediatric cancer genome project. *Nat Genet.* 2012;44(6):619-22.
24. Zhang J, Mullighan CG, Harvey RC, et al. Key pathways are frequently mutated in high-risk childhood acute lymphoblastic leukemia: a report from the Children's Oncology Group. *Blood.* 2011;118(11):3080-7.
25. Zhang J, Ding L, Holmfeldt L, et al. The genetic basis of early T-cell precursor acute lymphoblastic leukaemia. *Nature.* 2012;481(7380):157-63.
26. Linet MS, Devesa SS, Morgan GJ. The leukemias. In: Schottenfeld D, Fraumeni JF, editors. Epidemiology and Prevention. 3rd ed. New York: Oxford University Press; 2008. p. 841-71.
27. Papaemmanuil E, Hosking FJ, Vijayakrishnan J, et al. Loci on 7p12.2, 10q21.2 and 14q11.2 are associated with risk of childhood acute lymphoblastic leukemia. *Nat Genet.* 2009;41(9):1006-10.
28. Trevino LR, Yang W, French D, et al. Germline genomic variants associated with childhood acute lymphoblastic leukemia. *Nat Genet.* 2009;41(9):1001-5.
29. Prasad RB, Hosking FJ, Vijayakrishnan J, et al. Verification of the susceptibility loci on 7p12.2, 10q21.2, and 14q11.2 in precursor B-cell acute lymphoblastic leukemia of childhood. *Blood.* 2010;115(9):1765-7.
30. Sherborne AL, Hosking FJ, Prasad RB, et al. Variation in CDKN2A at 9p21.3 influences childhood acute lymphoblastic leukemia risk. *Nat Genet.* 2010;42(6):492-4.
31. Xu H, Cheng C, Devidas M, et al. ARID5B genetic polymorphisms contribute to racial disparities in the incidence and treatment outcome of childhood acute lymphoblastic leukemia. *J Clin Oncol.* 2012;30(7):751-7.
32. National Comprehensive Cancer Network. (2012) NCCN guidelines for acute lymphoblastic leukemia, Version 1.2012. [online] Available from: www.nccn.org. [Accessed August, 2013].
33. Harrison CJ, Haas O, Harbott J, et al. Detection of prognostically relevant genetic abnormalities in childhood B-cell precursor acute lymphoblastic leukaemia: recommendations from the Biology and Diagnosis Committee of the International Berlin-Frankfurt-Munster study group. *Br J Haematol.* 2010;151(2):132-42.
34. Shaffer LG, Slovak ML, Campell LJ. An International System for Human Cytogenetic Nomenclature. Basel, Switzerland: Karger; 2009.
35. Schouten JP, McElgunn CJ, Waaijer R, et al. Relative quantification of 40 nucleic acid sequences by multiplex ligation-dependent probe amplification. *Nucleic Acids Res.* 2002;30(12):e57.
36. Moorman AV, Richards SM, Martineau M, et al. Outcome heterogeneity in childhood high-hyperdiploid acute lymphoblastic leukemia. *Blood.* 2003;102(8):2756-62.
37. Sutcliffe MJ, Shuster JJ, Sather HN, et al. High concordance from independent studies by the Children's Cancer Group (CCG) and Pediatric Oncology Group (POG) associating favorable prognosis with combined trisomies 4, 10, and 17 in children with NCI Standard-Risk B-precursor Acute Lymphoblastic Leukemia: a Children's Oncology Group (COG) initiative. *Leukemia.* 2005;19(5):734-40.
38. Paulsson K, Heidenblad M, Morse H, et al. Identification of cryptic aberrations and characterization of translocation breakpoints using array CGH in high hyperdiploid childhood acute lymphoblastic leukemia. *Leukemia.* 2006;20(11):2002-7.
39. Tabernero MD, Bortoluci AM, Alaejos I, et al. Adult precursor B-ALL with BCR/ABL gene rearrangements displays a unique immunophenotype based on the pattern of CD10, CD34, CD13 and CD38 expresssion. *Leukemia.* 2001;15(3):406-14.
40. Borkhardt A, Cazzaniga G, Viehmann S, et al. Incidence and clinical relevance of TEL/AML1 fusion genes in children with acute lymphoblastic leukemia enrolled in the German and

Italian multicenter therapy trials. Associazione Italiana Ematologia Oncologia Pediatrica and the Berlin-Frankfurt-Munster Study Group. *Blood.* 1997;90(2):571-7.

41. Harrison CJ, Moorman AV, Broadfield ZJ, et al. Three distinct subgroups of hypodiploidy in acute lymphoblastic leukaemia. *Br J Haematol.* 2004;125(5):552-9.
42. Armstrong SA, Staunton JE, Silverman LB, et al. MLL translocations specify a distinct gene expression profile that distinguishes a unique leukemia. *Nat Genet.* 2002;30(1):41-7.
43. Yeoh EJ, Ross ME, Shurtleff SA, et al. Classification, subtype discovery, and prediction of outcome in pediatric acute lymphoblastic leukemia by gene expression profiling. *Cancer Cell.* 2002;1(2):133-43.
44. Juric D, Lacayo NJ, Ramsey MC, et al. Differential gene expression patterns and interaction networks in BCR-ABL-positive and -negative adult acute lymphoblastic leukemias. *J Clin Oncol.* 2007;25(11):1341-9.
45. Harvey RC, Mullighan CG, Wang X, et al. Identification of novel cluster groups in pediatric high-risk B-precursor acute lymphoblastic leukemia with gene expression profiling: correlation with genome-wide DNA copy number alterations, clinical characteristics, and outcome. *Blood.* 2010;116(23):4874-84.
46. Pui CH, Relling MV, Downing JR. Acute lymphoblastic leukemia. *N Engl J Med.* 2004; 350(15):1535-48.
47. Borowitz ML, Chan JK. Precursor lymphoid neoplasms. In: Swerdlow SH, Campo E, Harris NL, Pileri SA, Stein H, Thiele J, editors. Classification of Tumours of Haematopoietic and Lymphoid Tissue. 4th ed. Lyon, France: IARC; 2008. pp. 167-78.
48. Mulligan CG, Miller CB, Radtke I, et al. BCR-ABL1 lymphoblastic leukaemia is characterized by the deletion of Ikaros. *Nature.* 2008;453(7191):110-4.
49. Iacobucci I, Ferrari A, Lonetti A, et al. CDKN2A/B alterations impair prognosis in adult BCR-ABL1-positive acute lymphoblastic leukemia patients. *Clin Cancer Res.* 2011;17(23):7413-23.
50. Lundin C, Heldrup J, Ahlgren T, et al. B-cell precursor t(8;14)(q11;q32)-positive acute lymphoblastic leukemia in children is strongly associated with Down syndrome or with a concomitant Philadelphia chromosome. *Eur J Haematol.* 2009;82(1):46-53.
51. Schultz KR, Bowman WP, Aledo A, et al. Improved early event-free survival with imatinib in Philadelphia chromosome-positive acute lymphoblastic leukemia: a children's oncology group study. *J Clin Oncol.* 2009;27(31):5175-81.
52. Rives S, Estella J, Gomez P, et al. Intermediate dose of imatinib in combination with chemotherapy followed by allogeneic stem cell transplantation improves early outcome in paediatric Philadelphia chromosome-positive acute lymphoblastic leukaemia (ALL): results of the Spanish Cooperative Group SHOP studies ALL-94, ALL-99 and ALL-2005. *Br J Haematol.* 2011;154(5):600-11.
53. Ottmann OG, Pfeifer H. Management of Philadelphia chromosome-positive acute lymphoblastic leukemia (Ph+ ALL). Hematology *Am Soc Hematol Educ Program.* 2009;371-81.
54. Johansson B, Moorman AV, Haas OA, et al. Hematologic malignancies with t(4;11) (q21;q23)—a cytogenetic, morphologic, immunophenotypic and clinical study of 183 cases. European 11q23 Workshop participants. *Leukemia.* 1998;12(5):779-87.
55. Zandvliet DW, Hanby AM, Austin CA, et al. Analysis of foetal expression sites of human type II DNA topoisomerase alpha and beta mRNAs by in situ hybridisation. *Biochim Biophys Acta.* 1996;1307(2):239-47.
56. Strick R, Strissel PL, Borgers S, et al. Dietary bioflavonoids induce cleavage in the MLL gene and may contribute to infant leukemia. *Proc Natl Acad Sci U S A.* 2000;97(9):4790-5.
57. Rubnitz JE, Camitta BM, Mahmoud H, et al. Childhood acute lymphoblastic leukemia with the MLL-ENL fusion and t(11;19)(q23;p13.3) translocation. *J Clin Oncol.* 1999;17(1):191-6.
58. Romana SP, Le CM, Berger R. t(12;21): a new recurrent translocation in acute lymphoblastic leukemia. Genes Chromosomes *Cancer.* 1994;9(3):186-91.
59. Romana SP, Mauchauffe M, Le CM, et al. The t(12;21) of acute lymphoblastic leukemia results in a tel-AML1 gene fusion. *Blood.* 1995;85(12):3662-70.

60. Kobayashi H, Montgomery KT, Bohlander SK, et al. Fluorescence in situ hybridization mapping of translocations and deletions involving the short arm of human chromosome 12 in malignant hematologic diseases. *Blood.* 1994;84(10):3473-82.

61. Bateman CM, Colman SM, Chaplin T, et al. Acquisition of genome-wide copy number alterations in monozygotic twins with acute lymphoblastic leukemia. *Blood.* 2010;115(17): 3553-8.

62. Raynaud S, Mauvieux L, Cayuela JM, et al. TEL/AML1 fusion gene is a rare event in adult acute lymphoblastic leukemia. *Leukemia.* 1996;10(9):1529-30.

63. Shurtleff SA, Buijs A, Behm FG, et al. TEL/AML1 fusion resulting from a cryptic t(12;21) is the most common genetic lesion in pediatric ALL and defines a subgroup of patients with an excellent prognosis. *Leukemia.* 1995;9(12):1985-9.

64. Sulong S, Moorman AV, Irving JA, et al. A comprehensive analysis of the CDKN2A gene in childhood acute lymphoblastic leukemia reveals genomic deletion, copy number neutral loss of heterozygosity, and association with specific cytogenetic subgroups. *Blood.* 2009;113(1):100-7.

65. Lilljebjorn H, Soneson C, Andersson A, et al. The correlation pattern of acquired copy number changes in 164 ETV6/RUNX1-positive childhood acute lymphoblastic leukemias. *Hum Mol Genet.* 2010;19(16):3150-8.

66. van Delft FW, Horsley S, Colman S, et al. Clonal origins of relapse in ETV6-RUNX1 acute lymphoblastic leukemia. *Blood.* 2011;117(23):6247-54.

67. Bhojwani D, Pei D, Sandlund JT, et al. ETV6-RUNX1-positive childhood acute lymphoblastic leukemia: improved outcome with contemporary therapy. *Leukemia.* 2012;26(2):265-70.

68. Kuster L, Grausenburger R, Fuka G, et al. ETV6-RUNX1-positive relapses evolve from an ancestral clone and frequently acquire deletions of genes implicated in glucocorticoid signaling. *Blood.* 2011;117(9):2658-67.

69. Pui CH, Raimondi SC, Hancock ML, et al. Immunologic, cytogenetic, and clinical characterization of childhood acute lymphoblastic leukemia with the t(1;19) (q23; p13) or its derivative. *J Clin Oncol.* 1994;12(12):2601-6.

70. Hunger SP. Chromosomal translocations involving the E2A gene in acute lymphoblastic leukemia: clinical features and molecular pathogenesis. *Blood.* 1996;87(4):1211-24.

71. Kager L, Lion T, Attarbaschi A, et al. Incidence and outcome of TCF3-PBX1-positive acute lymphoblastic leukemia in Austrian children. *Haematologica.* 2007;92(11):1561-4.

72. Hunger SP, Sun T, Boswell AF, et al. Hyperdiploidy and E2A-PBX1 fusion in an adult with t(1;19)+ acute lymphoblastic leukemia: case report and review of the literature. *Genes Chromosomes Cancer.* 1997;20(4):392-8.

73. Hunger SP, Devaraj PE, Foroni L, et al. Two types of genomic rearrangements create alternative E2A-HLF fusion proteins in t(17;19)-ALL. *Blood.* 1994;83(10):2970-7.

74. Busson-Le CM, Nguyen KF, Daniel MT, et al. Chromosome 21 abnormalities with AML1 amplification in acute lymphoblastic leukemia. *Genes Chromosomes Cancer.* 2001;32(3): 244-9.

75. Harewood L, Robinson H, Harris R, et al. Amplification of AML1 on a duplicated chromosome 21 in acute lymphoblastic leukemia: a study of 20 cases. *Leukemia.* 2003;17(3):547-53.

76. Moorman AV, Richards SM, Robinson HM, et al. Prognosis of children with acute lymphoblastic leukemia (ALL) and intrachromosomal amplification of chromosome 21 (iAMP21). *Blood.* 2007;109(6):2327-30.

77. Robinson HM, Harrison CJ, Moorman AV, et al. Intrachromosomal amplification of chromosome 21 (iAMP21) may arise from a breakage-fusion-bridge cycle. *Genes Chromosomes Cancer.* 2007;46(4):318-26.

78. Rand V, Parker H, Russell LJ, et al. Genomic characterization implicates iAMP21 as a likely primary genetic event in childhood B-cell precursor acute lymphoblastic leukemia. *Blood.* 2011;117(25):6848-55.

79. Russell LJ, Capasso M, Vater I, et al. Deregulated expression of cytokine receptor gene, CRLF2, is involved in lymphoid transformation in B-cell precursor acute lymphoblastic leukemia. *Blood.* 2009;114(13):2688-98.

80. Dyer MJ, Akasaka T, Capasso M, et al. Immunoglobulin heavy chain locus chromosomal translocations in B-cell precursor acute lymphoblastic leukemia: rare clinical curios or potent genetic drivers? *Blood.* 2010;115(8):1490-9.

81. Akasaka T, Balasas T, Russell LJ, et al. Five members of the CEBP transcription factor family are targeted by recurrent IGH translocations in B-cell precursor acute lymphoblastic leukemia (BCP-ALL). *Blood.* 2007;109(8):3451-61.

82. Harrison CJ. Cytogenetics of paediatric and adolescent acute lymphoblastic leukaemia. *Br J Haematol.* 2009;144(2):147-56.

83. Meeker TC, Hardy D, Willman C, et al. Activation of the interleukin-3 gene by chromosome translocation in acute lymphocytic leukemia with eosinophilia. *Blood.* 1990;76(2):285-9.

84. Bellido M, Aventin A, Lasa A, et al. Id4 is deregulated by a t(6;14)(p22;q32) chromosomal translocation in a B-cell lineage acute lymphoblastic leukemia. *Haematologica.* 2003;88(9): 994-1001.

85. Russell LJ, Akasaka T, Majid A, et al. t(6;14)(p22;q32): a new recurrent IGH@ translocation involving ID4 in B-cell precursor acute lymphoblastic leukemia (BCP-ALL). *Blood.* 2008; 111(1):387-91.

86. Russell LJ, De Castro DG, Griffiths M, et al. A novel translocation, t(14;19)(q32;p13), involving IGH@ and the cytokine receptor for erythropoietin. *Leukemia.* 2009;23(3):614-7.

87. Mullighan CG, Collins-Underwood JR, Phillips LA, et al. Rearrangement of CRLF2 in B-progenitor- and Down syndrome-associated acute lymphoblastic leukemia. *Nat Genet.* 2009;41(11):1243-6.

88. Hertzberg L, Vendramini E, Ganmore I, et al. Down syndrome acute lymphoblastic leukemia, a highly heterogeneous disease in which aberrant expression of CRLF2 is associated with mutated JAK2: a report from the International BFM Study Group. *Blood.* 2010;115(5): 1006-17.

89. Harvey RC, Mullighan CG, Chen IM, et al. Rearrangement of CRLF2 is associated with mutation of JAK kinases, alteration of IKZF1, Hispanic/Latino ethnicity, and a poor outcome in pediatric B-progenitor acute lymphoblastic leukemia. *Blood.* 2010;115(26):5312-21.

90. Cario G, Zimmermann M, Romey R, et al. Presence of the P2RY8-CRLF2 rearrangement is associated with a poor prognosis in non-high-risk precursor B-cell acute lymphoblastic leukemia in children treated according to the ALL-BFM 2000 protocol. *Blood.* 2010; 115(26):5393-7.

91. Ensor HM, Schwab C, Russell LJ, et al. Demographic, clinical, and outcome features of children with acute lymphoblastic leukemia and CRLF2 deregulation: results from the MRC ALL97 clinical trial. *Blood.* 2011;117(7):2129-36.

92. Medvedovic J, Ebert A, Tagoh H, et al. Pax5: a master regulator of B cell development and leukemogenesis. *Adv Immunol.* 2011;111:179-206.

93. Strehl S, Konig M, Dworzak MN, et al. PAX5/ETV6 fusion defines cytogenetic entity dic(9;12) (p13;p13). *Leukemia.* 2003;17(6):1121-3.

94. Familiades J, Bousquet M, Lafage-Pochitaloff M, et al. PAX5 mutations occur frequently in adult B-cell progenitor acute lymphoblastic leukemia and PAX5 haploinsufficiency is associated with BCR-ABL1 and TCF3-PBX1 fusion genes: a GRAALL study. *Leukemia.* 2009;23(11):1989-98.

95. Coyaud E, Struski S, Prade N, et al. Wide diversity of PAX5 alterations in B-ALL: a Groupe Francophone de Cytogenetique Hematologique study. *Blood.* 2010;115(15):3089-97.

96. An Q, Wright SL, Konn ZJ, et al. Variable breakpoints target PAX5 in patients with dicentric chromosomes: a model for the basis of unbalanced translocations in cancer. *Proc Natl Acad Sci U S A.* 2008;105(44):17050-4.

97. Put N, Deeren D, Michaux L, et al. FOXP1 and PAX5 are rare but recurrent translocations partners in acute lymphoblastic leukemia. *Cancer Genet.* 2011;204(8):462-4.

98. Zachariadis V, Gauffin F, Kuchinskaya E, et al. The frequency and prognostic impact of dic(9;20)(p13.2;q11.2) in childhood B-cell precursor acute lymphoblastic leukemia: results from the NOPHO ALL-2000 trial. *Leukemia.* 2011;25(4):622-8.

99. Forestier E, Gauffin F, Andersen MK, et al. Clinical and cytogenetic features of pediatric dic(9;20)(p13.2;q11.2)-positive B-cell precursor acute lymphoblastic leukemias: a Nordic series of 24 cases and review of the literature. *Genes Chromosomes Cancer.* 2008;47(2): 149-58.

100. Pichler H, Moricke A, Mann G, et al. Prognostic relevance of dic(9;20)(p11;q13) in childhood B-cell precursor acute lymphoblastic leukaemia treated with Berlin-Frankfurt-Munster (BFM) protocols containing an intensive induction and post-induction consolidation therapy. *Br J Haematol.* 2010;149(1):93-100.

101. Behrendt H, Charrin C, Gibbons B, et al. Dicentric (9;12) in acute lymphocytic leukemia and other hematological malignancies: report from a dic(9;12) study group. *Leukemia.* 1995;9(1):102-6.

102. Forestier E, Izraeli S, Beverloo B, et al. Cytogenetic features of acute lymphoblastic and myeloid leukemias in pediatric patients with Down syndrome: an iBFM-SG study. *Blood.* 2008;111(3):1575-83.

103. Bercovich D, Ganmore I, Scott LM, et al. Mutations of JAK2 in acute lymphoblastic leukaemias associated with Down's syndrome. *Lancet.* 2008;372(9648):1484-92.

104. Hasle H, Clemmensen IH, Mikkelsen M. Risks of leukaemia and solid tumours in individuals with Down's syndrome. *Lancet.* 2000;355(9199):165-9.

105. Maloney KW. Acute lymphoblastic leukaemia in children with Down syndrome: an updated review. *Br J Haematol.* 2011;155(4):420-5.

106. Linabery AM, Ross JA. Childhood and adolescent cancer survival in the US by race and ethnicity for the diagnostic period 1975-1999. *Cancer.* 2008;113(9):2575-96.

107. Hilden JM, Dinndorf PA, Meerbaum SO, et al. Analysis of prognostic factors of acute lymphoblastic leukemia in infants: report on CCG 1953 from the Children's Oncology Group. *Blood.* 2006;108(2):441-51.

108. Nagayama J, Tomizawa D, Koh K, et al. Infants with acute lymphoblastic leukemia and a germline MLL gene are highly curable with use of chemotherapy alone: results from the Japan Infant Leukemia Study Group. *Blood.* 2006;107(12):4663-5.

109. Sam TN, Kersey JH, Linabery AM, et al. MLL gene rearrangements in infant leukemia vary with age at diagnosis and selected demographic factors: a Children's Oncology Group (COG) study. *Pediatr Blood Cancer.* 2012;58(6):836-9.

110. Pieters R, Schrappe M, de LP, et al. A treatment protocol for infants younger than 1 year with acute lymphoblastic leukaemia (Interfant-99): an observational study and a multicentre randomised trial. *Lancet.* 2007;370(9583):240-50.

111. Stam RW, Schneider P, Hagelstein JA, et al. Gene expression profiling-based dissection of MLL translocated and MLL germline acute lymphoblastic leukemia in infants. *Blood.* 2010;115(14):2835-44.

112. Kang H, Wilson CS, Harvey RC, et al. Gene expression profiles predictive of outcome and age in infant acute lymphoblastic leukemia: a Children's Oncology Group study. *Blood.* 2012;119(8):1872-81.

113. Kuiper RP, Schoenmakers EF, van Reijmersdal SV, et al. High-resolution genomic profiling of childhood ALL reveals novel recurrent genetic lesions affecting pathways involved in lymphocyte differentiation and cell cycle progression. *Leukemia.* 2007;21(6):1258-66.

114. Kawamata N, Ogawa S, Zimmermann M, et al. Molecular allelokaryotyping of pediatric acute lymphoblastic leukemias by high-resolution single nucleotide polymorphism oligonucleotide genomic microarray. *Blood.* 2008;111(2):776-84.

115. Paulsson K, Horvat A, Strombeck B, et al. Mutations of FLT3, NRAS, KRAS, and PTPN11 are frequent and possibly mutually exclusive in high hyperdiploid childhood acute lymphoblastic leukemia. *Genes Chromosomes Cancer.* 2008;47(1):26-33.

116. Den Boer ML, van SM, de Menezes RX, et al. A subtype of childhood acute lymphoblastic leukaemia with poor treatment outcome: a genome-wide classification study. *Lancet Oncol.* 2009;10(2):125-34.

117. Collins-Underwood JR, Mullighan CG. Genomic profiling of high-risk acute lymphoblastic leukemia. *Leukemia.* 2010;24(10):1676-85.

118. Buitenkamp TD, Pieters R, Gallimore NE, et al. Outcome in children with Down's syndrome and acute lymphoblastic leukemia: role of IKZF1 deletions and CRLF2 aberrations. *Leukemia.* 2012;26(10):2204-11.

119. Graux C, Cools J, Michaux L, et al. Cytogenetics and molecular genetics of T-cell acute lymphoblastic leukemia: from thymocyte to lymphoblast. *Leukemia.* 2006;20(9):1496-510.

120. Armstrong SA, Look AT. Molecular genetics of acute lymphoblastic leukemia. *J Clin Oncol.* 2005;23(26):6306-15.

121. Van Vlierberghe P, Pieters R, Beverloo HB, et al. Molecular-genetic insights in paediatric T-cell acute lymphoblastic leukaemia. *Br J Haematol.* 2008;143(2):153-68.

122. Van Vlierberghe P, van GM, Beverloo HB, et al. The cryptic chromosomal deletion del(11) (p12p13) as a new activation mechanism of LMO2 in pediatric T-cell acute lymphoblastic leukemia. *Blood.* 2006;108(10):3520-9.

123. Ferrando AA, Neuberg DS, Staunton J, et al. Gene expression signatures define novel oncogenic pathways in T cell acute lymphoblastic leukemia. *Cancer Cell.* 2002;1(1):75-87.

124. Ferrando AA, Armstrong SA, Neuberg DS, et al. Gene expression signatures in MLL-rearranged T-lineage and B-precursor acute leukemias: dominance of HOX dysregulation. *Blood.* 2003;102(1):262-8.

125. Ferrando AA, Neuberg DS, Dodge RK, et al. Prognostic importance of TLX1 (HOX11) oncogene expression in adults with T-cell acute lymphoblastic leukaemia. *Lancet.* 2004; 363(9408):535-6.

126. De KK, Marynen P, Cools J. Genetic insights in the pathogenesis of T-cell acute lymphoblastic leukemia. *Haematologica.* 2005;90(8):1116-27.

127. Clappier E, Cuccuini W, Kalota A, et al. The C-MYB locus is involved in chromosomal translocation and genomic duplications in human T-cell acute leukemia (T-ALL), the translocation defining a new T-ALL subtype in very young children. *Blood.* 2007;110(4): 1251-61.

128. Clappier E, Cuccuini W, Cayuela JM, et al. Cyclin D2 dysregulation by chromosomal translocations to TCR loci in T-cell acute lymphoblastic leukemias. *Leukemia.* 2006; 20(1):82-6.

129. Cauwelier B, Cave H, Gervais C, et al. Clinical, cytogenetic and molecular characteristics of 14 T-ALL patients carrying the TCRbeta-HOXA rearrangement: a study of the Groupe Francophone de Cytogenetique Hematologique. *Leukemia.* 2007;21(1):121-8.

130. Bernard OA, Busson-LeConiat M, Ballerini P, et al. A new recurrent and specific cryptic translocation, t(5;14)(q35;q32), is associated with expression of the Hox11L2 gene in T acute lymphoblastic leukemia. *Leukemia.* 2001;15(10):1495-504.

131. Berger R, Dastugue N, Busson M, et al. t(5;14)/HOX11L2-positive T-cell acute lymphoblastic leukemia. A collaborative study of the Groupe Francais de Cytogenetique Hematologique (GFCH). *Leukemia.* 2003;17(9):1851-7.

132. Su XY, Busson M, Della Valle V, et al. Various types of rearrangements target TLX3 locus in T-cell acute lymphoblastic leukemia. *Genes Chromosomes Cancer.* 2004;41(3):243-9.

133. Su XY, Della Valle V, Andre-Schmutz I, et al. HOX11L2/TLX3 is transcriptionally activated through T-cell regulatory elements downstream of BCL11B as a result of the t(5;14)(q35;q32). *Blood.* 2006;108(13):4198-201.

134. Xia Y, Brown L, Yang CY, et al. TAL2, a helix-loop-helix gene activated by the (7;9)(q34;q32) translocation in human T-cell leukemia. *Proc Natl Acad Sci U S A.* 1991;88(24):11416-20.
135. Soulier J, Clappier E, Cayuela JM, et al. HOXA genes are included in genetic and biologic networks defining human acute T-cell leukemia (T-ALL). *Blood.* 2005;106(1):274-86.
136. Nagel S, Scherr M, Kel A, et al. Activation of TLX3 and NKX2-5 in t(5;14)(q35;q32) T-cell acute lymphoblastic leukemia by remote 3'-BCL11B enhancers and coregulation by PU.1 and HMGA1. *Cancer Res.* 2007;67(4):1461-71.
137. Van Vlierberghe P, Homminga I, Zuurbier L, et al. Cooperative genetic defects in TLX3 rearranged pediatric T-ALL. *Leukemia.* 2008;22(4):762-70.
138. Homminga I, Pieters R, Meijerink JP. NKL homeobox genes in leukemia. *Leukemia.* 2012; 26(4):572-81.
139. Hayette S, Tigaud I, Maguer-Satta V, et al. Recurrent involvement of the MLL gene in adult T-lineage acute lymphoblastic leukemia. *Blood.* 2002;99(12):4647-9.
140. Asnafi V, Radford-Weiss I, Dastugue N, et al. CALM-AF10 is a common fusion transcript in T-ALL and is specific to the TCRgammadelta lineage. *Blood.* 2003;102(3):1000-6.
141. Groupe Français de Cytogénétique Hématologique (GFCH). t(10;11)(p13-14;q14-21): a new recurrent translocation in T-cell acute lymphoblastic leukemias. Groupe Francais de Cytogenetique Hematologique (GFCH). *Genes Chromosomes Cancer.* 1991;3(6):411-5.
142. Dreyling MH, Schrader K, Fonatsch C, et al. MLL and CALM are fused to AF10 in morphologically distinct subsets of acute leukemia with translocation t(10;11): both rearrangements are associated with a poor prognosis. *Blood.* 1998;91(12):4662-7.
143. Dik WA, Brahim W, Braun C, et al. CALM-AF10+ T-ALL expression profiles are characterized by overexpression of HOXA and BMI1 oncogenes. *Leukemia.* 2005;19(11):1948-57.
144. Park IK, Qian D, Kiel M, et al. Bmi-1 is required for maintenance of adult self-renewing haematopoietic stem cells. *Nature.* 2003;423(6937):302-5.
145. Jacobs JJ, Kieboom K, Marino S, et al. The oncogene and Polycomb-group gene bmi-1 regulates cell proliferation and senescence through the ink4a locus. *Nature.* 1999;397(6715):164-8.
146. van Grotel M, Meijerink JP, Beverloo HB, et al. The outcome of molecular-cytogenetic subgroups in pediatric T-cell acute lymphoblastic leukemia: a retrospective study of patients treated according to DCOG or COALL protocols. *Haematologica.* 2006;91(9):1212-21.
147. Graux C, Stevens-Kroef M, Lafage M, et al. Heterogeneous patterns of amplification of the NUP214-ABL1 fusion gene in T-cell acute lymphoblastic leukemia. *Leukemia.* 2009; 23(1):125-33.
148. Hagemeijer A, Graux C. ABL1 rearrangements in T-cell acute lymphoblastic leukemia. *Genes Chromosomes Cancer.* 2010;49(4):299-308.
149. Yu L, Slovak ML, Mannoor K, et al. Microarray detection of multiple recurring submicroscopic chromosomal aberrations in pediatric T-cell acute lymphoblastic leukemia. *Leukemia.* 2011; 25(6):1042-6.
150. Graux C, Cools J, Melotte C, et al. Fusion of NUP214 to ABL1 on amplified episomes in T-cell acute lymphoblastic leukemia. *Nat Genet.* 2004;36(10):1084-9.
151. Quintas-Cardama A, Tong W, Manshouri T, et al. Activity of tyrosine kinase inhibitors against human NUP214-ABL1-positive T cell malignancies. *Leukemia.* 2008;22(6):1117-24.
152. Kleppe M, Lahortiga I, El CT, et al. Deletion of the protein tyrosine phosphatase gene PTPN2 in T-cell acute lymphoblastic leukemia. *Nat Genet.* 2010;42(6):530-5.
153. Lahortiga I, De KK, Van VP, et al. Duplication of the MYB oncogene in T cell acute lymphoblastic leukemia. *Nat Genet.* 2007;39(5):593-5.
154. Remke M, Pfister S, Kox C, et al. High-resolution genomic profiling of childhood T-ALL reveals frequent copy-number alterations affecting the TGF-beta and PI3K-AKT pathways and deletions at 6q15-16.1 as a genomic marker for unfavorable early treatment response. *Blood.* 2009;114(5):1053-62.

155. Flotho C, Coustan-Smith E, Pei D, et al. Genes contributing to minimal residual disease in childhood acute lymphoblastic leukemia: prognostic significance of CASP8AP2. *Blood.* 2006;108(3):1050-7.

156. Homminga I, Pieters R, Langerak AW, et al. Integrated transcript and genome analyses reveal NKX2-1 and MEF2C as potential oncogenes in T cell acute lymphoblastic leukemia. *Cancer Cell.* 2011;19(4):484-97.

157. Stehling-Sun S, Dade J, Nutt SL, et al. Regulation of lymphoid versus myeloid fate 'choice' by the transcription factor Mef2c. *Nat Immunol.* 2009;10(3):289-96.

158. Coustan-Smith E, Mullighan CG, Onciu M, et al. Early T-cell precursor leukaemia: a subtype of very high-risk acute lymphoblastic leukaemia. *Lancet Oncol.* 2009;10(2):147-56.

159. Gutierrez A, Dahlberg SE, Neuberg DS, et al. Absence of biallelic TCRgamma deletion predicts early treatment failure in pediatric T-cell acute lymphoblastic leukemia. *J Clin Oncol.* 2010;28(24):3816-23.

160. Van Vlierberghe P, Ambesi-Impiombato A, Perez-Garcia A, et al. ETV6 mutations in early immature human T cell leukemias. *J Exp Med.* 2011;208(13):2571-9.

161. Cave H, Suciu S, Preudhomme C, et al. Clinical significance of HOX11L2 expression linked to t(5;14)(q35;q32), of HOX11 expression, and of SIL-TAL fusion in childhood T-cell malignancies: results of EORTC studies 58881 and 58951. *Blood.* 2004;103(2):442-50.

162. Asnafi V, Buzyn A, Le NS, et al. NOTCH1/FBXW7 mutation identifies a large subgroup with favorable outcome in adult T-cell acute lymphoblastic leukemia (T-ALL): a Group for Research on Adult Acute Lymphoblastic Leukemia (GRAALL) study. *Blood.* 2009;113(17):3918-24.

163. Breit S, Stanulla M, Flohr T, et al. Activating NOTCH1 mutations predict favorable early treatment response and long-term outcome in childhood precursor T-cell lymphoblastic leukemia. *Blood.* 2006;108(4):1151-7.

164. Mansour MR, Sulis ML, Duke V, et al. Prognostic implications of NOTCH1 and FBXW7 mutations in adults with T-cell acute lymphoblastic leukemia treated on the MRC UKALLXII/ECOG E2993 protocol. *J Clin Oncol.* 2009;27(26):4352-6.

165. Clappier E, Collette S, Grardel N, et al. NOTCH1 and FBXW7 mutations have a favorable impact on early response to treatment, but not on outcome, in children with T-cell acute lymphoblastic leukemia (T-ALL) treated on EORTC trials 58881 and 58951. *Leukemia.* 2010;24(12):2023-31.

166. Zuurbier L, Homminga I, Calvert V, et al. NOTCH1 and/or FBXW7 mutations predict for initial good prednisone response but not for improved outcome in pediatric T-cell acute lymphoblastic leukemia patients treated on DCOG or COALL protocols. *Leukemia.* 2010; 24(12):2014-22.

167. Palomero T, Sulis ML, Cortina M, et al. Mutational loss of PTEN induces resistance to NOTCH1 inhibition in T-cell leukemia. *Nat Med.* 2007;13(10):1203-10.

168. Van Vlierberghe P, Palomero T, Khiabanian H, et al. PHF6 mutations in T-cell acute lymphoblastic leukemia. *Nat Genet.* 2010;42(4):338-42.

Chemotherapy of Childhood Acute Lymphoblastic Leukemia

Kristen Eisenman, Ashley Rogers, Stephen P Hunger

INTRODUCTION AND OVERVIEW

Childhood acute lymphoblastic leukemia (ALL) was incurable 50 years ago. Today, 5-year survival rates exceed 90% and continue to increase, and it is anticipated that at least 85% of patients will be cured.[1] These dramatic improvements have occurred because of advances in chemotherapy with the development of new combinations of chemotherapeutic agents, optimization of treatment duration, and improved treatment of sanctuary sites. To date, the introduction of new agents has contributed little to improved outcome, as the agents used today have been used routinely in clinical trials since the mid to late 1970s, with the exception of imatinib and related tyrosine kinase inhibitors (TKI) that are used only for the 3–4% of patients with Philadelphia chromosome positive (Ph⁺) ALL.[2,3] The efforts of many different groups have contributed to these remarkable advances, including the Berlin-Frankfurt-Münster (BFM) group, Children's Oncology Group (COG), Dana-Farber Cancer Institute (DFCI) consortium, St Jude Children's Research Hospital (SJCRH), and many others.[4-8] Other chapters deal with many important aspects of ALL epidemiology, biology, classification, response assessment, and late effects. In this chapter, we will discuss chemotherapy treatment for pediatric ALL, focusing on features of treatment that are common to all groups while also emphasizing some of the important differences that exist.

TREAMENT OF NEWLY DIAGNOSED ALL

There are several phases in the treatment of newly diagnosed ALL patients including induction, consolidation or postinduction intensification (PII), and maintenance or continuation. Presymptomatic or prophylactic treatment of the central nervous system (CNS) is a critical component of therapy that spans all of these phases. During these phases, chemotherapy drugs are given intravenously (IV), intramuscularly (IM), orally (PO), and via intrathecal (IT) administration. Radiation of the CNS and sometimes testicles was a key component of the first effective ALL treatment regimens, but this has now largely been replaced by intensified IV and IT chemotherapy.

Induction Therapy

The goal of the first 4–6 weeks of therapy is to induce remission, defined as attaining an M1 marrow (<5% blasts), resolution of extramedullary involvement, and marrow recovery with restoration of normal hematopoiesis as reflected by peripheral blood counts. Most contemporary induction regimens include either 3 [corticosteroid, vincristine (VCR) and asparaginase (ASNase)] or 4 (addition of an anthracycline to the 3-drug regimen) agents given over 4 weeks and allow for count recovery and response assessment before the next phase of treatment is started. Others may include additional agents, such as cyclophosphamide (CPM) and assess response after 6–7 weeks. With this approach, 97–99% of patients enter complete remission (CR), with about half of failures due to resistant disease and about half due to death during induction.[9]

For several decades, the COG has taken a different approach than many other groups and used only 3-drugs to induce remission for patients with National Cancer Institute (NCI)/Rome standard risk (SR) features [age 1–9.99 years and initial white blood cell count (WBC) <50,000/μL].[10] This approach derives from results of the Children's Cancer Group (CCG) 105 trial conducted in the mid 1980s that investigated components of BFM-based treatment in children with intermediate risk (similar but not identical to NCI SR) ALL and showed similar outcomes for 3- and 4-drug induction as long as all patients received a delayed intensification (DI) or Protocol II phase (see below).[11] The COG uses a 4-drug induction for patients with NCI high risk (HR; age 10+ years or initial WBC ≥ 50,000/μL) features and most other groups use a 4-drug induction for all patients.

Use of a Prednisone Prephase

In the initial BFM trials, multiagent chemotherapy was started immediately.[12] ALL-BFM 83 introduced a 7-day course of prednisone (PRED) (60 mg/m^2/day) with a single dose of IT methotrexate (MTX) given on day 1 with the goals of decreasing complications related to tumor lysis syndrome and providing time to stabilize the patient.[13] The PRED prephase (also termed prophase) was found to be an indicator of rapid response to therapy.[14] About 90% of patients have less than 1,000 blasts/μL at the end of the prophase [termed prednisone good responders (PGR)], and have an excellent outcome. In contrast, the remaining 10% of prednisone poor responders (PPR) have a markedly inferior outcome. The prephase has been retained in all subsequent BFM trials, with PPR patients frequently assigned to receive more intensive therapy than PGR patients.

Corticosteroid Choice during Induction

One very important issue regarding induction therapy is the choice and dose of corticosteroid. Historically, PRED was used at a dose of 40–60 mg/m^2/day for 4 weeks (initially with a dose taper over 7–10 days, often now without a taper). However, there are important theoretical reasons suggesting that dexamethasone (DEX) may be superior to PRED for treatment of ALL, including better CNS penetration, different half-lives and potentially better antileukemic response at presumably "equitoxic" doses. The CCG showed that SR ALL patients had superior long-term results when treated with DEX 6 mg/m^2/day as compared to PRED 40 mg/m^2/day in the context of a 3-drug induction, with improved event-free survival (EFS) and decreased rates of isolated CNS relapse.[15] The United Kingdom Medical Research Council ALL97 trial similarly showed significantly improved EFS and decreased CNS relapse with DEX 6.5 mg/m^2/day as compared to PRED 40 mg/m^2/day during induction and maintenance therapy.[16]

Despite improved antileukemic efficacy with DEX, incorporating this agent into 4-drug induction regimens, particularly at 10 mg/m^2/day (presumed equitoxic to PRED 60 mg/m^2/day, which is the dose often used for higher risk patients) has proved problematic in many studies with increased rates of significant infectious toxicity and death during induction.[17] The BFM group recently completed a trial comparing (after a PRED prephase) 21 days (plus taper) of DEX 10 mg/m^2/day and PRED 60 mg/m^2/day in the context of a 4-drug induction.[18] Results showed decreased relapse and improved EFS, but increased severe toxicity with DEX. Patients with T-cell ALL, particularly those with a PGR, had the most substantial benefit to DEX with a one-third reduction in the risk of relapse. The EFS benefit was less clear for other patients, many of whom can be salvaged by other approaches. Hence, the BFM group elected to treat PGR T-ALL patients with DEX during induction in their current AIEOP (Associazione Italiana Ematologia Oncologia Pediatrica)-BFM ALL 2009 trial, while retaining PRED for all other patients.

The results of completed induction steroid randomizations were summarized recently in a meta-analysis by Teuffel and colleagues who found that DEX decreased CNS relapse, improved EFS, and increased toxicity but that results on overall survival (OS) were uncertain.[19] They also noted that trial results were dependent upon the PRED: DEX dose ratio studied.

Because of concerns about the toxicity of 28 consecutive days of DEX in a 4-drug induction and good results with pulse steroid administration in relapse ALL protocols,[20] the COG AALL0232 trial compared DEX 10 mg/m^2/day days 1–14 (Dex14) with PRED 60 mg/m^2/day days 1–28 (Pred28) in a 4-drug induction regimen for HR ALL patients. Early in the conduct of this trial, a significantly higher rate of osteonecrosis (ON) was observed in patients 10$^+$ years old randomized to the Dex14 arm and the randomization was stopped for patients of this age, but continued for patients less than 10 years old.[21] Longer-term results of AALL0232 showed significantly higher EFS for patients less than 10 years randomized to Dex14 without any appreciable incidence of ON in this age group.[22] With longer follow-up, the EFS was equivalent for patients 10$^+$ years old randomized to Dex14 versus Pred28, but the Dex14 group still had a higher rate of ON. Based on these results, the COG now uses three different induction regimens for children with B-cell precursor ALL. Patients with SR ALL receive a 3-drug DEX (6 mg/m^2/day) based induction. The HR patients with ALL receive a 4-drug induction, with those less than 10 years receiving Dex14 and those greater than or equal to 10 years receiving Pred28.

Asparaginase Use in Induction

There are three formulations of ASNase available: (1) the native *Escherichia coli* enzyme (generally termed L-asparaginase); (2) a pegylated version of native ASNase (PEG-L-asparaginase); and (3) Erwinia ASNase. The pegylated form was developed to decrease immunogenicity and increase half-life such that a single dose can be substituted for 2–3 weeks of two to three times per week dosing using the native form. All forms appear to be equally well tolerated without major differences in the side effects of hypersensitivity, pancreatitis, coagulopathy and stroke, or hepatitis.[23] Dose intensity and duration of activity are more important than product type,[23] and most groups have transitioned to using PEG-asparaginase with one to two doses given during a 4-week induction. There has been some variability in mode of administration until recently, but the COG now uses IV PEG-asparaginase as has been done for many years by other groups. Erwinia ASNase is now Food and Drug Administration (FDA)-approved in the United States (US) for use in patients who have had an allergic reaction to other ASNase preparations. ASNase use in ALL therapy is discussed in detail in chapter 8.

Toxicity during Induction

Unlike the case for acute myeloid leukemia, ALL induction chemotherapy is not profoundly myelosuppressive. However, ALL induction therapy is quite immunosuppressive, which is confounded by the fact that patients generally have complete marrow replacement at the time they are diagnosed and treatment is initiated. The major concern during induction is infection, and signs and symptoms of infection can be masked by corticosteroids, especially DEX. Thus, aggressive supportive care is critical during this phase of therapy, and should include some form of prophylaxis against candidal infection. Other potential toxicities and complications that can occur during induction include steroid (and ASNase) induced hyperglycemia which may require treatment, mood and behavioral disturbances, steroid myopathy, gastric disturbance, hepatotoxicity, and coagulopathy due to ASNase which can cause bleeding, thrombosis, or stroke. Prior to the advent of modern blood banks, bleeding was a major cause of complications during induction, and often led to death. Thankfully this is now extremely rare in higher income countries, but remains a significant issue in low-income countries that do not have easy access to blood products needed for supportive care, particularly platelets. As noted above, the toxic death rate during induction is generally less than 2% in higher income countries, although some patients, particularly those with Down syndrome (DS; constitutional trisomy 21) are at much higher risk (see below).

Postinduction Therapy

Following remission induction, contemporary pediatric ALL treatment typically involves 6–8 months of PII. In the past two decades, more intense PII has demonstrated improved outcomes in HR and SR subsets of ALL.[1,4-8] Most treatment groups use risk-adapted therapy whereby the intensity of postinduction treatment is based upon the risk of relapse, with patients at lower risk of relapse receiving less intensive therapy than those at higher risk of relapse. A number of different factors are used to assess risk, including clinical features, such as age and initial WBC (reflected by the NCI risk group), presence/absence of key sentinel cytogenetic/ genetic lesions, and early response as measured by response to the PRED prophase, early marrow morphology, or subclinical levels of minimal residual disease (MRD) present at end-induction.[24] These issues are discussed in depth in other chapters and will be considered only briefly here.

There have now been several very large studies published involving thousands of patients showing that end-induction MRD burden, as measured either by polymerase chain reaction (PCR) amplification of leukemia-specific immunoglobulin or T-cell receptor gene rearrangements or multiparameter flow cytometry, is the single strongest predictor of outcome in pediatric ALL.[25,26] Based on this, most groups intensify postinduction therapy for poor MRD responders. The BFM group also reassesses MRD at week 12 of therapy, and uses results, in part, to allocate patients to receive hematopoietic stem cell transplant (HSCT) in first remission.[26,27]

As most children with ALL are treated with BFM- or COG-based regimens, we will focus our discussion on the approaches taken by these groups, with limited discussion of other approaches (Table 6-1). It is important to emphasize that the outcomes attained by the different major North American and European groups with contemporary therapies are quite similar.[4-8] The differences that exist are relatively minor and it is uncertain if they are reflective of different treatment efficacies, different patient populations, or other reasons.

BFM-based Postinduction Intensification

The initial BFM trials of the early 1970s used an 8-week 8-drug intensive induction/ consolidation regimen that was revolutionary at that time.[12] This was divided into two 4-week blocks termed Protocols Ia and Ib, with Ia being what we termed induction in the above discussion. Protocol Ib consisted of weekly IT MTX, two doses

Table 6-1 Standard ALL Systemic Treatment Backbones for Selected Pediatric Oncology Groups

	COG		BFM	DFCI	SJCRH
	SR	HR			
Induction (Ia)	(4 weeks), no prophase 3-drugs: DEX, VCR, ASNase	(4 weeks), no prophase 4-drugs: DEX (<10 years) or PRED (10+ years), VCR, ASNase, DAUNO	(4 weeks), PRED prophase 4-drugs for all patients: PRED (DEX for T-ALL PGR), VCR, ASNase, DAUNO	(4 weeks), methyl PRED prophase 4-drugs for all patients: PRED, VCR, ASNase, DOXO IV MTX	(7 weeks; combines Ia/Ib), no prophase 4-drugs for all patients: PRED, VCR, ASNase, DAUNO HD MTX × 1, PO 6-MP, CPM, Ara-C
Consolidation (Ib)	(4 weeks), PO 6-MP, VCR	(8 weeks), PO 6-MP, CPM, Ara-C, PEG-ASNase, VCR	(8 weeks), PO 6-MP CPM, Ara-C	(3 weeks), PO 6-MP, VCR, HD MTX × 1 For HR patients: Above + DOXO For VHR patients: 3 multiagent blocks	Included in induction
Interim maintenance (IM) (Protocol M, CNS therapy, consolidation)	(8 weeks), Capizzi IV MTX, VCR	(8 weeks), PO 6-MP, HD-MTX × 4, VCR	(8 weeks), PO 6-MP, HD-MTX × 4 For HR patients: 3 multiagent blocks	(3 weeks), PO 6-MPVCR, DEX, ASNase For HR patients: Above + DOXO, C-XRT	(8 weeks), PO 6-MP HD-MTX × 4
Delayed intensification (DI) (Protocol II, consolidation II, reinduction)	(8 weeks), DEX, DOXO, ASNase, VCR PO 6-TG, CPM, Ara-C	(8 weeks), DEX, DOXO, ASNase, VCR PO 6-TG, CPM, Ara-C, VCR, ASNase	(8 weeks), DEX, DOXO, ASNase, VCR PO 6-TG, CPM, Ara-C	(30 weeks), DEX ASNase, VCRPO 6-MP IV MTX HR patients: Above + DOXO	(24 weeks), DEX, DOXO, ASNase, VCR PO 6-MP, CPM, Ara-C, IV MTX
Interim maintenance II	(8 weeks), VCR, Capizzi IV MTX	Only for VHR patients: (8 weeks), VCR, Capizzi IV MTX, ASNase	Only for HR patients: (4 weeks), PO 6-MP, PO MTX	Not given	Not given

Continued

Continued

| | COG | | BFM | DFCI | SJCRH |
	SR	HR			
Delayed intensification II	Not given	Not given	*Only for HR patients:* (8 weeks), DEX, DOXO, ASNase, VCR PO 6-TG, CPM, Ara-C	Not given	Not given
Maintenance (continuation)	[Until 26 months (girls) or 38 months (boys)] PO MTX, PO 6-MP, DEX, VCR	[Until 27 months (girls) or 39 months (boys)] PO MTX, PO 6-MP, PRED, VCR	[Until 24 months (girls) or 36 months (boys)] PO MTX, PO 6-MP	(Until 25 months) PO 6-MP, IV MTX, DEX, VCR	[Until 120 weeks (girls) or 146 weeks (boys)] *For LR patients:* PO MTX, PO 6-MP, DEX, VCR *SR or HR patients:* PO MTX, PO 6-MP, DEX, VCR, CPM, Ara-C

ALL, acute lymphoblastic leukemia; Ara-C, cytarabine; ASNase, asparaginase; BFM, Berlin-Frankfurt-Münster; COG, Children's Oncology Group; CPM, cyclophosphamide; C-XRT, cranial radiation therapy; DAUNO, daunorubicin; DEX, dexamethasone; DFCI, Dana-Farber Cancer Institute; DOXO, doxorubicin; HD, high dose; HR, high risk; IV, intravenous; LR, low risk; MTX, methotrexate; PO, oral; PRED, prednisone; PGR, prednisone good responder; SJCRH, St Jude Children's Research Hospital; SR, standard risk; T-ALL, T-cell acute lymphocytic leukemia; VCR, vincristine; VHR, very high risk; 6-MP, 6-mercaptopurine; 6-TG, 6-thioguanine.

of CPM at days 1 and 28, four 4-day cycles of cytarabine (Ara-C) (75 mg/m^2/day for 4 days) given weekly, and daily PO 6-mercaptopurine (6-MP). In the BFM 76/79 study, outcomes were improved by adding a second application of Protocol I (with some modifications) that was referred to as Protocol II. The modifications included substituting DEX for PRED, doxorubicin (DOXO) for daunorubicin (DAUNO), and 6-thioguanine (6-TG) for 6-MP. The best results were seen when there was an 8-week gap of maintenance type therapy [termed interim maintenance (IM)] given between Protocols I and II.[28] In the ALL-BFM-86 trial, the IM phase was replaced by an 8-week phase that consisted of four courses of high dose (HD) MTX (5 g/m^2 over 24 hours) followed by leucovorin rescue given at 2 week intervals plus PO 6-MP (Protocol M).[29] Thus, modern BFM therapy includes the PRED prephase, Protocols Ia and Ib, Protocol M, Protocol II (a and b), followed by maintenance (see below). Because some patients did not do well with this approach, particularly those with a PPR or adverse genetic features, the BFM later replaced Protocol M with three pulses of short, intensive multiagent chemotherapy termed high-risk (HR) blocks 1–3 for the highest risk patient subsets.[4]

COG-based Postinduction Intensification

In the 1980s, the CCG recognized that their results did not appear to be as good as those reported by the BFM. They then conducted two pivotal randomized clinical trials, CCG 105 for intermediate risk patients and CCG 106 for HR patients, comparing contemporary CCG and BFM therapies.[11,30] Both trials found that the BFM approach was superior and these became the baseline CCG regimens used in subsequent trials. Because there were some differences in the BFM regimens tested, CCG (later COG) therapy evolved separately for SR and HR patients and has diverged from the parent BFM regimens.

Children's Oncology Group therapy for SR patients has evolved through several successive trials. All SR patients receive a 3-drug DEX-based (6 mg/m^2/day for 28 days) induction. Those with a poor response, now defined by end-induction MRD burden, are crossed over to receive postinduction treatment analogous to that given to HR patients (see below). Those with a good response do not receive the BFM Ib consolidation, but rather receive 4 weeks of maintenance-like therapy with PO 6-MP and weekly IT MTX. Based on results of the CCG 1991 randomized trial, they then received an 8-week IM block that now consists of escalating dose IV MTX without leucovorin rescue, followed by a single DI phase and a second IM block followed by maintenance therapy.[31]

In contrast, HR patients are treated with a so-called "augmented BFM" (ABFM) regimen that has evolved over a series of clinical trials. In CCG 1882, HR ALL patients with a slow response to initial induction therapy (>25% marrow blasts at day 8) were randomized to either an augmented intensive regimen of postinduction chemotherapy that included both intensified therapy (more VCR, ASNase, MTX, and DEX) and more prolonged intensive treatment with a second IM and DI phase, or the standard regimen of PII.[32] Those randomized to the augmented regimen had significantly better EFS and OS. The toxic effects of augmented therapy were considerable but manageable. The successor CCG 1961 trial randomized HR ALL patients with a good early response (<25% marrow blasts at day 8) in a 2 × 2 manner to standard or longer duration and standard or increased intensity PII. Stronger intensity PII improved EFS and OS, while longer duration PII provided no benefit demonstrating that the augmented intensity but not the prolonged duration of PII was the critical component of the ABFM regimen.[33]

Pharmacokinetic data demonstrate that there is a great deal of variability in MTX levels and clearance,[34] and HR ALL patients with lower MTX levels are at increased risk of relapse,[35] leading to great interest in investigating the optimal dosing and regimen for MTX. The successor COG HR ALL trial AALL0232 was limited to patients with B-cell precursor ALL and studied induction steroid (see above) and mode of MTX administration in a 2 × 2 design. The ABFM regimen utilized Capizzi I MTX (escalating IV MTX without leucovorin rescue, followed by ASNase), while the BFM group uses HD MTX during the same 8-week IM block. In COG AALL0232, these two approaches were compared and HD MTX was shown to be superior.[36] Thus, modern COG HR ALL therapy has evolved to resemble BFM treatment with key differences in Ib (COG consolidation) and IIb (COG DI part 2).

Presymptomatic Central Nervous System Therapy

In the mid 1960s, chemotherapy regimens were developed that led to relatively high rates of CR and short-term disease control in the marrow, but most patients relapsed within 6–12 months with many of these relapses being "isolated" CNS relapses without marrow involvement. Based on this, the CNS was viewed as a "sanctuary site" for lymphoblasts and CNS directed therapy was implemented with presymptomatic CNS radiation, leading to significant improvement in cure rates in the early 1970s.[37] Initially, whole brain irradiation was given to all patients, with many groups also using spinal irradiation. While effective at preventing CNS relapse and improving cure rates, this was associated with significant adverse events including learning difficulties, endocrine disorders, and secondary brain tumors.[38] Because of this, all groups have greatly decreased the percentage of patients receiving cranial irradiation; the dose has been reduced from 2,400 cGy to 1,200–1,800 cGy and spinal irradiation has largely abandoned. This has been accomplished by intensifying systemic therapy with agents with improved CNS penetration (DEX rather than PRED, IV MTX) and more intensive use of IT chemotherapy (either MTX alone or triple IT therapy that also includes Ara-C and hydrocortisone). Most groups now administer cranial irradiation to only a minority

(10–25%) of ALL patients, and some do not radiate any newly diagnosed ALL patients or reserve irradiation for those with overt CNS disease at presentation.[39,40] Therapy of the CNS is discussed further in chapter 10.

Other Approaches to Postinduction Intensification

The DFCI consortium trials regimens have several major differences as compared to BFM/COG therapies. The most notable is that DFCI trials include 30 weeks of HD ASNase (25,000 units/m^2/dose) starting immediately after induction is complete.[41] In the DFCI 91-01 trial, patients who tolerated 25 or fewer doses had an inferior outcome to that obtained by patients who tolerated 26 or more doses.[42] In recent trials, the DFCI has compared weekly HD native ASNase to every other week pegylated ASNase.[43] DFCI trials have also included frequent VCR/steroid pulses during all phases of postinduction therapy, and relatively high cumulative doses of anthracyclines in higher risk patients.

The contemporary SJCRH total therapy trials have incorporated many elements found to be effective by other groups, with the major focus of recent trials being the complete elimination of presymptomatic cranial irradiation.[39] The initial 7 weeks of therapy on SJCRH trials is an intensive induction/consolidation phase similar to the BFM Protocol I, but with the second block of therapy starting earlier before count recovery occurs. The next phase utilizes HD MTX similar to the BFM Protocol M, but with MTX doses individualized to obtain prespecified target blood concentrations. Patients then receive an early continuation/reinduction phase that includes two reinduction treatments and current trials are testing the use of intensive ASNase treatment, similar to that used by the DFCI, during this phase.

Maintenance Therapy

In many ways, maintenance therapy is the "black box" of ALL treatment. The overwhelming majority of patients start maintenance with no detectable leukemia, even using sensitive MRD testing, but attempts to shorten total treatment to less than 24 months and maintenance to less than 12–18 months have resulted in a significantly higher incidence of relapse.[13,44] Most groups, therefore, continue to use a total duration of ALL therapy that ranges from about 2 years to almost 3.5 years, with about 16–30 months of this being maintenance therapy. The backbone of maintenance therapy is daily PO 6-MP (50–75 mg/m^2/day) and weekly MTX (20–40 mg/m^2/dose), with doses adjusted up or down based on blood count parameters and toxicity. Most groups now administer MTX PO, although some use IV MTX to assure compliance, which is an important issue in ALL treatment.[45] Bhatia and colleagues recently reported that nonadherence to PO maintenance chemotherapy occurs frequently in pediatric ALL, is more common in teenagers and Hispanics, and is associated with an increased risk of relapse.[46]

While the 6-MP/MTX backbone is a universal component of maintenance therapy, there are important differences between groups in the use of VCR/ corticosteroid pulses, intensity of IT therapy, duration of maintenance therapy, and whether or not this differs for males and females.

A number of reports showed that intermittent pulses of VCR and a glucocorticoid during maintenance improved outcomes.[44] Typical regimens include 5–7 days of corticosteroid with a single dose of VCR on the first day of the pulse with or without a second dose at the end of the pulse. However, the studies that showed such pulses to improve outcome were generally conducted in the 1970s and 1980s when therapy was less intensive and outcomes were not as good as they are today, and there is debate over whether or not pulses improve outcome in the context of contemporary therapy.[47] The international BFM group conducted a prospective meta-analysis trial that randomized patients to receive or not receive six pulses of 7 days of DEX (6 mg/m^2/day) plus VCR 1.5 mg/m^2 on days 1 and 8 during maintenance therapy in the context of contemporary BFM therapy.[48] Outcomes of the two groups were essentially identical; based on this, current BFM regimens do not include maintenance VCR/corticosteroid pulses. In contrast, COG regimens include 5-day pulses of DEX (SR) or PRED (HR) plus a single dose of VCR every 4 weeks during maintenance therapy, and DFCI and SJCRH regimens also use pulses. The COG is currently conducting a randomized trial of every 4-week versus every 12-week pulses during maintenance for children with SR ALL.

Another significant difference between BFM and COG trials is the intensity of IT therapy during maintenance. BFM studies generally do not give IT chemotherapy during maintenance and include only about 11–13 total doses of IT therapy. In contrast, COG trials give IT chemotherapy at least every 12 weeks during maintenance and include a total of 21–25 IT treatments. Both BFM and COG use IT MTX alone, while SJCRH trials use IT triple therapy throughout. In CCG 1952, patients with SR ALL were randomized to receive IT MTX versus IT triple chemotherapy. While there was a significantly lower rate of CNS relapse in those randomized to receive IT triple therapy, there were ultimately more marrow relapses in this arm leading to inferior long-term survival.[49] This trial used PRED rather than DEX as the corticosteroid and also had a relatively nonintensive backbone, leading to results that are inferior to those obtained in subsequent CCG/COG SR ALL trials. Thus, it is possible that better CNS control with IT triples might translate to improved outcomes in the context of more intensive therapy. The COG is currently testing IT MTX versus IT triple therapy in children with HR ALL treated with a more intensive treatment backbone.

The different treatment groups use therapies of different length. Perhaps the biggest difference is that the COG treats males with 1 year longer maintenance therapy than females. In older trials, when the length of therapy was the same for both sexes, females had a 20% higher 2-year EFS than boys, reaching a 38% difference at 5 years.[50] In subsequent studies, males were treated for a year longer than females and obtained outcomes that were almost as good, though small differences still remain.[1,7,8] However, it is not clear whether the improved relative outcome for males is due to longer maintenance therapy or improved overall treatment.

Special ALL Subsets

Treatment of T-ALL

T-cell ALL was identified in the 1970s to be associated with unique clinical features including older age, higher initial WBC, thymic involvement, male sex, and an inferior outcome as compared to what we now know to be B-cell precursor ALL.[51] While outcomes for T-ALL are now much better than they were 30 years ago, T-cell immunophenotype continues to be associated with an increased risk of relapse in contemporary pediatric ALL trials.[1] It has also become clear that while low-risk patients with B-cell precursor ALL can be treated quite successfully with relatively less intensive therapy, children with T-ALL require more intensive treatment to obtain good outcomes regardless of clinical features.[32,52] A goal of contemporary therapy is to test "targeted" therapies in HR groups. Nelarabine, a prodrug of ara-G, is a synthetic deoxyguanosine derivative that is cytotoxic to T-lymphoblasts at micromolar concentrations. The cytotoxicity is mediated via accumulation of ara-G nucleotides in T-cells greater than in B-cells, resulting in inhibition of ribonucleotide reductase and inhibition of deoxyribonucleic acid (DNA) synthesis. Nelarabine showed very promising responses in patients with relapsed T-ALL, but was associated with significant and sometimes fatal CNS toxicity. In contrast, the COG showed that nelarabine could be incorporated into intensive treatment regimens for newly diagnosed ALL with little toxicity,[53] and is currently conducting a trial that randomizes newly diagnosed patients with T-ALL to ABFM therapy with/ without nelarabine.

Treatment of Ph[+] ALL

While a number of different sentinel lesions are associated with either an excellent [ETV6-RUNX1 (TEL-AML1) fusion, hyperdiploidy and/or favorable chromosome trisomies] or inferior [mixed-lineage leukemia (MLL) translocations, hypodiploidy, Ph[+] ALL] prognosis, at this time, truly specific therapy is available only for those with Ph[+] ALL. This subtype accounts for 3–4% of pediatric ALL and was associated with a dismal prognosis until the past decade.[2,3] Patients with Ph[+] ALL have BCR-ABL1 fusion analogous to that present in patients with chronic myeloid leukemia (CML), which produces a chimeric BCR-ABL1 protein with constitutive tyrosine kinase (TK) activity. The development of imatinib revolutionized treatment of CML and monotherapy with imatinib or a second generation TKI, such as dasatinib or nilotinib is now the treatment of choice for CML.[54-57] The COG showed that addition of imatinib to intensive chemotherapy led to dramatic improvements in early EFS/OS for patients with Ph[+] ALL and other groups have also shown very encouraging results.[58,59] Based on these and other findings, most groups now screen all patients with ALL for BCR-ABL1 fusion at initial diagnosis and assign those found to be positive to receive chemotherapy plus a TKI (imatinib or dasatinib).

Recently, a subset of ALL patients has been identified that has a gene expression profile similar to that of Ph[+] ALL, but lacks BCR-ABL1 fusion.[60,61] Among children with ALL, patients with this so-called BCR-ABL1-like phenotype are about three times as common as those with Ph[+] ALL and also have a poor prognosis.[62] Recent studies have shown that a subset (perhaps a third) of these patients have genomic rearrangements that create novel *ABL1* and platelet-derived growth factor receptor beta (PDGFRB) fusion genes that are responsive *in vitro* to ABL class TKIs, suggesting that targeted therapy with such drugs may be applicable to a larger subgroup than simply those with Ph[+] ALL.[63]

Treatment of Infant ALL

Infants less than 1 year of age account for less than 5% of childhood ALL cases.[64] Rearrangements of the *MLL* gene on chromosome 11q23 occur in 70–80% of infants with ALL.[65] Infants with ALL have a poor prognosis, with the most adverse prognostic features being young age (neonates and those <3 months at diagnosis tend to fare most poorly), elevated WBC at diagnosis, lack of CD10 expression, MLL rearrangement, and poor early response to therapy.[64,66] CNS leukemia is common in infant ALL at the time of diagnosis, but it can be adequately treated without cranial irradiation and with intensive IT and systemic chemotherapy.[67] Overall, only half or fewer of infants with ALL are cured with contemporary therapies that are often extremely intensive.[68,69] There is some controversy over the relative benefits of HSCT in first remission for infants with ALL, with the Europe-based INTERFANT-99 trial showing an advantage of transplant for a HR subset, while a COG study showed no advantage.[70,71] MLL-rearranged infant leukemia patients have demonstrated high level Fms-like tyrosine kinase 3 (FLT3) expression[72,73] and increased FLT3 expression in this population has been associated with adverse prognosis.[74] Preclinical data show sequence-dependent synergy between chemotherapy and FLT3 inhibitors in infant ALL patient samples,[75] leading the COG to conduct a trial testing the FLT3 inhibitor lestaurtinib in infants with MLL-rearranged ALL.

Treatment of Adolescents and Young Adults with ALL

An important ALL subgroup to consider is adolescents and young adults (AYA) 16–21 years of age. Patients of this age have generally had an inferior outcome as compared to younger children.[76,77] There are changes in leukemia biology with increasing age that may explain some of these differences, as fewer AYA patients have favorable genetic features, such as hyperdiploidy or ETV6-RUNX1 fusion, and more have unfavorable genetic features, such as Ph$^+$ ALL and MLL translocations. Because AYA patients may be treated by either adult or pediatric oncologists, there have been a number of retrospective studies that compared outcomes obtained in these different settings showing markedly better outcomes for AYA patients treated on pediatric as opposed to adult oncology trials.[78-81] The reasons that underlie these differences are likely multifactorial and include differences in the chemotherapy itself, differences in patient (and perhaps physician) treatment adherence, and perhaps the preferential inclusion of AYA patients living with parents in the pediatric trials and emancipated AYA patients in the adult trials.[78,82] In any case, the best approach for AYA patients is treatment with a pediatric ALL regimen and a number of groups have reported excellent results with such therapies.[83-85] The US adult cooperative groups are now testing pediatric ALL treatments in patients 16–39 years of age in the C10403 trial.

Treatment of Children with Down Syndrome and ALL

Patients with constitutional trisomy 21 (DS) have a 10–20 times increased risk of developing leukemia.[86] ALL in DS has unique biological features with a lower incidence of the common sentinel cytogenetic features and an increased incidence of mutations in Janus kinase 2 (JAK2) and cytokine receptor-like factor 2 (CRLF2).[87,88] When comparing DS and non-DS ALL, the CR rate is equivalent; however, the risk of death in induction and the risk of toxic complications and mortality is increased for patients with DS-ALL.[89] This creates a need to balance efforts to reduce toxic mortality with those to decrease relapse. In the future, it is possible that targeted therapies directed at the CRLF2/JAK2 axis will be tested in children with DS-ALL.

TREAMENT OF RELAPSED ALL

Unfortunately, outcomes for ALL following relapse are far worse than those for newly diagnosed ALL and because of the high frequency of ALL, relapsed ALL is the most common cause of cancer death in children.[90-92] A number of studies have shown that the most important prognostic factors for relapsed ALL are time to relapse, site of relapse, and immunophenotype.[92-95] The highest risk subgroup includes patients with marrow relapse occurring within 36 months of initial diagnosis or T-ALL and marrow relapse at any point in time. Remission reinduction rates are only about 70% for such patients (even lower for those who relapse within 12–18 months of diagnosis) and there is general agreement that allogeneic HSCT is the best consolidation therapy for those that attain remission. However, the long-term survival is generally less than 20% for these patients.[92] Patients with marrow relapse occurring more than 36 months postdiagnosis have a 40–50% cure rate with a number of different treatments. There is some controversy about the relative merits of chemotherapy versus HSCT for this subgroup, with MRD at the end of reinduction now used by many groups to allocate therapies.

The cure rate is better for patients with isolated extramedullary relapse, except for those that relapse within 12–18 months of initial diagnosis. The most common sites of extramedullary relapse are the CNS and the testes. Because the major cause of treatment failure for patients with isolated extramedullary relapse is subsequent marrow relapse, these patients are typically treated with regimens similar to those used to treat marrow relapse. Most groups include cranial irradiation in the treatment of patients with CNS relapse, typically using doses of 18–24 Gy, although some still utilize craniospinal irradiation with a lower dose to the spine than delivered to the cranium. If HSCT is used to treat the relapse, then the radiation therapy is usually included as a boost that precedes total body irradiation to attain a total cranial dose of 18–24 Gy. The role of irradiation in the treatment of testicular relapse is uncertain and hard to define, given the very low rate of this site of relapse with contemporary therapy. Most centers do not radiate the testicle(s) if the leukemia responds completely within 4–6 weeks, reserving testicular irradiation (usual dose 2,400 Gy) for those that do not have a rapid and complete response of the testicular leukemia.

SUMMARY AND PERSPECTIVES

Over the past few decades, substantial progress has been made in improving the survival of children, adolescents and young adults with ALL. To date, this progress has been almost entirely due to optimization of the same chemotherapy agents used since the mid 1970s. Future efforts will likely expand the use of therapies targeted at the underlying genetic changes that drive leukemogenesis as exemplified by dramatic improvements in outcome for Ph+ ALL with the addition of imatinib to chemotherapy.[58] New technologies have led to new major insights into the genomic landscape of ALL, with many more anticipated as additional ALL genomes are sequenced.[96,97] It is hoped that these developments will lead to new therapies that will improve cure rates for HR patients and also allow other patients to be cured with less noxious therapy with fewer short- and long-term toxicities.

REFERENCES

1. Hunger SP, Lu X, Devidas M, et al. Improved survival for children and adolescents with acute lymphoblastic leukemia between 1990 and 2005: a report from the children's oncology group. *J Clin Oncol*. 2012;30(14):1663-9.
2. Aricò M, Valsecchi MG, Camitta B, et al. Outcome of treatment in children with Philadelphia chromosome-positive acute lymphoblastic leukemia. *N Engl J Med*. 2000;342(14):998-1006.
3. Aricò M, Schrappe M, Hunger SP, et al. Clinical outcome of children with newly diagnosed Philadelphia chromosome-positive acute lymphoblastic leukemia treated between 1995 and 2005. *J Clin Oncol*. 2010;28(31):4755-61.
4. Möricke A, Zimmermann M, Reiter A, et al. Long-term results of five consecutive trials in childhood acute lymphoblastic leukemia performed by the ALL-BFM study group from 1981 to 2000. *Leukemia*. 2010;24(2):265-84.

5. Pui CH, Pei D, Sandlund JT, et al. Long-term results of St Jude Total Therapy Studies 11, 12, 13A, 13B, and 14 for childhood acute lymphoblastic leukemia. *Leukemia.* 2010;24(2): 371-82.

6. Silverman LB, Stevenson KE, O'Brien JE, et al. Long-term results of Dana-Farber Cancer Institute ALL Consortium protocols for children with newly diagnosed acute lymphoblastic leukemia (1985-2000). *Leukemia.* 2010;24(2):320-34.

7. Gaynon PS, Angiolillo AL, Carroll WL, et al. Long-term results of the children's cancer group studies for childhood acute lymphoblastic leukemia 1983-2002: a Children's Oncology Group Report. *Leukemia.* 2010;24(2):285-97.

8. Salzer WL, Devidas M, Carroll WL, et al. Long-term results of the pediatric oncology group studies for childhood acute lymphoblastic leukemia 1984-2001: a report from the children's oncology group. *Leukemia.* 2010;24(2):355-70.

9. Schrappe M, Hunger SP, Pui CH, et al. Outcomes after induction failure in childhood acute lymphoblastic leukemia. *N Engl J Med.* 2012;366(15):1371-81.

10. Smith M, Bleyer A, Crist W, et al. Uniform criteria for childhood acute lymphoblastic leukemia risk classification. *J Clin Oncol.* 1996;14(2):680-1.

11. Tubergen DG, Gilchrist GS, O'Brien RT, et al. Improved outcome with delayed intensification for children with acute lymphoblastic leukemia and intermediate presenting features: a Childrens Cancer Group phase III trial. *J Clin Oncol.* 1993;11(3):527-37.

12. Schrappe M. Evolution of BFM trials for childhood ALL. *Ann Hematol.* 2004;83(Suppl 1): S121-3.

13. Riehm H, Gadner H, Henze G, et al. Results and significance of six randomized trials in four consecutive ALL-BFM studies. *Haematol Blood Transfus.* 1990;33:439-50.

14. Schrappe M, Reiter A, Riehm H. Cytoreduction and prognosis in childhood acute lymphoblastic leukemia. *J Clin Oncol.* 1996;14(8):2403-6.

15. Bostrom BC, Sensel MR, Sather HN, et al. Dexamethasone versus prednisone and daily oral versus weekly intravenous mercaptopurine for patients with standard-risk acute lymphoblastic leukemia: a report from the Children's Cancer Group. *Blood.* 2003;101(10):3809-17.

16. Mitchell CD, Richards SM, Kinsey SE, et al. Benefit of dexamethasone compared with prednisolone for childhood acute lymphoblastic leukaemia: results of the UK Medical Research Council ALL97 randomized trial. *Br J Haematol.* 2005;129(6):734-45.

17. Hurwitz CA, Silverman LB, Schorin MA, et al. Substituting dexamethasone for prednisone complicates remission induction in children with acute lymphoblastic leukemia. *Cancer.* 2000;88(8):1964-9.

18. Schrappe M, Zimmermann M, Moricke A, et al. Dexamethasone in induction can eliminate one third of all relapses in childhood acute lymphoblastic leukemia (ALL): results of an international randomized trial in 3655 patients (trial AIEOP-BFM ALL 2000). *Blood.* 2008; 112(11):9.

19. Teuffel O, Kuster SP, Hunger SP, et al. Dexamethasone versus prednisone for induction therapy in childhood acute lymphoblastic leukemia: a systematic review and meta-analysis. *Leukemia.* 2011;25(8):1232-8.

20. Parker C, Waters R, Leighton C, et al. Effect of mitoxantrone on outcome of children with first relapse of acute lymphoblastic leukaemia (ALL R3): an open-label randomised trial. *Lancet.* 2010;376(9757):2009-17.

21. Mattano LA, Nachman JB, Devidas M, et al. Increased incidence of osteonecrosis (ON) with a dexamethasone (DEX) induction for high-risk acute lymphoblastic leukemia (HR-ALL): a report from the Children's Oncology Group (COG). *Blood.* 2008;112(898):333-4.

22. Winick NJ, Salzer WL, Devidas M, et al. Dexamethasone (DEX) versus prednisone (PRED) during induction for children with high-risk acute lymphoblastic leukemia (HR-ALL): a report from the Children's Oncology Group study AALL0232. *J Clin Oncol.* 2011;29(15 Suppl):586s.

23. Asselin BL. L-asparaginase for treatment of childhood acute lymphoblastic leukemia: what have we learned? *Pediatr Blood Cancer.* 2011;57(3):357-8.

24. Schultz KR, Pullen DJ, Sather HN, et al. Risk- and response-based classification of childhood B-precursor acute lymphoblastic leukemia: a combined analysis of prognostic markers from the Pediatric Oncology Group (POG) and Children's Cancer Group (CCG). *Blood.* 2007;109(3):926-35.

25. Borowitz MJ, Devidas M, Hunger SP, et al. Clinical significance of minimal residual disease in childhood acute lymphoblastic leukemia and its relationship to other prognostic factors: a Children's Oncology Group study. *Blood.* 2008;111(12):5477-85.

26. Conter V, Bartram CR, Valsecchi MG, et al. Molecular response to treatment redefines all prognostic factors in children and adolescents with B-cell precursor acute lymphoblastic leukemia: results in 3184 patients of the AIEOP-BFM ALL 2000 study. *Blood.* 2010;115(16): 3206-14.

27. Schrappe M, Valsecchi MG, Bartram CR, et al. Late MRD response determines relapse risk overall and in subsets of childhood T-cell ALL: results of the AIEOP-BFM-ALL 2000 study. *Blood.* 2011;118(8):2077-84.

28. Henze G, Langermann HJ, Brämswig J, et al. [The BFM 76/79 acute lymphoblastic leukemia therapy study (author's transl)]. *Klin Padiatr.* 1981;193(3):145-54.

29. Reiter A, Schrappe M, Ludwig WD, et al. Chemotherapy in 998 unselected childhood acute lymphoblastic leukemia patients. Results and conclusions of the multicenter trial ALL-BFM 86. *Blood.* 1994;84(9):3122-33.

30. Gaynon PS, Steinherz PG, Bleyer WA, et al. Improved therapy for children with acute lymphoblastic leukemia and unfavorable presenting features: a follow-up report of the Childrens Cancer Group Study CCG-106. *J Clin Oncol.* 1993;11(11):2234-42.

31. Matloub Y, Bostrom BC, Hunger SP, et al. Escalating intravenous methotrexate improves event-free survival in children with standard-risk acute lymphoblastic leukemia: a report from the Children's Oncology Group. *Blood.* 2011;118(2):243-51.

32. Nachman JB, Sather HN, Sensel MG, et al. Augmented post-induction therapy for children with high-risk acute lymphoblastic leukemia and a slow response to initial therapy. *N Engl J Med.* 1998;338(23):1663-71.

33. Seibel NL, Steinherz PG, Sather HN, et al. Early postinduction intensification therapy improves survival for children and adolescents with high-risk acute lymphoblastic leukemia: a report from the Children's Oncology Group. *Blood.* 2008;111(5):2548-55.

34. Borsi J, Révész T, Schuler D. [Prognostic significance of systemic clearance of methotrexate in acute lymphoid leukemia in childhood]. *Orv Hetil.* 1986;127(8):439-42.

35. Camitta B, Mahoney D, Leventhal B, et al. Intensive intravenous methotrexate and mercapto-purine treatment of higher-risk non-T, non-B acute lymphocytic leukemia: A Pediatric Oncology Group study. *J Clin Oncol.* 1994;12(7):1383-9.

36. Larsen EC, Salzer WL, Devidas M, et al. High dose methotrexate (HD-MTX) as compared to Capizzi methotrexate plus asparaginase (C-MTX/ASNase) improves event-free survival (EFS) in children and young adults with high-risk acute lymphoblastic leukemia (HR-ALL): a report from the Children's Oncology Group study AALL0232. *J Clin Oncol.* 2011;29:6s.

37. Aur RJ, Simone JV, Hustu HO, et al. A comparative study of central nervous system irradiation and intensive chemotherapy early in remission of childhood acute lymphocytic leukemia. *Cancer.* 1972;29(2):381-91.

38. Pui CH, Howard SC. Current management and challenges of malignant disease in the CNS in paediatric leukaemia. *Lancet Oncol.* 2008;9(3):257-68.

39. Pui CH, Campana D, Pei D, et al. Treating childhood acute lymphoblastic leukemia without cranial irradiation. *N Engl J Med.* 2009;360(26):2730-41.

40. Veerman AJ, Kamps WA, van den Berg H, et al. Dexamethasone-based therapy for childhood acute lymphoblastic leukaemia: results of the prospective Dutch Childhood Oncology Group (DCOG) protocol ALL-9 (1997-2004). *Lancet Oncol.* 2009;10(10):957-66.

41. Sallan SE, Hitchcock-Bryan S, Gelber R, et al. Influence of intensive asparaginase in the treatment of childhood non-T-cell acute lymphoblastic leukemia. *Cancer Res.* 1983;43(11):5601-7.

42. Silverman LB, Gelber RD, Dalton VK, et al. Improved outcome for children with acute lymphoblastic leukemia: results of Dana-Farber Consortium Protocol 91-01. *Blood.* 2001; 97(5):1211-8.

43. Silverman LB, Supko JG, Stevenson KE, et al. Intravenous PEG-asparaginase during remission induction in children and adolescents with newly diagnosed acute lymphoblastic leukemia. *Blood.* 2010;115(7):1351-3.

44. Duration and intensity of maintenance chemotherapy in acute lymphoblastic leukaemia: overview of 42 trials involving 12,000 randomised children. Childhood ALL Collaborative Group. *Lancet.* 1996;347(9018):1783-8.

45. Pritchard MT, Butow PN, Stevens MM, et al. Understanding medication adherence in pediatric acute lymphoblastic leukemia: a review. *J Pediatr Hematol Oncol.* 2006;28(12):816-23.

46. Bhatia S, Landier W, Shangguan M, et al. Nonadherence to oral mercaptopurine and risk of relapse in Hispanic and non-Hispanic white children with acute lymphoblastic leukemia: a report from the children's oncology group. *J Clin Oncol.* 2012;30(17):2094-101.

47. Eden T, Pieters R, Richards S. Systematic review of the addition of vincristine plus steroid pulses in maintenance treatment for childhood acute lymphoblastic leukaemia - an individual patient data meta-analysis involving 5,659 children. *Br J Haematol.* 2010;149(5):722-33.

48. Conter V, Valsecchi MG, Silvestri D, et al. Pulses of vincristine and dexamethasone in addition to intensive chemotherapy for children with intermediate-risk acute lymphoblastic leukaemia: a multicentre randomised trial. *Lancet.* 2007;369(9556):123-31.

49. Matloub Y, Lindemulder S, Gaynon PS, et al. Intrathecal triple therapy decreases central nervous system relapse but fails to improve event-free survival when compared with intrathecal methotrexate: results of the Children's Cancer Group (CCG) 1952 study for standard-risk acute lymphoblastic leukemia, reported by the Children's Oncology Group. *Blood.* 2006;108(4):1165-73.

50. Shuster JJ, Wacker P, Pullen J, et al. Prognostic significance of sex in childhood B-precursor acute lymphoblastic leukemia: a Pediatric Oncology Group Study. *J Clin Oncol.* 1998;16(8): 2854-63.

51. Sen L, Borella L. Clinical importance of lymphoblasts with T markers in childhood acute leukemia. *N Engl J Med.* 1975;292(16):828-32.

52. Goldberg JM, Silverman LB, Levy DE, et al. Childhood T-cell acute lymphoblastic leukemia: the Dana-Farber Cancer Institute acute lymphoblastic leukemia consortium experience. *J Clin Oncol.* 2003;21(19):3616-22.

53. Dunsmore KP, Devidas M, Linda SB, et al. Pilot study of nelarabine in combination with intensive chemotherapy in high-risk T-cell acute lymphoblastic leukemia: a report from the Children's Oncology Group. *J Clin Oncol.* 2012;30(22):2753-9.

54. Kantarjian H, Shah NP, Hochhaus A, et al. Dasatinib versus imatinib in newly diagnosed chronic-phase chronic myeloid leukemia. *N Engl J Med.* 2010;362(24):2260-70.

55. Saglio G, Kim DW, Issaragrisil S, et al. Nilotinib versus imatinib for newly diagnosed chronic myeloid leukemia. *N Engl J Med.* 2010;362(24):2251-9.

56. Druker BJ, Sawyers CL, Kantarjian H, et al. Activity of a specific inhibitor of the BCR-ABL tyrosine kinase in the blast crisis of chronic myeloid leukemia and acute lymphoblastic leukemia with the Philadelphia chromosome. *N Engl J Med.* 2001;344(14):1038-42.

57. Druker BJ, Talpaz M, Resta DJ, et al. Efficacy and safety of a specific inhibitor of the BCR-ABL tyrosine kinase in chronic myeloid leukemia. *N Engl J Med.* 2001;344(14):1031-7.

58. Schultz KR, Bowman WP, Aledo A, et al. Improved early event-free survival with imatinib in Philadelphia chromosome-positive acute lymphoblastic leukemia: a children's oncology group study. *J Clin Oncol.* 2009;27(31):5175-81.

59. Biondi A, Schrappe M, De Lorenzo P, et al. Imatinib after induction for treatment of children and adolescents with Philadelphia-chromosome-positive acute lymphoblastic leukaemia (EsPhALL): a randomised, open-label, intergroup study. *Lancet Oncol.* 2012;13(9):936-45.

60. Mullighan CG, Su X, Zhang J, et al. Deletion of IKZF1 and prognosis in acute lymphoblastic leukemia. *N Engl J Med.* 2009;360(5):470-80.
61. Den Boer ML, van Slegtenhorst M, De Menezes RX, et al. A subtype of childhood acute lymphoblastic leukaemia with poor treatment outcome: a genome-wide classification study. *Lancet Oncol.* 2009;10(2):125-34.
62. Loh ML, Zhang J, Harvey RC, Roberts K, Payne-Turner D, Kang H, et al. Tyrosine kinome sequencing of pediatric acute lymphoblastic leukemia: A report from the children's Oncology Group TARGET Project. *Blood.* 2013;121(3):485-8.
63. Roberts KG, Morin RD, Zhang J, et al. Genetic alterations activating kinase and cytokine receptor signaling in high-risk acute lymphoblastic leukemia. *Cancer Cell.* 2012;22(2):153-66.
64. Pui CH, Ribeiro RC, Campana D, et al. Prognostic factors in the acute lymphoid and myeloid leukemias of infants. *Leukemia.* 1996;10(6):952-6.
65. Biondi A, Cimino G, Pieters R, et al. Biological and therapeutic aspects of infant leukemia. *Blood.* 2000;96(1):24-33.
66. Dördelmann M, Reiter A, Borkhardt A, et al. Prednisone response is the strongest predictor of treatment outcome in infant acute lymphoblastic leukemia. *Blood.* 1999;94(4):1209-17.
67. Isaacs H. Fetal and neonatal leukemia. *J Pediatr Hematol Oncol.* 2003;25(5):348-61.
68. Pieters R, Schrappe M, De Lorenzo P, et al. A treatment protocol for infants younger than 1 year with acute lymphoblastic leukaemia (Interfant-99): an observational study and a multicentre randomised trial. *Lancet.* 2007;370(9583):240-50.
69. Salzer WL, Jones TL, Devidas M, et al. Modifications to induction therapy decrease risk of early death in infants with acute lymphoblastic leukemia treated on Children's Oncology Group P9407. *Pediatr Blood Cancer.* 2012;59(5):834-9.
70. Mann G, Attarbaschi A, Schrappe M, et al. Improved outcome with hematopoietic stem cell transplantation in a poor prognostic subgroup of infants with mixed-lineage-leukemia (MLL)-rearranged acute lymphoblastic leukemia: results from the Interfant-99 Study. *Blood.* 2010;116(15):2644-50.
71. Dreyer ZE, Dinndorf PA, Camitta B, et al. Analysis of the role of hematopoietic stem-cell transplantation in infants with acute lymphoblastic leukemia in first remission and MLL gene rearrangements: a report from the Children's Oncology Group. *J Clin Oncol.* 2011;29(2):214-22.
72. Armstrong SA, Kung AL, Mabon ME, et al. Inhibition of FLT3 in MLL. Validation of a therapeutic target identified by gene expression based classification. *Cancer Cell.* 2003;3(2):173-83.
73. Levis M, Small D. FLT3: ITDoes matter in leukemia. *Leukemia.* 2003;17(9):1738-52.
74. Kang H, Wilson CS, Harvey RC, et al. Gene expression profiles predictive of outcome and age in infant acute lymphoblastic leukemia: a Children's Oncology Group study. *Blood.* 2012;119(8):1872-81.
75. Brown P, Levis M, McIntyre E, et al. Combinations of the FLT3 inhibitor CEP-701 and chemotherapy synergistically kill infant and childhood MLL-rearranged ALL cells in a sequence-dependent manner. *Leukemia.* 2006;20(8):1368-76.
76. Chessells JM, Hall E, Prentice HG, et al. The impact of age on outcome in lymphoblastic leukaemia; MRC UKALL X and XA compared: a report from the MRC Paediatric and Adult Working Parties. *Leukemia.* 1998;12(4):463-73.
77. Pulte D, Gondos A, Brenner H. Improvement in survival in younger patients with acute lymphoblastic leukemia from the 1980s to the early 21st century. *Blood.* 2009;113(7):1408-11.
78. Stock W, La M, Sanford B, et al. What determines the outcomes for adolescents and young adults with acute lymphoblastic leukemia treated on cooperative group protocols? A comparison of Children's Cancer Group and Cancer and Leukemia Group B studies. *Blood.* 2008;112(5):1646-54.
79. Ramanujachar R, Richards S, Hann I, et al. Adolescents with acute lymphoblastic leukaemia: emerging from the shadow of paediatric and adult treatment protocols. *Pediatr Blood Cancer.* 2006;47(6):748-56.

80. de Bont JM, Holt Bv, Dekker AW, et al. Significant difference in outcome for adolescents with acute lymphoblastic leukemia treated on pediatric vs adult protocols in the Netherlands. *Leukemia.* 2004;18(12):2032-5.

81. Boissel N, Auclerc MF, Lhéritier V, et al. Should adolescents with acute lymphoblastic leukemia be treated as old children or young adults? Comparison of the French FRALLE-93 and LALA-94 trials. *J Clin Oncol.* 2003;21(5):774-80.

82. Schafer ES, Hunger SP. Optimal therapy for acute lymphoblastic leukemia in adolescents and young adults. *Nat Rev Clin Oncol.* 2011;8(7):417-24.

83. Barry E, DeAngelo DJ, Neuberg D, et al. Favorable outcome for adolescents with acute lymphoblastic leukemia treated on Dana-Farber Cancer Institute Acute Lymphoblastic Leukemia Consortium Protocols. *J Clin Oncol.* 2007;25(7):813-9.

84. Pui CH, Pei D, Campana D, et al. Improved prognosis for older adolescents with acute lymphoblastic leukemia. *J Clin Oncol.* 2011;29(4):386-91.

85. Nachman JB, La MK, Hunger SP, et al. Young adults with acute lymphoblastic leukemia have an excellent outcome with chemotherapy alone and benefit from intensive postinduction treatment: a report from the children's oncology group. *J Clin Oncol.* 2009;27(31):5189-94.

86. Maloney KW. Acute lymphoblastic leukaemia in children with Down syndrome: an updated review. *Br J Haematol.* 2011;155(4):420-5.

87. Hertzberg L, Vendramini E, Ganmore I, et al. Down syndrome acute lymphoblastic leukemia, a highly heterogeneous disease in which aberrant expression of CRLF2 is associated with mutated JAK2: a report from the International BFM Study Group. *Blood.* 2010;115(5):1006-17.

88. Mullighan CG, Collins-Underwood JR, Phillips LA, et al. Rearrangement of CRLF2 in B-progenitor- and Down syndrome-associated acute lymphoblastic leukemia. *Nat Genet.* 2009;41(11):1243-6.

89. Maloney KW, Carroll WL, Carroll AJ, et al. Down syndrome childhood acute lymphoblastic leukemia has a unique spectrum of sentinel cytogenetic lesions that influences treatment outcome: a report from the Children's Oncology Group. *Blood.* 2010;116(7):1045-50.

90. Henze G. Childhood acute lymphoblastic leukaemia. *Eur J Cancer.* 1997;33(1):8-9.

91. Roy L, Guilhot J, Martineau G, et al. Unexpected occurrence of second malignancies in patients treated with interferon followed by imatinib mesylate for chronic myelogenous leukemia. *Leukemia.* 2005;19(9):1689-92.

92. Nguyen K, Devidas M, Cheng SC, et al. Factors influencing survival after relapse from acute lymphoblastic leukemia: a Children's Oncology Group study. *Leukemia.* 2008;22(12):2142-50.

93. Schroeder H, Garwicz S, Kristinsson J, et al. Outcome after first relapse in children with acute lymphoblastic leukemia: a population-based study of 315 patients from the Nordic Society of Pediatric Hematology and Oncology (NOPHO). *Med Pediatr Oncol.* 1995;25(5):372-8.

94. Gaynon PS, Qu RP, Chappell RJ, et al. Survival after relapse in childhood acute lymphoblastic leukemia: impact of site and time to first relapse—the Children's Cancer Group Experience. *Cancer.* 1998;82(7):1387-95.

95. Wheeler K, Richards S, Bailey C, et al. Comparison of bone marrow transplant and chemotherapy for relapsed childhood acute lymphoblastic leukaemia: the MRC UKALL X experience. Medical Research Council Working Party on Childhood Leukaemia. *Br J Haematol.* 1998;101(1):94-103.

96. Hunger SP, Raetz EA, Loh ML, et al. Improving outcomes for high-risk ALL: translating new discoveries into clinical care. *Pediatr Blood Cancer.* 2011;56(6):984-93.

97. Zhang J, Ding L, Holmfeldt L, et al. The genetic basis of early T-cell precursor acute lymphoblastic leukaemia. *Nature.* 2012;481(7380):157-63.

Chemotherapy of Adult Acute Lymphoblastic Leukemia

Ibrahim Aldoss, Vinod Pullarkat

INTRODUCTION

Management of acute lymphoblastic leukemia (ALL) has substantially evolved over the last 3 decades, and the disease has become one of the most curable cancers in children. Despite dramatic improvement in outcomes in the pediatric age group, ALL in adults remains a challenging illness where progress has been sluggish even with the adoption of intensive "pediatric-like" regimens.

The disparity in outcomes between childhood and adult ALL can be attributed to several factors. These include (1) differences in disease biology—adverse cytogenetic features like Philadelphia (Ph) chromosome are more common in adults and favorable cytogenetic abnormalities like *TEL-AML* fusion are rare, (2) differences in therapy—generally less intensive therapy is given to adults compared to children due to decreased tolerability and comorbidities, (3) pharmacokinetic factors—drug metabolism and distribution vary with age, (4) omission of some valuable drugs in adult regimens, most notably, asparaginase (Asp), (5) paucity of randomized clinical trial data in adults—unlike in children such data are not available to guide refinements of existing regimens, partly due to rarity of adult ALL, and (6) the generally poor compliance in adults to therapy as well as less stringent adherence to intense protocols by physicians treating adult ALL.

Therapy in adults generally follows the same principles as pediatric ALL outlined in chapter 6. As in pediatric regimens, prolonged use of non-cross resistant conventional chemotherapeutic agents is the mainstay of therapy for adult ALL. Active agents like Asp are less consistently used in adult ALL regimens. Use of Asp in ALL is discussed in chapter 8. Imatinib or a later generation tyrosine kinase inhibitor (TKI) for Philadelphia-positive (Ph+) ALL are the only molecularly targeted agents that are currently used in ALL regimens.

Most modern regimens for ALL include one to two cycles of induction therapy with combination of an anthracycline, vincristine (V), and prednisone (PSE), with or without agents like cyclophosphamide (CY) and Asp. The goal of induction therapy is to achieve complete remission (CR), defined as less than 5% blasts on bone marrow (BM) morphology, BM cellularity greater than 20%, and maturation of all cell lines. The highest risk for treatment-related mortality (TRM) is usually encountered during the induction phase of therapy, and aggressive supportive care should be applied to reduce this risk. Due to the intensive follow-up and close monitoring required, therapy of ALL is best delegated to specialized centers with expertise in this disease.

Following a successful induction phase, most current regimens employ six to eight courses of post-remission consolidation therapy with or without treatment intensification, and usually incorporate high-doses of methotrexate (MTX) and cytosine arabinoside (Ara-C) for systemic and central nervous system (CNS) disease control. CNS prophylaxis is an integral part of therapy. There is a tendency in modern regimens to use less myelosuppressive agents in order to decrease risk of neutropenia without compromising treatment efficacy. Consolidation therapy is usually followed by maintenance treatment with daily oral 6-mercaptopurine (6-MP) and weekly MTX for 2–3 years, sometimes with periodic doses of V and steroids.

The goal of consolidation, intensification, and maintenance therapy is to eradicate minimal residual disease (MRD) and prevent relapse. MRD monitoring is increasingly being used to guide therapy in pediatric ALL since it has been shown in various studies to predict relapse risk. Again partly due to technical complexities, MRD monitoring is not universally used and its utilization varies between centers treating adult ALL. MRD monitoring and its role in guiding therapy are discussed in detail in chapter 9.

This chapter will mainly focus on results of cooperative group studies of combination chemotherapy in adult ALL. High quality cytogenetic studies are critical for accurate prognostication of ALL (see chapter 5). No clear guidelines exist for use of hematopoietic stem cell transplantation (HSCT) in CR1. HSCT for ALL is discussed in chapter 12.

COOPERATIVE GROUP STUDIES IN ADULT ALL
Modified Berlin-Frankfurt-Munster and German Study Group for Adult ALL Regimens

Between 1978 and 1981, Hoelzer et al. conducted a trial using a modified version of the pediatric Berlin-Frankfurt-Munster (BFM) regimen, and prospectively treated 162 patients (median age 25 years, range 15–65 years) with ALL. The regimen included two phases of induction [phase I with PSE, V, daunorubicin (DNR), and L-asparaginase (L-Asp) and phase II with CY, Ara-C and 6-MP] given over 8 weeks, and two phases of consolidation starting at week 20, and consisting of dexamethasone (DEX), V and doxorubicin (DOX) in phase I and CY, Ara-C and 6-thioguanine (6-TG) in phase II. Patients received maintenance therapy consisting of 6-MP and weekly MTX between induction and consolidation (weeks 10–20), and after completing consolidation therapy (weeks 28–130). Patients with bulky disease or initial leukocyte count greater than 25,000/µL also received V and PSE prephase therapy (see chapter 6 for discussion of prephase therapy). The CNS prophylaxis included cranial irradiation (24 Gy) and intrathecal (IT) MTX. CR was achieved in 78% of enrolled patients, and median overall survival (OS) and median remission duration for patients achieving CR were 26 months and 20 months, respectively. Time to achieve CR (4 weeks vs 8 weeks) was predictive of remission duration.[1] The study was the largest prospective study in adult ALL at that time, and it did prove the feasibility of intensified "pediatric-like" therapy in adults.

Subsequent German Study Group for Adult ALL (GMALL) studies (02/84 and 03/87) used the same induction, reinduction, and maintenance protocol but with minor modifications to the original Hoelzer study. These studies stratified adult ALL into defined-risk groups, and they applied the concept of tailoring treatment according to the patient's risk status. The GMALL 05/93 was a large multicenter study that enrolled 1,200 patients and stratified them into four groups: (1) standard-risk (SR) B-precursor ALL, (2) high-risk (HR) B-precursor ALL, (3) T-ALL, and (4) elderly ALL (defined as age >50 years). Risk adapted intensified therapy was employed during consolidation as follows; high-dose MTX for SR B-cell acute lymphoblastic leukemia (B-ALL), CY and Ara-C for T-cell acute lymphoblastic leukemia (T-ALL), and high-doses of MTX and Ara-C followed by HSCT for HR B-ALL. The CR rate was 83% for all patients. CR and 5-year leukemia-free survival (LFS) for SR, HR, elderly, and T-ALL were 87% and 47%, 85% and 27%, 70% and 16%, and 86% and 51%, respectively.[2]

Goekbuget et al. have reported the preliminary results of the ongoing GMALL 07/2003 study at the 2010 American Society of Hematology (ASH) meeting. This study reported outcomes of 1,226 patients with ALL (aged 15–55 years) treated on a BFM-like protocol that included various doses of polyethylene glycol (PEG)-ylated asparaginase (PEG-Asp).[3] Patients in this study received two cycles of induction therapy with DEX, V, DNR, and PEG-Asp in phase I, and 6-MP, CY, and Ara-C in phase-II followed by consolidation with PEG-Asp, 6-MP, and high-dose MTX. The dose of PEG-Asp was escalated in the study from 1,000 U/m^2 to 2,000 U/m^2 during induction phase and from 500 U/m^2 to 1,000 U/m^2 during consolidation phase in the more recent cohort. Although CR (91%) and MRD after induction (79% vs 82%) were not significantly different among the study cohorts, higher doses of PEG-Asp was associated with trend toward superior 3-year OS (67% vs 60%; $p > 0.05$) in all patients compared to lower doses. The benefit of escalated PEG-Asp dose was most prominent in SR patients (3-year OS; 80% vs 68%, $p = 0.02$) and younger patients (15–45 years) (3-year OS; 82% vs 71%; $p = 0.02$). This study demonstrates that escalated dose of PEG-Asp is feasible in adults and might be associated with improved outcomes at least in the SR subgroup.

At the University of Southern California (USC), Douer et al. have tested a modified version of the original BFM regimen that included six doses of PEG-Asp during induction and consolidation phases (Table 7-1). Among 51 adults with untreated

| Table 7-1 | University of Southern California–ALL Regimen |

Induction phase I

Daunorubicin 60 mg/m^2, IV days 1,2,3

Vincristine 1.4 mg/m^2, IV (max 2 mg) days 1, 8, 15, 22

Pegasparaginase 2,000 U/m^2, IV day 16

Prednisone 60 mg/m^2, PO days 1–28

Methotrexate 12 mg, intrathecal (IT) days 8, 15

Induction phase II

Cyclophosphamide 1 g/m^2, IV days 1, 29

Cytarabine 75 mg/m^2, days 1–4, 8–11, 29–32, 36–39

Vincristine 1.4 mg/m^2 (max 2 mg), days 15, 22, 43, 50

Pegasparaginase 2,000 U/m^2, IV day 15

Prednisone 20 mg/m^2, PO days 15–22

6-Mercaptopurine 60 mg/m^2, PO days 1–14, 29–43

Methotrexate 12 mg, IT days 1, 8, 15, 22

Intensification

Methotrexate 1 g/m^2, IV (T-ALL 2.5 g/m^2) days 1, 15

Leucovorin 15 mg, q6h IV, start 36 hours from start of methotrexate

Pegasparaginase 2,000 U/m^2, IV day 15

Prednisone 20 mg/m^2, PO days 16–23

Consolidation

Ara-C 75 mg/m^2, IV days 1–5

Teniposide 60 mg/m^2, IV days 1–5

Delayed reinduction

Daunorubicin 25 mg/m^2, IV days 1, 8, 15

Vincristine 1.4 mg/m^2, IV days 1, 8, 15, 43, 50

Dexamethasone 10 mg/m^2, PO days 15–22, 43–50

Pegaspargase 2,000 U/m^2, IV day 15

Cyclophosphamide 1 g/m^2, IV day 29

Cytarabine 75 mg/m^2, IV days 29–32, 36–39

6-Thioguanine 60 mg/m^2, PO days 29–42

Methotrexate 12 mg, IT days 1, 29, 36

Maintenance (24 months from end of all consolidations)

Prednisone 60 mg/m^2, PO days 1–5 (monthly–1 year; every 2 months–2 years)

Vincristine 2 mg/m^2 (max 2 mg), IV day 1 (monthly–1 year; every 2 months–2 years)

6-Mercaptopurine 60 mg/m^2, PO days 1–28

Methotrexate 20 mg/m^2, PO days 1, 8, 15, 22 Methotrexate 12 mg, IT once every 3 months–1 year

Continued

Continued

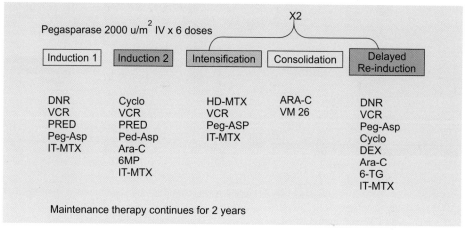

ALL, acute lymphoblastic leukemia.

ALL enrolled in the study, 98% achieved CR, and the 7-year OS and LFS were 51% and 58%, respectively, for all patients (Figure 7-1). These encouraging results were observed despite the fact that 67% of patients in the study were classified as high-risk (based on Ph positivity, t(4;11), elevated white blood cell count, age >30 years) and the rate of HSCT in CR1 was as low as 20%. Almost half of the patients (n = 23) in the study were able to receive all six doses of PEG-Asp.[4]

Hyper-CVAD Regimen

Investigators at MD Anderson Cancer Center (MDACC) have tested the hyper-cyclophosphamide, vincristine, adriamycin, and dexamethasone (CVAD) regimen in treatment of adult ALL.[5,6] This regimen was originally developed by Murphy et al. for treatment of advanced-stage Burkitt's lymphoma and B-ALL in children.[7]

The regimen consisted of four cycles of Hyper-CVAD (CY, DOX, V, and DEX) alternating with four cycles of high-dose of MTX (1 g/m^2) and Ara-C (3 g/m^2 every 12 hours × 4 doses), followed by 2 years of maintenance therapy with 6-MP, MTX, V, and PSE, except in patients with mature B-ALL (11% of all patients). Cyclophosphamide dose was fractionated and given as 300 mg/m^2 every 12 hours for six doses. Intrathecal MTX and Ara-C were given in risk-adapted fashion for CNS prophylaxis and support with granulocyte colony-stimulating factor (G-CSF) was used. Of 204 patients treated between 1992 and 1998, 185 patients (91%) achieved CR and 12 patients (6%) died during induction therapy. The estimated 5-year OS was 39% and estimated 5-year CR rate was 36%. The median age of patients in this study was 39.5 years.[5,6] Hyper-CVAD regimen demonstrated superiority when compared to the vincristine, adriamycin, and dexamethasone (VAD) regimen which was used previously at the same institution.[8]

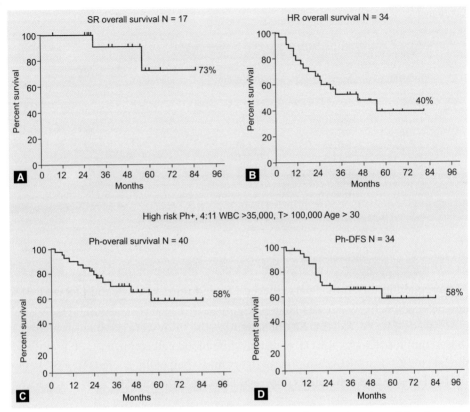

Figure 7-1 Outcome of 51 adult ALL patients treated on University of Southern California-Acute Lymphoblastic Leukemia protocol. SR, standard risk; HR, high risk (defined as having any of the following features: Philadelphia chromosome positive, t(4;11), WBC count over 35,000 for B-ALL and over 100,000 for T-ALL, and age over 30 years).

Between 1992 and 2009, 282 Philadelphia-negative ALL patients were treated in non-randomized manner based on the year of diagnosis at MDACC with either standard hyper-CVAD (n = 109) or modified hyper-CVAD with (n = 47) or without (n = 126) early anthracycline intensification in combination with Ara-C.[9] This modified regimen incorporated the anti-CD20 monoclonal antibody, rituximab, (for patients in whom >20% of blasts expressed CD20), in addition to early and late intensifications of therapy, prolongation of maintenance therapy, and tailoring CNS prophylaxis therapy according to CNS-relapse risk. The overall CR was 95%, and there was no difference based on regimen type or CD20 expression. Three-year CR duration was superior in the modified hyper-CVAD without anthracycline intensification in comparison to the modified hyper-CVAD with anthracycline intensification or standard hyper-CVAD (78% vs 54% and 53%, p < 0.01). The addition of rituximab to modified hyper-CVAD improved CR duration but not OS in all patients. In subset analysis, the addition of rituximab in CD20-positive patients improved CR duration and OS in younger patients but not in patients older than 60 years of age. Early anthracycline intensification in combination with Ara-C has failed to enhance outcomes in 68 patients treated in the modified hyper-CVAD arm between 2000 and 2001.[9,10] The incorporation of rituximab in ALL regimens is being currently tested in other studies.

Cancer and Leukemia Group B Studies

The Cancer and Leukemia Group B (CALGB) group prospectively randomized 98 previously untreated adults with ALL either to intensive induction therapy with V, PSE, and L-Asp or to the same regimen in addition to DNR. CR increased from 47% to 83% with addition of DNR (p = 0.003). Subsequently, another 78 patients were treated in the anthracycline arm in non-randomized fashion, and they achieved a 76% CR rate. Patients who attained CR subsequently received 3 years of maintenance therapy with 6-MP, MTX, and V. Three-year LFS was 25% for the all patients and it was not significantly different between patients who received DNR and who did not. The addition of DNR to three-drug induction therapy improved CR in patient with ALL but not LFS.[11] Higher CR rates with anthracycline-containing induction regimen was reported in subsequent studies.[12]

The CALGB-8011 study randomized patients who achieved CR after induction with DNR, PSE, V, MTX, and Asp to either intensive therapy with Ara-C and DNR or cycles of lower intensity with 6-MP, MTX, V, and PSE. Following induction therapy, 64% (177 of 277) achieved CR. For the 151 patients randomized for post-remission therapy, intensive therapy was associated with increased risk of myelosuppression without significant improvement in outcomes. The rate of LFS for patients who achieved CR was 29%.[13]

The CALGB-8811 was a multicenter phase II study that evaluated the role of intensive induction and post-remission chemotherapy in adults with newly diagnosed ALL. The regimen consisted of 5-drug induction therapy with CY, DNR, V, L-Asp, and PSE. Patients who achieved CR received early intensification (CY, 6-MP, Ara-C, V, and L-Asp), consolidation (6-MP and MTX), late intensification (DNR, V, CY, 6-TG, and Ara-C), and 2 years of maintenance therapy with PSE, MTX, and 6-MP. The CNS prophylaxis included cranial radiation and IT MTX. Median age of patients in the study was 32 years. The study enrolled 197 patients and reported a CR rate of 85% and a 9% induction-related death rate. The 3-year LFS for patients who achieved CR was 46%, and 3-year OS was 50%.[14] This study achieved higher CR and long-term outcomes compared to previous CALGB studies (8011 and 8513).[11,13]

University of California San Francisco Protocols

Linker et al. at University of California San Francisco (UCSF) treated 109 patients with ALL in the 1980s with their protocol-8001, which included 4-drug induction (DNR, V, PSE, and L-Asp), followed by eight alternative cycles of consolidation with (DNR, V, PSE, and L-Asp) and [teniposide (VM-26) and Ara-C], followed by a ninth cycle with a moderate-dose of MTX. Subsequently, patients received 30 months of oral maintenance with 6-MP and MTX. The regimen included prophylactic cranial-spinal irradiation and IT MTX. The reported CR rate was 88%, and 6-year LFS and OS were 35% and 40%, respectively.[15] The median age of patients was 25 years. Like CALGB 8811 discussed previously, this study validated the role of intensive cyclical multiagent chemotherapy in improving LFS in adult ALL.

In a subsequent study (protocol-8707), Linker et al. omitted cranial radiation from their previous protocol, while delivering IT and repeated doses of systematic chemotherapy with CNS penetration. The CR rate in this study was 93% in 84 patients, and the 5-year event-free survival (EFS) was 52%. Only one case of CNS relapse was reported and it was accompanied by simultaneous BM relapse.[16] This study provided proof of concept that craniospinal irradiation can be safely removed from adult ALL regimens without compromising outcomes if adequate IT and systemic chemotherapy is given.

Southwest Oncology Group Protocols

The L-10 and L-10M protocols were developed initially by Memorial Sloan-Kettering Cancer Center (MSKCC) investigators in the 1970s and they achieved a CR rate of 85% and 84%, respectively, in untreated adult patients with ALL.[17] These regimens consisted of 3-drug induction therapy (V, PSE, and DOX), followed by consolidation therapy with MTX alternating with 6-TG and Ara-C and a final cycle of L-Asp and CY. Subsequently, patients received a maintenance therapy program [V, PSE, DOX/CY, 6-MP, MTX, carmustine (BCNU), and actinomycin-D] for 3 years.

The encouraging results from the L-10/L-10M study led the Southwest Oncology Group (SWOG) to investigate the efficacy of this regimen in a multicenter fashion. In the SWOG-8001 study, 168 eligible patients were treated prospectively between 1980 and 1985 with the original L-10M regimen, and 68% of all patients attained a CR, but only 35% of those older than 50 years of age achieved CR. The 5-year OS was approximately 30%. TRM was high in this study and reached 50% in patients older than 50 years. The rate of CR was lower than what was seen in the original MSKCC study.[18]

In searching for more effective and less toxic regimen, the SWOG-8417/8419 protocols randomized 195 patients after successful induction therapy into either the original L10 consolidation arm or experimental consolidation with DAT

(DNR, Ara-C, and 6-TG) and escalating doses of MTX and L-Asp. No significant difference in LFS (5-year; 32% vs 25%, p = 0.46), OS, or toxicity was seen among the study arms. TRM was 4% in both arms during consolidation phase. The induction therapy for these patients was given as per the newer SWOG-8417 protocol which treated 353 patients with a four-drug regimen (V, PSE, DOX, and CY), and 218 (62%) patients of treated patients achieved a CR, and the 5-year OS for all patients was 25%.[19] The study therefore failed to improve overall outcome compared to the previous SWOG study.

The SWOG 9400 was a phase II study of combination chemotherapy regimen for induction and post-remission consolidation followed by either allogeneic HSCT or prolonged maintenance therapy depending on whether the patient is a suitable candidate with a histocompatible sibling donor. The regimen consisted of two cycles of induction therapy with DNR, V, PSE, and Asp followed by one cycle of consolidation with CY, Ara-C, 6-MP, MTX, and subsequently four cycles of maintenance therapy. Of 200 eligible patients treated on the protocol, 159 (80%) achieved CR after two cycles of induction therapy, and the 5-year LFS and OS for all patients were 29% and 33%, respectively. The study highlighted the value of cytogenetics as the most important independent prognostic factor in adult ALL. Interestingly, age ceased to be a prognostic factor when cytogenetics was accounted for.[20]

Japan Adult Leukemia Study Group

The Japan Adult Leukemia Study Group (JALSG) has conducted a series of studies in adult ALL, and the key premise of their studies was response-oriented further therapy. In the JALSG-ALL87 study, 116 adults were treated with a response-oriented five-drug induction therapy regimen, followed by three courses of intensive post-remission and maintenance. CR rate was 84%, and 6-year OS was 23%.[21] In the subsequent JALSG study, ALL90, mitoxantrone was added to induction therapy (6-drug regimen) in 180 patients, but the study failed to enhance outcomes, with CR rate and 5-year OS rate being 69% and 15%, respectively.[22]

In the JALSG-ALL93, frequent administration of anthracycline was added to a 4-drug induction regimen, followed by three courses of consolidation and maintenance therapy. Therapy regimen could be modified based on BM response and toxicity. Patients were then randomized to early sequential or intermittent intensification courses. Of 263 evaluable patients, 78% attained CR, and 6-year disease-free survival (DFS) and OS were 30% and 33%, respectively. No significant difference in outcomes was observed among the randomized arms (p = 0.85). Among patients who achieved CR and were younger than 40 years of age, 6-year survival was not different between the allocated related HSCT group and chemotherapy group. Ph+ patients on the other hand patients who actually received HSCT had superior survival compared to those who received chemotherapy.[23] Escalated DOX doses during consolidation courses did not improve outcomes in 404 patients in the JALSG-ALL97, with CR, 5-year DFS, and OS of 74%, 33%, and 32%, respectively.[24]

UK Medical Research Council/Eastern Cooperative Oncology Group Trial

The Medical Research Council (MRC) UKALL XII/Eastern Cooperative Oncology Group (ECOG) E2993 is one of the largest adult ALL studies and was a multinational study conducted between 1993 and 2006 that enrolled 1,913 patients. All patients received induction with two cycles; cycle I with DNR, V, L-Asp, and PSE; and cycle II with CY, Ara-C, and 6-MP. Subsequently, patients received intensified therapy with high-dose intravenous MTX and L-Asp, and then underwent allogeneic HSCT if sibling-donor was available, or were randomized to autologous HSCT or consolidation/maintenance therapy if no sibling-donor was identified. Consolidation therapy consisted of four cycles and followed by 2.5 years of maintenance therapy. Ninety-one percent of patients achieved CR and 5-year OS was 39% for all patients. Patients who were allocated to allogeneic HSCT achieved superior OS compared to patients who were continued on consolidation/maintenance therapy, while patients randomized to autologous HSCT had the worst survival. Surprisingly, among Ph chromosome-negative patients, significantly better OS for patients with matched donors was seen only in the SR group but not in the HR group. In HR older patients, the lower relapse risk was offset by the high HSCT mortality.[25,26] This study has shown in a randomized fashion that autologous HSCT is inferior to conventional chemotherapy in any risk group.

Leucémie Aiguës Lymphoblastique de l'Adulte/Group for Research on Adult ALL Studies

In the Leucémie Aiguës Lymphoblastique de l'Adulte (LALA)-87 trial, survival benefit was observed in patients who underwent allogeneic HSCT compared to patients who continued on chemotherapy or received autologous HSCT. The survival advantage was seen in the HR group but it did not reach statistical significance in the SR group.[27] Therefore, in the LALA-94 trial, patients were stratified into defined-risk groups, and patients who were identified as SR group were randomized to intensive post-remission consolidation (Ara-C and mitoxantrone) or less intensive therapy (CY, Ara-C, and 6-MP), while all HR groups received allogeneic HSCT if they had a matched sibling donor or autologous HSCT if no matched sibling was available. Of the 922 eligible patients, CR was achieved in 84% of all patients after 4-drug induction therapy, and 5-year DFS and OS were 30% and 33%, respectively. The 5-year OS according to disease risk was 44% and 38% in SR and HR patients, respectively. No significant difference was observed among patients randomized to post-remission therapy (p = 0.78). Allogeneic but not autologous HSCT improved DFS in HR patients compared to chemotherapy.[28]

The Group for Research on Adult Acute Lymphoblastic Leukemia (GRAALL) conducted a phase II trial with an intensive regimen inspired from pediatric treatment regimen in the GRAALL-2003. The regimen includes 1 week of pretreatment with corticosteroid, 5-drug induction therapy, nine cycles of consolidation, and late intensification, followed by maintenance therapy. Of the 225 enrolled patients with Ph⁻ ALL, 94% achieved CR, and 3.5-year DFS and OS were 55% and 60% respectively. Results of the study were reported as superior to the LALA-94 study when the studies were compared retrospectively.[29]

Gruppo Italiano Malattie Ematologiche Ddell'Adulto

In the Gruppo Italiano Malattie Ematologiche Ddell'Adulto (GIMEMA) ALL 0288 study, 778 patients received 1 week of pretreatment with PSE, and were then randomized to 4-drug induction (DNR, V, PSE, and L-Asp) with or without CY, and patients who achieved CR had second randomization to early intensified consolidation therapy with eight drugs followed by maintenance or to maintenance therapy alone. Single agent PSE produced 65% response rate (response was defined as circulating blasts at day 0 of ≤1000/μL), and response to PSE was an independent predictor for CR and OS. CR was achieved in 82%, and there was no difference in CR or induction death between 4- or 5-drugs induction arms. Nine-year DFS and OS were 29% and 27%, respectively, and intensification of post-remission therapy did not improve outcomes.[30]

Programa para el Estudio de la Terapéutica en Hemopatía Maligna

The Programa para el Estudio de la Terapéutica en Hemopatía Maligna (PETHEMA) ALL-87 study assessed the role of late intensification in adults with ALL. Of 108 enrolled patients, 92 (86%) attained CR after 5-drug induction therapy. Following consolidation, 55 patients were available for randomization to 6-week late intensification cycle or maintenance therapy at the end of the 1st year. Five-year LFS and OS were 41% and 47%, respectively. Late intensification therapy failed to improve outcome in the study.[31]

The PETHEMA ALL93 study enrolled 222 high-risk ALL patients, which was defined as one of the following features; age 30–50 years, elevated white blood cells (WBC ≥25,000/μL), Ph+ ALL or the presence of the mixed-lineage leukemia (*MLL*) gene rearrangement. After achieving CR with 5-drug induction therapy (V, DNR, PSE, L-Asp, and CY) and receiving three courses of early intensification therapy, patients were assigned to allogeneic HSCT if they have matched-sibling donor or randomized to autologous HSCT or three courses of late intensification and maintenance chemotherapy. Eighty-two percent of patients achieved CR, and 5-year

DFS and OS were 35% and 34%, respectively. There was no significant difference in outcomes among the study cohorts.[32] The outcomes of selected major adult ALL trials are summarized in table 7-2.

Table 7-2	Outcome of Selected Large Adult ALL Studies					
Study	Reference	Reported year	Patients	CR %	LFS	OS
GMALL 01/81	1	1984	162	78	20 months	26 months
GMALL 05/93	2	2001	1,200	83		
GMALL 07/03	3	2010	1,226	91	3-yr 74% vs 61%	3-yr 67% vs 60%
MDACC	5	2004	288	92	38%, 5 yrs	38%, 5 yrs
CALGB 8011	13	1991	277	64	29%	
CALGB 8811	14	1995	197	85	3-yr 46%	3-yr 50%
UCSF-8001	15	1991	109	88	6-yr 35%	6-yr 40%
UCSF-8707	16	2002	84	93	5-yr 52%	
SWOG-8001	18	1989	168	68		5-yr 30%
SWOG-8419/8417	19	2001	353	62		5-yr 25%
SWOG-9400	20	2008	200	80	5-yr 29%	5-yr 33%
JALSG-87	21	1998	116	84		6-yr 23%
JALSG-90	22	1998	180	69		5-yr 15%
JALSG 93	23	2002	263	78	6-yr 30%	6-yr 33%
JALSG 97	22	2010	404	74	5-yr 33%	5-yr 32%
MRC UKXII / ECOG E2993	25, 26	2008	1,913	91		5-yr 39%
LALA-94	28	2004	922	84	5-yr, 30%	5-yr, 33%
GRAALL 2003	29	2009	225	94	3.5-yr, 55%	3.5-yr, 60%
GIMEMA 02/88	30	2002	767	82	33%, 9 yrs	27%, 9 yrs
PETHEMA 87	31	1998	108	86	5-yr, 41%	5-yr, 47%
PETHEMA ALL93	32	2005	222	82	35%, 5yrs	34%, 5 yrs
HOVON	77	2009	433	67	NR	37%, 5 yrs
EORTC ALL3	78	2004	340	74	34%, 6 yrs	36%, 6 yrs
GOELAMS 02	79	2004	198	86	NR	41%, 6 yrs

ALL, acute lymphoblastic leukemia; CR, complete remission; LFS, leukemia-free survival; OS, overall survival; GMALL, German Study Group for Adult ALL; MDACC, MD Anderson Cancer Center; CALGB, Cancer and Leukemia Group B; UCSF, University of California San Francisco; SWOG, Southwest Oncology Group; JALSG, Japan Adult Leukemia Study Group; MRC, Medical Research Council; ECOG, Eastern Cooperative Oncology Group; LALA, Leucemie Aigues Lymphoblastique del'Adulte; GRALL, Group Research on Adult Acute Lymphoblastic Leukemia; GIMEMA, Gruppo Italiano Malattie Ematologiche Ddell'Adulto; PETHEMA, Programa para el Tratamiento de Hemopatÿas Malignas; ALL, acute lymphoblastic leukemia; HOVON, Dutch-Belgian Cooperative Trial Group for Hematology Oncology; EORTC, European Organization for Research and Treatment of Cancer; GOELAMS, Groupe Ouest Est d'Etude des Leucemies et Autres Maladies du Sang; NR, not reported.

PHILADELPHIA-POSITIVE ALL AND THE ROLE OF TYROSINE-KINASE INHIBITORS

Philadelphia chromosome is a translocation between chromosome 9 and 22 [t(9;22)] that results in formation of the BCR-ABL fusion gene. The product of this fusion gene is a constitutively activated protein tyrosine kinase, which plays a critical role in leukemogenesis.

Philadelphia-positive ALL is a unique disease and it is worth discussing it separately. The incidence of Ph+ ALL increases with age, and it approaches 50% in patients older than 40 years, and thus, Ph+ ALL is essentially an adult disease. The finding of Ph chromosome is one of the worst prognostic factors in ALL, and it was associated with dismal outcomes in the pre-TKI era. Prior to the introduction of TKIs, treatment of Ph+ ALL with intensive prolonged multiagent cytotoxic therapies produced median survivals of less than 1 year, and 5-year OS around 10%.[5,33-36] The only modality that was shown to improve long-term outcomes was allogeneic HSCT.[37]

Remission rates for patients with Ph+ ALL have markedly improved with the introduction of TKIs. Imatinib is a potent selective inhibitor of the BCR-ABL protein kinase. Single-agent imatinib induces response in a substantial proportion of Ph+ ALL patients, however, responses are usually short-lived and the malignant cells eventually develop resistance to imatinib, with median time to relapse of around 2 months in relapsed ALL.[38,39] On the other hand, combining imatinib with cytotoxic chemotherapies produces CR in the majority of patients with newly diagnosed Ph+ ALL and responses are usually sustained.

Feilding et al. have presented the results of 441 patients with Ph+ ALL treated since 1993, with induction therapy and allogeneic HSCT whenever possible in the UKALLXII/ECOG 2993 trial. Consistent with evolution of Ph+ ALL therapy resulting from the development of TKIs, the study underwent amendments during the course of enrolment; (1) from 1993 to 2003 (n = 226), no imatinib was given, (2) from 2003 to 2005 (n = 86), imatinib was given after induction and HSCT, and continued for 2 years, and (3) 2005 and after (n = 89), imatinib was started with induction therapy. Inclusion of imatinib during treatment was associated with higher total CR rate (including those who achieved CR later than postinduction) compared to no imatinib (92% vs 82%), and more patients were able to undergo allogeneic HSCT (44% vs 28%). In 3-year OS, EFS and relapse-free survival (RFS) were significantly superior in patients who received imatinib during anytime of therapy compared to no imatinib (42% vs 25%, 36% vs 19%, and 54% vs 36%, respectively), and improved outcomes were most prominent in patients started on imatinib therapy early during induction. The 3-year survival for patients received imatinib and underwent allogeneic HSCT was 59% versus 28% for those who received imatinib and no allogeneic HSCT was done, without plateau in the survival curve, which emphasizes the need of allogeneic HSCT at the present time to cure Ph+ ALL.[40]

The GMALL investigated the optimal timing for imatinib administration in newly diagnosed Ph+ ALL in a prospective non-randomized fashion, either alternating with chemotherapy after completing induction therapy (n = 47) or concurrently started with chemotherapy during induction phase (n = 45). Both schedules were reported to be feasible and allow large percentage of patients to undergo allogeneic HSCT (77%), but higher number of patients in the simultaneous treatment cohort achieved polymerase chain reaction (PCR) negativity for BCR-ABL compared to the alternative group (52% vs 19%, p = 0.01).[41]

One-hundred and three patients were treated with concurrent imatinib and combination chemotherapy on the JALSG ALL 2002 study, with imatinib given on days 8–62 during induction, and alternatively with chemotherapy during consolidation. Subsequently, patients were recommended to undergo allogeneic HSCT if matched-sibling donor was available. CR rate was 97% and 3-year OS for all patients was 57% (75% for patients <55 years and underwent allogeneic HSCT vs 36% for non-transplanted patients).[42] When compared to a historical cohort of patients with Ph+ ALL who underwent allogeneic HSCT, patients received imatinib prior to transplant had superior 3-year survival (65% vs 44%, p = 0.005).[43]

The addition of imatinib to hyper-CVAD regimen yielded a CR rate of 93% of patients with de novo or minimally treated Ph+ ALL (n = 54). When compared to a historical cohort of Ph+ patients treated with hyper-CVAD alone, the addition of imatinib produced significantly higher 3-year DFS and OS (68% vs 25% and 55% vs 15%, respectively, p < 0.001) compared to the historical arm, irrespective of allogeneic HSCT status.[44] Several other studies validated the feasibility and efficacy of imatinib in Ph+ ALL treatment as well.[45-48]

Therefore, the standard of care for treating patients with Ph+ ALL is to combine TKIs (imatinib or a later generation TKIs if imatinib is intolerable or ineffective) simultaneously with chemotherapy, and subsequently performing an allogeneic HSCT in first CR. The main role of TKIs during Ph+ ALL treatment is to bridge the patient to allogeneic HSCT, whereas historically, many patients with Ph+ ALL did not reach CR or relapsed before undergoing allogeneic HSCT in the pre-TKI era. Allogeneic HSCT currently remains a key component of Ph+ ALL therapy as most patients relapse if transplant is not performed and studies have shown no plateau in remission rate with time, even when TKIs are included in the regimen.

Dasatinib is a dual SRC and ABL kinase inhibitor which has a 325-fold greater potency than imatinib that is active against various BCR-ABL mutations that confer imatinib resistance. The addition of dasatinib to intensive chemotherapy in Ph+ ALL has yielded promising results in phase II studies.[49,50] In patients who failed imatinib, dasatinib 70 mg twice a day was found to have the same efficacy and safety of 140 mg daily dose.[51] Nilotinib is another potent second-generation TKI that has shown promising results in Ph+ ALL as well.[52] Later generation TKIs should be used when patients fail initial TKI therapy or are intolerant to the initial agent, however, more studies are shifting use of newer TKIs to the first-line setting given their higher potency.

Ponatinib has recently been granted Food and Drug Administration (FDA) approval for treating Ph+ ALL that is resistant or if patient is intolerant to previous TKIs. The approval was based on studies showing activity in this setting. Ponatinib is potent pan-BCR/ABL inhibitor, and it has a unique activity against the gatekeeper mutation, T315I. In the phase II Ponatinib Ph ALL and CML Evaluation (PACE) trial, 32 patients with Ph+ ALL were enrolled, including 10 patients who were resistant or intolerant (R/I) to dasatinib or nilotinib and 22 patients who harbored the T315I mutation. The major and complete hematological response rates were 41% and 34%, respectively. A major cytogenetic response was observed in 50% and 32% among patients with R/I and T315I Ph+ ALL, respectively.[53,54]

RELAPSED/REFRACTORY ALL

Relapsed/refractory (R/R) ALL is a challenging disease to treat and has dismal outcomes which highlight the need for optimizing first-line therapy to prevent relapse. The goal of salvage therapy for R/R ALL is to achieve CR2 in order to proceed to an allogeneic HSCT if the patient is a suitable candidate. Allogeneic HSCT remains the only curative therapy at the present time. Overall, the median OS for relapsed ALL is less than 6 months, and independent factors correlated with decreased survival observed in studies are increased age and short duration of first CR.

A retrospective review of 609 patients who relapsed after they were treated on the MRC UKALL12/ECOG 2993 study yielded a median survival of 6 months, and 1- and 5-year OS of 22% and 7%, respectively. Patients were treated with diverse salvage regimens according to the treating physician's judgment. Among patients who were able to undergo allogeneic HSCT, the 5-year OS was 23%. Multivariate analysis showed that younger age and longer first remission duration (>2 years) were associated with better outcomes.[55]

The GIMEMA ALL-Rescue 97 study prospectively treated 135 patients with refractory/relapsed ALL with a salvage regimen that consisted of high-doses of Ara-C (3 g/m^2/day × 3 days) and idarubicin (40 mg/m^2) followed by HSCT (allogeneic or autologous) if feasible or continuing chemotherapy if no transplant was performed. Patients were given consolidation therapy every 2–3 weeks until they were ready for transplant. The overall CR rate was 55%, and median OS and LFS were 6.4 and 5 months, respectively, with no significant difference in outcomes between patients with refractory (n = 28) or relapsed disease (n = 107). However, OS was higher in patients who relapsed beyond 2 years after achieving CR compared to those who relapsed before 2 years. Fifty patients (37%) underwent transplant, and the reported TRM was 16% for matched sibling HSCT, 31% for matched-unrelated HSCT, and 57% for haploidentical donor HSCT. After a median follow-up of 40 months, 10 patients were alive and disease-free, 9 of them were transplanted as salvage therapy. Although the regimen achieved a reasonable CR that facilitated transplant, the TRM was high.[56]

An analysis of 263 patients with relapsed ALL treated in four PETHEMA trials showed a median OS of only 4.5 months and 5-year OS of only 10%. Of patients treated with intensive second-line regimen, 45% of them achieved a CR2, and 5-year LFS for patients attained CR2 was 22%. Again, age and duration of first CR were predictors for long-term survival in this study.[57]

Using an augmented version of hyper-CVAD (containing intensified doses of V, DEX, and Asp), investigators at MDACC treated 90 patients with relapsed ALL, among whom 47% attained CR, with a median LFS and OS of 6.2 and 6 months, respectively. Thirty-two percent of all patients underwent allogeneic HSCT.[58] In another analysis of 245 patients with relapsed ALL treated at MDACC, 31% achieved CR, with median CR and OS of 5 and 4.7 months, respectively. Using multivariate analysis, they showed that achieving CR was associated with improved survival, while increased age, high BM blasts, low platelets count, low albumin and high lactate dehydrogenase (LDH) were associated with decreased survival.[59]

Using the Centers for International Blood and Marrow Transplant Research (CIBMTR) database, 582 patients with relapsed or refractory ALL who underwent allogeneic HSCT were identified and outcomes were analyzed. The 3-year OS was 16% for all patients following transplant again highlighting the poor outcome for R/R ALL even when HSCT is performed.[60]

Nelarabine is a prodrug of the deoxyguanosine analogue, 9-β-D-arabino-furanosylguanine (Ara-G), and it was granted the FDA approval for treating R/R T-cell ALL after two lines of therapy. The approval was based on induction of CR rate in two phase II studies, one in pediatric ALL and another in adults.[61,62] In the CALGB-19801 study, 39 adults with R/R T-cell ALL (n = 26) and T-cell lymphoblastic lymphoma (T-LBL) (n = 13) were treated with single agent nelarabine (1.5 g/m^2/day on days 1–3 every 3 weeks). Overall response rate and CR were achieved in 41% and 31%, respectively. Median OS and LFS were 20 weeks. The drug was tolerable, and grade III and IV toxicities were mainly cytopenias, and one patient had grade IV neurotoxicity.[61]

In more recent larger study, Gokbuget and colleague reported the outcome of 126 evaluable patients with R/R T-cell ALL or LBL treated with salvage nelarabine. Thirty-six percent achieved CR and 80% of these patients subsequently underwent allogeneic HSCT. One-year OS was 24% for all patients, and 3-year LFS and OS for patients who underwent HSCT were 37% and 31%, respectively. There was one treatment-related death with nelarabine, and grade III/IV neurotoxicity was reported in 7% of the cohort.[63]

Clofarabine is another purine analog agent that was granted FDA approval for pediatric R/R ALL in combination with other cytotoxic agents. In adults, clofarabine in combination with other agents has shown activity in R/R ALL, with CR rates ranging between 17% and 41%.[64,65] In the SWOG S053 study, 37 adult patients with relapsed or refractory ALL were treated with clofarabine (40 mg/m^2/day) and Ara-C (1 g/m^2/day) for 5 days. CR with or without platelet recovery was 17%, and the median OS was only 3 months.[64] However, the CR rate was higher in the Group Research on Adult Acute Lymphoblastic Leukemia (GRALL) study where a different reinduction regimen is used with clofarabine.[65]

Blinatumimab is an antibody with dual specificity for CD19 and CD3 and belongs to a new class of agents termed bispecific T-cell engaging (BITE) antibodies. This agent has shown impressive activity in patients with relapse detected by MRD monitoring as well as overt disease. This and other novel agents for R/R ALL are discussed in chapter 14.

In conclusion, the goal of second-line therapy in R/R ALL is to achieve a second remission and proceed to an allogeneic HSCT as soon as possible if patient is a suitable candidate with a matched donor. Given poor outcomes of R/R disease with the current treatments, the priority relays on optimizing first-line regimens to avoid relapse. It is anticipated that novel active agents like blinatumimab that produce better disease control may allow more patients to undergo allogeneic HSCT. MRD monitoring represents a major advance towards optimizing frontline therapy as well as treating relapsed disease prior to development of clinical manifestations of leukemia.

ELDERLY PATIENTS WITH ALL

Acute lymphoblastic leukemia in the elderly is associated with dismal outcomes. In addition to increased unfavorable risk factors associated with age (such as Ph+ disease), treating elderly patient is complicated with increasing comorbidities, alterations in drug metabolism as well as physicians' fear of treatment tolerability. Elderly patients are usually under-represented in clinical studies and the reported outcomes in the majority of clinical studies do not reflect the reality in this age group.

In 33 patients aged greater than 55 years treated on the PETHEMA ALL-96 trial with a regimen that includes induction (V, DNR, PSE, CY, and Asp), consolidation and maintenance phases, CR of 58% with 2-year OS and LFS of 39% and 46%, respectively, were observed. The reported early death rate was 36% highlighting the toxicity of induction therapy in this age group. The study was amended in 1999 to remove Asp and CY from the induction phase due to increased toxicity, and omitting these agents was associated with decreased TRM and improved OS (20% vs 52%, p = 0.05). This study concluded that in general, less intensive therapy in the elderly is associated with better outcomes.[66]

Among 122 elderly patients (aged ≥60 years) treated with hyper-CVAD, CR, induction mortality, relapse rate, and 5-year OS were 84%, 10%, 40%, and 20%, respectively. When compared to elderly patients who received less intensive therapy, patients received hyper-CVAD had superior outcomes, except for death risk during CR (34% vs 15%).[67]

When compared with continuous infusion of DOX in elderly patients with ALL, the pegylated liposomal form of DOX was more tolerable but did not improve outcomes.[68] Interferon-α post-remission also did not improve outcomes in older patients (>60 years) with ALL.[69]

Philadelphia-positive ALL is more common in elderly patients and although single agent imatinib induces CR in the majority of patients, the response is not durable and relapse occurs almost invariably. When imatinib is combined with steroids with or without chemotherapy in elderly patients with Ph+ ALL, improvement in quality of life and outcomes were reported.[47,48] Thus, in elderly patients with Ph+ ALL who are not candidates for intensive therapy, combination of TKIs and steroids seems a reasonable option.

In conclusion, treating elderly patient with ALL is a complicated situation that requires careful assessment of an individual's ability to tolerate therapy as well as consideration of comorbidities. Less intensive therapy generally has shown to decrease treatment-related death but at the cost of increased relapse. It is critical to enroll older patients in clinical trials whenever possible. Given the dismal outcomes and poor tolerability of standard regimens, less toxic novel agents as well as reduced intensity HSCT have the potential to improve outcome of elderly patients with ALL.

ADOLESCENTS AND YOUNG ADULTS WITH ALL

Adolescents and young adults (AYA) with ALL represent a distinct subset with around half of these patients in the United States being treated by pediatric oncologists while the rest are treated by adult oncologists.[70] In spite of the substantial improvement in outcomes that has been observed in pediatric ALL, outcomes of ALL in AYA remains inferior with less striking improvements in long-term survival.[71] Recent retrospective studies have reviewed the outcomes of ALL in this unique subgroup and showed an advantage for patients treated on pediatric cooperative group protocols compared to patients treated by adult cooperative groups.

In a comparative analysis of age-matched AYA patients (aged 16–20 years) with newly diagnosed ALL treated in North America with either adult CALGB protocols (n = 124) or pediatric Children's Cooperative Group (CCG) protocols (n = 197), superior 7-year LFS (63% vs 34%, p < 0.001) and OS (67% vs 46%, p < 0.001) were seen in patients treated on the CCG protocols compared to those treated on the CALGB protocols, despite similar CR attained in both groups (90%).[72] Similar results were observed by other cooperative groups from France, United Kingdom, Netherlands, and Finland.[73-76]

In comparison to adults ALL protocols, pediatric regimens usually involve more intensive therapy including higher dose intensity of drugs like L-Asp and early incorporation of CNS directed prophylactic therapy which may be some factors that may account for the overall inferior outcomes for AYA patients with ALL.

SUMMARY

Treatment of ALL in adults should be individualized, and considerations for patient age, comorbidities, and disease risk should be made. Recognizing the poor outcome of adult ALL with the current treatment regimens, patients should be enrolled in clinical trials whenever possible. As ALL is an infrequent disease seen by adult oncologists in the community practice, early referral to specialized centers is crucial given the complexity of the treatment regimens. Moreover, such referral enables early human leukocyte antigen (HLA) typing and timely identification of matched donors in case HSCT is necessary. Better MRD assessment as well as cytogenetic and molecular risk assessment are not widely available outside of specialized centers and these tests are critical in developing a risk adapted treatment strategy.

Aggressive supportive care is critical in reducing non-relapse mortality, particularly in the early phases of treatment. This includes growth factor support, infection prophylaxis, as well as aggressive management of drug toxicities particularly of Asp. Excessive concerns about toxicity on the other hand may result in avoidance of some active drugs like Asp from adult ALL protocols which in turn may compromise efficacy. Studies have shown that fit, relatively younger adults (up to age 55–60 years) can tolerate intensive prolonged multiagent chemotherapy regimens. Pretreatment with steroids have been used in several studies and has shown to be feasible and can predict long-term outcomes but this practice is not often employed in adults. One to two cycles of induction therapy with three to five drugs have been used and are able to yield a high CR rate. If the patient does not achieve CR with the first cycle of induction therapy, a second cycle of induction therapy with non-cross resistant drugs should be administered while searching for matched-donor in preparing for allogeneic HSCT, as failing to achieve early CR after the first cycle is an indicator of chemoresistant disease and stratifies the patient to the high-risk group.

After successful induction therapy and achievement of morphologic CR, MRD is present, and without further treatment, disease relapse is imminent and guaranteed. Thus, consolidation therapy with either allogeneic HSCT or chemotherapy is required to ensure eradicating residual disease with either graft-versus-leukemia (GVL) effect or cytotoxic therapy or both. Patients with matched-sibling donor should undergo transplant as soon as achieving CR, and if delay occurs while search for unrelated donor is underway, cycles of consolidation should be given until the patient is ready for HSCT. Chemotherapies with potential toxicities that can preclude the patient from future transplant should be avoided in such situations or used with caution.

For patients allocated to consolidation with chemotherapy, many schedules and regimens were used with no proven superiority of one regimen over another. Considerations for patient factors should be made during consolidation phase and it should be borne in mind that some randomized studies have failed to prove that more intensified consolidation is superior to less intensified approach. Again, MRD monitoring during this phase is proving to be a critical prognostic factor and may allow risk-adapted therapy as discussed in detail in chapter 9.

Prolonged maintenance therapy has been used in most protocols. The backbone of maintenance therapy is oral 6-MP and MTX, pulses of other agents and/or steroids, given for 2 years or more. CNS prophylaxis is an integral part of ALL treatment that is vital to ensure cure and is discussed in detail in chapter 10.

REFERENCES

1. Hoelzer D, Thiel E, Löffler H, et al. Intensified therapy in acute lymphoblastic and acute undifferentiated leukemia in adults. *Blood.* 1984;64:38-47.
2. Gökbuget N, Hoelzer D, Arnold R, et al. Treatment of adult ALL according to protocols of the German Multicenter Study Group for Adult ALL (GMALL). *Hematol Oncol Clin North Am.* 2000;14:1307-25.
3. Goekbuget N, Baumann A, Beck J, et al. PEG-asparaginase intensification in adult acute lymphoblastic leukemia (ALL): significant improvement of outcome with moderate increase of liver toxicity in the German Multicenter Study Group for Adult ALL (GMALL) Study 07/2003. ASH Annual Meeting Abstracts. 2010;116:494.
4. Douer D, Aldoss I, Lunning MA, et al. Pharmacokinetics-based modification of intravenous Pegylated asparaginase dosing in the context of a "Pediatric-inspired" protocol in adults with newly diagnosed acute lymphoblastic leukemia. *ASH Annual Meeting.* 2012;120:1495.
5. Kantarjian H, O'Brian S, Smith TL, et al. Results of treatment with hyper-CVAD, a dose-intensive regimen in adult acute lymphoblastic leukemia. *J Clin Oncol.* 2000;18:547-61.
6. Kantarjian H, Thomas D, O'Brian S, et al. long-term follow-up results of hyperfractionated CY, V, doxorubicin, and dexamethasone (Hyper-CVAD), a dose-intensive regimen, in adult acute lymphocytic leukemia. *Cancer.* 2004;101:2788-801.
7. Murphy SB, Bowman WP, Abromowitch M, et al. Results of the treatment of advanced-stage Burkitt's lymphoma and B cell (Sig1) acute lymphoblastic leukemia with high-dose fractionated cyclophosphamide and coordinated high-dose methotrexate and cytarabine. *J Clin Oncol.* 1986;4:1732-9.
8. Kantarjian HM, Walters RS, Keating MJ, et al. Results of the vincristine, doxorubicin and dexamethasone regimen in adults with standard- and high-risk acute lymphocytic leukemia. *J Clin Oncol.* 1990;8:994-1004.
9. Thomas DA, O'Brien S, Faderl S, et al. Chemoimmunotherapy with a modified hyper-CVAD and rituximab regimen improves outcome in de novo Philadelphia chromosome-negative precursor B-lineage acute lymphoblastic leukemia. *J Clin Oncol.* 2010;28:3880-9.
10. Thomas D, O'Brien S, Faderl S, et al. Anthracycline dose intensification in adult acute lymphoblastic leukemia: lack of benefit in the context of the fractionated cyclophosphamide, vincristine, doxorubicin, and dexamethasone regimen. *Cancer.* 2010;116:4580-9.

11. Gottlieb AJ, Weinberg V, Ellison RR, et al. Efficacy of daunorubicin in the therapy of adult acute lymphocytic leukemia: a prospective randomized trial by Cancer and Leukemia Group B. *Blood.* 1984;64:267-74.

12. Schauer P, Arlin ZA, Mertelsmann R, et al. Treatment of acute lymphoblastic leukemia in adults: results of the L-10 and L-10M protocols. *J Clin Oncol.* 1983;1:462-70.

13. Ellison RR, Mick R, Cuttner J, et al. The effects of post-induction intensification treatment with cytarabine and daunorubicin in adult acute lymphocytic leukemia: a prospective randomized clinical trial by Cancer and Leukemia Group B. *J Clin Oncol.* 1991;9:2002-15.

14. Larson RA, Dodge RK, Burns CP, et al. A five-drug remission induction regimen with intensive consolidation for adults with acute lymphoblastic leukemia: Cancer and Leukemia Group B Study 8811. *Blood.* 1995;85;2025-37.

15. Linker CA, Levitt LJ, O'Donnell M, et al. Treatment of adult acute lymphoblastic leukemia with intensive cyclical chemotherapy: a follow-up report. *Blood.* 1991;78:2814-22.

16. Linker C, Damon L, Ries C, et al. Intensified and shortened cyclical chemotherapy for adult acute lymphoblastic leukemia. *J Clin Oncol.* 2002;20:2464-71.

17. Schauer P, Arlin ZA, Miertelsmann R, et al. Treatment of acute lymphoblastic leukemia in adults: results of the L-10 and L-I0M protocols. *J Clin Oncol.* 1983;1:462-70.

18. Hussein KK, Dahlberg S, Head D, et al. Treatment of acute lymphoblastic leukemia in adults with intensive induction, consolidation and maintenance chemotherapy. *Blood.* 1989;73:57-63.

19. Petersdorf SH, Kopecky KJ, Head DR, et al. Comparison of the L10M consolidation regimen to an alternative regimen including escalating methotrexate/L-asparaginase for adult acute lymphoblastic leukemia: a Southwest Oncology Group Study. *Leukemia.* 2001;15:208-16.

20. Pullarkat V, Slovak ML, Kopecky KJ, et al. Impact of cytogenetics on the outcome of adult acute lymphoblastic leukemia: results of Southwest Oncology Group 9400 study. *Blood.* 2008;111:2563-72.

21. Tanimoto M, Miyawaki S, Ino T, et al. Response-oriented individualized induction therapy followed by intensive consolidation and maintenance for adult patients with acute lymphoblastic leukemia: the ALL-87 study of Japan Adult Leukemia Study Group (JALSG). *Int J Hematol.* 1998;68:421-9.

22. Ueda T, Miyawaki S, Asou N, et al. Response-oriented individualized induction therapy with 6 drugs followed by 4 courses of intensive consolidation, one-year maintenance and intensification therapy: the ALL90 study of the Japan Adult Leukemia Study Group. *Int J Hematol.* 1998;68:279-89.

23. Takeuchi J, Kyo T, Naito K, et al. Induction therapy by frequent administration of doxorubicin with four other drugs, followed by intensive consolidation and maintenance therapy for adult acute lymphoblastic leukemia: the JALSG-ALL93 study. *Leukemia.* 2002;16:1259-66.

24. Jinnai I, Sakura T, Tsuzuki M, et al. Intensified consolidation therapy with dose-escalated doxorubicin did not improve the prognosis of adults with acute lymphoblastic leukemia: the JALSG-ALL97 study. *Int J Hematol.* 2010;92:490-502.

25. Rowe JM, Buck G, Burnett AK, et al. Induction therapy for adults with acute lymphoblastic leukemia: results of more than 1500 patients from the international ALL trial: MRC UKALL XII/ECOG E2993. *Blood.* 2005;106:3760-7.

26. Goldstone AH, Richards SM, Lazarus HM, et al. In adults with standard-risk acute lymphoblastic leukemia, the greatest benefit is achieved from a matched sibling allogeneic transplantation in first complete remission, and an autologous transplantation is less effective than conventional consolidation/ maintenance chemotherapy in all patients: Final results of the International ALL trial (MRC UKALL XII/ECOG E2993). *Blood.* 2008;111:1827-33.

27. Thiebaut A, Vernant JP, Degos L, et al. Adult acute lymphocytic leukemia study testing chemotherapy and autologous and allogeneic transplantation. A follow-up report of the French protocol LALA 87. *Hematol Oncol Clin North Am.* 2000;14:1353-66.

28. Thomas X, Boiron JM, Huguet F, et al. Outcome of treatment in adults with acute lymphoblastic leukemia: analysis of the LALA-94 trial. *J Clin Oncol.* 2004;22:4075-86.

29. Huguet F, Leguay T, Raffoux E, et al. Pediatric-inspired therapy in adults with Philadelphia chromosome-negative acute lymphoblastic leukemia: the GRAALL-2003 study. *J Clin Oncol.* 2009;27:911-8.

30. Annino L, Vegna ML, Camera A, et al. Treatment of adult acute lymphoblastic leukemia (ALL): long-term follow-up of the GIMEMAALL 0288 randomized study. *Blood.* 2002;99:863-871.

31. Ribera JM, Ortega JJ, Oriol A, et al. Late intensification chemotherapy has not improved the results of intensive chemotherapy in adult acute lymphoblastic leukemia. Results of a prospective multicenter randomized trial (PETHEMA ALL-89). Spanish Society of Hematology. *Haematologica.* 1998;83:222-30.

32. Ribera JM, Oriol A, Bethencourt C, et al. Comparison of intensive chemotherapy, allogeneic or autologous stem cell transplantation as postremission treatment for adult patients with high-risk acute lymphoblastic leukemia: Results of the PETHEMA ALL-93 trial. *Haematologica.* 2005;90:1346-56.

33. Wetzler M, Dodge RK, Mrózek K, et al. Prospective karyotype analysis in adult acute lymphoblastic leukemia: the cancer and leukemia Group B experience. *Blood.* 1999;93:3983-93.

34. Westbrook CA, Hooberman AL, Spino C, et al. Clinical significance of the BCR-ABL fusion gene in adult acute lymphoblastic leukemia: a Cancer and Leukemia Group B Study (8762). *Blood.* 1992;80:2983-90.

35. Secker-Walker LM, Prentice HG, Durrant et al. Cytogenetics adds independent prognostic information in adults with acute lymphoblastic leukaemia on MRC trial UKALL XA. MRC Adult Leukaemia Working Party. *Br J Haematol.* 1997;96:601-10.

36. Gleissner B, Gökbuget N, Bartram CR, et al. Leading prognostic relevance of the BCR-ABL translocation in adult acute B-lineage lymphoblastic leukemia: a prospective study of the German Multicenter Trial Group and confirmed polymerase chain reaction analysis. *Blood.* 2002;99:1536-43.

37. Fielding AK, Rowe JM, Richards SM, et al. Prospective outcome data on 267 unselected adult patients with Philadelphia chromosome–positive acute lymphoblastic leukemia confirms superiority of allogeneic transplantation over chemotherapy in the pre-imatinib era: results from the International ALL Trial MRC UKALLXII/ECOG2993. *Blood.* 2009;113:4489-96.

38. Druker BJ, Sawyers CL, Kantarjian H, et al. Activity of a specific inhibitor of the BCR-ABL tyrosine kinase in the blast crisis of chronic myeloid leukemia and acute lymphoblastic leukemia with the Philadelphia chromosome. *N Engl J Med.* 2001;344:1038-42.

39. Ottmann OG, Druker BJ, Sawyers CL, et al. A phase 2 study of imatinib in patients with relapsed or refractory Philadelphia chromosome-positive acute lymphoid leukemias. *Blood.* 2002;100:1965-71.

40. Fielding AK, Buck G, Lazarus HM, et al. Imatinib significantly enhances long-term outcomes in philadelphia positive acute lymphoblastic leukaemia; final results of the UKALLXII/ECOG2993 Trial ASH Annual Meeting Abstracts. 2010;116:169.

41. Eassmann B, Pfeifer H, Goekbuget N, et al. Alternating versus concurrent schedules of imatinib and chemotherapy as front-line therapy for Philadelphia-positive acute lymphoblastic leukemia (Ph+ ALL). *Blood.* 2006;108:1469-77.

42. Hatta Y, Mizuta S, Ohtake S, et al. Promising outcome of imatinib-combined chemotherapy followed by allogeneic hematopoietic stem cell transplantation for Philadelphia chromosome-positive acute lymphoblastic leukemia: results of the Japan Adult Leukemia Study Group (JALSG) Ph+ALL202 Regimen. *ASH Annual Meeting Abstracts.* 2009;114:3090.

43. Mizuta S, Matsuo K, Yagasaki F, et al. Pre-transplant imatinib-based therapy improves the outcome of allogeneic hematopoietic stem cell transplantation for BCR–ABL-positive acute lymphoblastic leukemia. *Leukemia.* 2011;25:41-7.

44. Thomas DA, O'Brien SM, Faderl S, et al. Long-term outcome after hyper-CVAD and imatinib (IM) for de novo or minimally treated Philadelphia chromosome-positive acute lymphoblastic leukemia (Ph-ALL). *J Clin Oncol.* 2010;28:15s.

45. Ribera JM, Oriol A, González M, et al. Concurrent intensive chemotherapy and imatinib before and after stem cell transplantation in newly diagnosed Philadelphia chromosome-positive acute lymphoblastic leukemia. Final results of the CSTIBES02 trial. *Haematologica.* 2010;95:87-95.
46. de Labarthe A, Rousselot P, Huguet-Rigal F, et al. Imatinib combined with induction or consolidation chemotherapy in patients with de novo Philadelphia chromosome-positive acute lymphoblastic leukemia: results of the GRAAPH-2003 study. *Blood.* 2007;109:1408-13.
47. Vignetti M, Fazi P, Cimino G, et al. Imatinib plus steroids induces complete remissions and prolonged survival in elderly Philadelphia chromosome-positive patients with acute lymphoblastic leukemia without additional chemotherapy: results of the Gruppo Italiano Malattie Ematologiche dell'Adulto (GIMEMA) LAL0201-B protocol. *Blood.* 2007;109:3676-8.
48. Delannoy A, Delabesse E, Lhéritier V, et al. Imatinib and methylprednisolone alternated with chemotherapy improve the outcome of elderly patients with Philadelphia-positive acute lymphoblastic leukemia: results of the GRAALL AFR09 study. *Leukemia.* 2006;20:1526-32.
49. Ravandi F, O'Brien S, Thomas D, et al. First report of phase 2 study of dasatinib with hyper-CVAD for the frontline treatment of patients with Philadelphia chromosome-positive (Ph+) acute lymphoblastic leukemia. *Blood.* 2010;116:2070-7.
50. Foà R, Vitale A, Vignetti M, et al. Dasatinib as first-line treatment for adult patients with Philadelphia chromosome-positive acute lymphoblastic leukemia. *Blood.* 2011;118:6521-8.
51. Lilly MB, Ottmann OG, Shah NP, et al. Dasatinib 140 mg once daily versus 70 mg twice daily in patients with Ph-positive acute lymphoblastic leukemia who failed imatinib: results from a phase 3 study. *Am J Hematol.* 2010;85:164-70.
52. Kim DY, Joo YD, Lee JH, et al. Nilotinib combined with multi-agent chemotherapy for adult patients with newly diagnosed Philadelphia chromosome-positive acute lymphoblastic leukemia: interim results of Korean Adult ALL Working Party Phase 2 Study. *ASH Meeting.* 2011:1517.
53. Kantarjian HM, Kim DW, Pinilla-Ibarz J, et al. Efficacy and safety of ponatinib in patients with accelerated phase of blast phase chronic myeloid leukemia (AP-CML or BP-CML) or Philadelphia chromosome-positive acute lymphoblastic leukemia (Ph+ ALL): 12-month follow-up of the PACE trial. *ASH Meeting Abstracts.* 2012;120:915.
54. Iclusig™. [online] Available from iclusig.com/wp-content/uploads/2013/02/Iclusig-Letter-for-Healthcare-Professionals.pdf [Accessed August, 2013].
55. Fielding AK, Richards SM, Chopra R, et al. Outcome of 609 adults after relapse of acute lymphoblastic leukemia (ALL); an MRC UKALL12/ECOG 2993 study. *Blood.* 2007;109:944-50.
56. Camera A, Annino L, Chiurazzi F, et al. GIMEMA ALL - Rescue 97: a salvage strategy for primary refractory or relapsed adult acute lymphoblastic leukemia. *Haematologica.* 2004;89:145-53.
57. Oriol A, Vives S, Hernández-Rivas JM, et al. Outcome after relapse of acute lymphoblastic leukemia in adult patients included in four consecutive risk-adapted trials by the PETHEMA Study Group. *Haematologica.* 2010;95:589-96.
58. Faderl S, Thomas DA, O'Brien S, et al. Augmented hyper-CVAD based on dose-intensified vincristine, dexamethasone, and asparaginase in adult acute lymphoblastic leukemia salvage therapy. *Clin Lymphoma Myeloma Leuk.* 2011;11:54-9.
59. Kantarjian HM, Thomas D, Ravandi F, et al. Defining the course and prognosis of adults with acute lymphocytic leukemia in first salvage after induction failure or short first remission duration. *Cancer.* 2010;116:5568-74.
60. Duval M, Klein JP, He W, et al. Hematopoietic stem-cell transplantation for acute leukemia in relapse or primary induction failure. *J Clin Oncol.* 2010;28:3730-8.
61. DeAngelo DJ, Yu D, Johnson JL, et al. Nelarabine induces complete remissions in adults with relapsed or refractory T-lineage acute lymphoblastic leukemia or lymphoblastic lymphoma: Cancer and Leukemia Group B study 1980. *Blood.* 2007;109:5136-42.

62. Berg SL, Blaney SM, Devidas M, et al. Phase II study of nelarabine (compound 506U78) in children and young adults with refractory T-cell malignancies: a report from the Children's Oncology Group. *J Clin Oncol.* 2005;23:3376-82.

63. Gokbuget N, Basara N, Baurmann H, et al. High single-drug activity of nelarabine in relapsed T-lymphoblastic leukemia/lymphoma offers curative option with subsequent stem cell transplantation. *Blood.* 2011;118:3504-11.

64. Advani AS, Gundacker HM, Sala-Torra O, et al. Southwest Oncology Group Study S0530: a phase 2 trial of clofarabine and cytarabine for relapsed or refractory acute lymphocytic leukaemia. *Br J Haematol.* 2010;151:430-4.

65. Pigneux A, Sauvezie M, Vey N, et al. Clofarabine Combinations in Adults with Refractory/ Relapsed Acute Lymphoblastic Leukemia (ALL): A GRAALL Report. ASH Meeting. 2011. 2586.

66. Sancho JM, Ribera JM, Xicoy B, et al. Results of the PETHEMA ALL-96 trial in elderly patients with Philadelphia chromosome-negative acute lymphoblastic leukemia. *Eur J Haematol.* 2007;78:102-10.

67. O'Brien S, Thomas DA, Ravandi F, et al. Results of the hyperfractionated cyclophosphamide, vincristine, doxorubicin, and dexamethasone regimen in elderly patients with acute lymphocytic leukemia. *Cancer.* 2008;113:2097-101.

68. Hunault-Berger M, Leguay T, Thomas X, et al. A randomized study of pegylated liposomal doxorubicin vs continuous-infusion doxorubicin in elderly patients with acute lymphoblastic leukemia: the GRAALL SA1 study. *Haematologica.* 2011;96:245-52.

69. Delannoy A, Cazin B, Thomas X, et al. Treatment of acute lymphoblastic leukemia in the elderly: an evaluation of interferon alpha given as a single agent after complete remission. *Leuk Lymphoma.* 2002;43:75-81.

70. Schafer ES, Hunger SP. Optimal therapy for acute lymphoblastic leukemia in adolescents and young adults. *Nat Rev Clin Oncol.* 2011;8:417-24.

71. Pulte D, Gondos A, Brenner H. Improvement in survival in younger patients with acute lymphoblastic leukemia from the 1980s to the early 21st century. *Blood.* 2009;113:1408-11.

72. Stock W, La Mei, Sanford B, et al. What determines the outcomes for adolescents and young adults with acute lymphoblastic leukemia treated on cooperative group protocols? A comparison of Children's Cancer Group and Cancer and Leukemia Group B studies. *Blood.* 2008;112:1646-54.

73. Boissel N, Auclerc MF, Lheritier V, et al. Should adolescents with acute lymphoblastic leukemia be treated as old children or young adults? Comparison of the French FRALLE-93 and LALA-94 trials. *J Clin Oncol.* 2003;21:774-80.

74. Ramanujachar R, Richards S, Hann I, et al. Adolescents with acute lymphoblastic leukaemia: outcome on UK national pediatric (ALL97) and adult (UKALLXII/E2993) trials. *Pediatr Blood Cancer.* 2007;48:254-61.

75. de Bont JM, van der Holt B, Dekker AW, et al. Significant difference in outcome for adolescents with acute lymphoblastic leukemia treated on pediatric vs adult protocols in the Netherlands. *Leukemia.* 2004;18:2032-35.

76. Usvasalo A, Raty R, Knuuitila S, et al. Acute lymphoblastic leukemia in adolescents and young adults in Finland. *Haematologica.* 2008;93:1161-8.

8 Use of Asparaginase in Acute Lymphoblastic Leukemia Therapy

Patrick W Burke, Justin M Watts, Martin S Tallman, Dan Douer

INTRODUCTION

Asparaginase is incorporated into all pediatric and many adult acute lymphoblastic leukemia (ALL) protocols, but reluctance exists when using it in adults since more toxicity occurs with advancing age.[1] Furthermore, data is more limited in adults, as no randomized trials with asparaginase have been performed in adults. Thus, the benefit of asparaginase is more difficult to define in this population. Also noteworthy is conflicting data demonstrating comparable outcomes between some adult regimens without asparaginase and regimens including the drug. However, as in pediatric trials, some adult protocols have shown improvement when using asparaginase. Nonetheless, given the multiple asparaginase preparations, various schedule permutations, related toxicities, and heterogeneity of ALL risk-stratification groups, the final verdict regarding asparaginase's importance in multi-agent front-line treatment in adult ALL is far from being issued. Currently, multiple trials are ongoing to help further delineate the role of asparaginase and possibly optimize its use in adult ALL. These investigations will advance the understanding of an enzyme that was first studied approximately 100 years ago.

HISTORICAL OVERVIEW

Early 20th Century Biochemical Discoveries

Through the early portion of the 20th century, forays into amino acid and protein biology and metabolism were made, including explorations of asparagine. Discoveries were made regarding nitrogen and ammonia liberation from certain amino acids, including, but not limited to, asparagine. Nonetheless, certain research was focused on asparagine. Initially, there was only strong suggestion, but without confirmation, of the *in vitro* and *in vivo* biochemical connection between asparagine and aspartic acid. In fact, initially, it was uncertain if ammonia liberation from asparagine occurred via deamination or deamidation (Figure 8-1).[2,3] Much of the initial work occurred in plants, but the presence of deamidases was confirmed in yeast and molds, such as *Aspergillus niger*, as well.

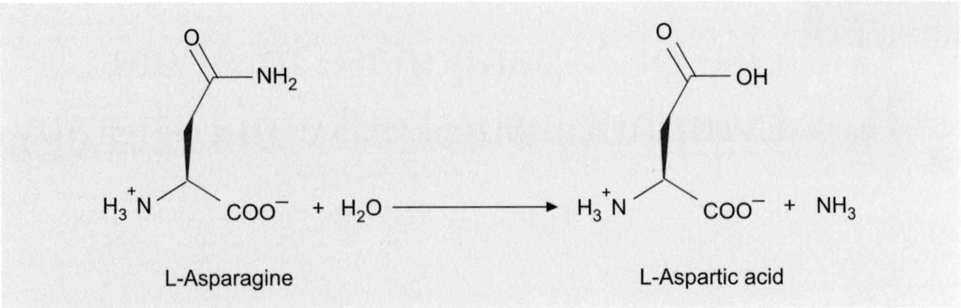

Figure 8-1 Hydrolytic deamidation of alpha-amino acid L-asparagine.[2] L-aspartate and ammonia are yielded. Nitrogen (in the form of ammonia) is liberated from the amide group attached to the beta carbon of the alpha-amino acid.

Animal studies also, at first, showed conflicting evidence between deamination and deamidation. Adding to the confusion, was that multiple experiments were performed using different animal extracts, with likely varying amounts of the viable enzyme of interest being isolated and tested. One notable report from Furth and Friedman in 1910 found that various animal organ extracts were able to hydrolyze the amide group (deamidation) of asparagine.[4] However, the most extensive initial work regarding enzymatic deamidation of asparagine by animal organ extracts was performed by Clementi, who found that only certain animals and certain tissue extracts contained the enzyme. In fact, Clementi's seminal 1922 paper coined the term "asparaginase".[5]

Early Landmark Preclinical Work

In 1953, John G Kidd reported a series of experiments where mice xenografts from two kinds of lymphoma cell lines injected subcutaneously into mice regressed after intraperitoneal injection of the mice with guinea pig serum. The particular efficacy of the guinea pig serum was highlighted by the fact that neither untreated mice xenograft controls nor xenograft mice treated with rabbit or horse serum showed lymphoma response, and in fact, they progressed and died. Furthermore, the guinea pig serum anticancer effect seemed to be unique to lymphoma, as additional experiments with different mice xenografts with mammary carcinoma and fibrosarcoma failed to show response.[6]

Building upon this, Broome, working in Kidd's laboratory, sought to elucidate the specific agent in guinea pig serum responsible for its anti-lymphoma activity. Previous hypotheses of the effective agent in guinea pig serum included complements since these proteins are very abundant in guinea pig serum. However, prior experiments had ruled out complements, and Broome focused his attention to L-asparaginase due to the previous work by Clementi. In a series of experiments, Broome showed that stepwise denaturing and inactivation of asparaginase activity, by either increased heating of guinea pig serum or altering pH, resulted in corresponding lowering of *in vivo* anti-lymphoma activity in the mice xenografts. The stepwise decline in anti-lymphoma effect correlated with stepwise decrements in L-asparaginase activity. Next, Broome further demonstrated L-asparaginase's anti-lymphoma activity through experiments with newborn guinea pig serum, which has only a small fraction of asparaginase compared to adult serum. Previous reports had demonstrated that sarcoma cell lines that were inhibited by adult guinea pig serum were not inhibited by newborn serum. Broome further demonstrated this to be true with lymphoma mouse xenografts. Lastly in this report, Broome definitively demonstrated that L-asparaginase was the effective anti-lymphoma agent, as successive purifications involving precipitation, electrophoresis, and chromatography demonstrated L-asparaginase as the definitive agent, with increasing concentrations having higher anti-lymphoma activity.[7]

Subsequently, Old reported the anti-leukemic effect of L-asparaginase in mice in 1963.[8]

Early Human Trials

In 1964, Mashburn and Wriston isolated *Escherichia coli* asparaginase, which provided a sufficient source of the enzyme, and human clinical trials ensued.[9] Among the initial reports, in 1967, Oettgen et al. and Hill et al. reported promising results in ALL.[10,11] L-asparaginase's effect on other leukemias was also subsequently assessed, as Ohnuma et al. described in a case report of a patient with acute myelogenous leukemia (AML) who achieved an 8-month complete remission, despite significant toxicity, after a single high dose of L-asparaginase. After relapse, remission was again achieved with L-asparaginase administration.[12] Beard et al. reported a trial of L-asparaginase in 40 patients with previously untreated or relapsed ALL, AML, or lymphosarcoma. Of the 15 patients with active ALL at enrollment, nine achieved a significant response with single-agent L-asparaginase, with five complete responses (CR) and four very good partial responses (PR). Of the 11 AML patients treated, none achieved a remission with either single-agent L-asparaginase or in L-asparaginase in combination with other chemotherapy. Impressive reductions in peripheral blasts counts were seen with L-asparaginase. However, these responses were very transient, as a quick onset of resistance was demonstrated.[13]

Given these initial trial results, enthusiasm for L-asparaginase treatment in AML was tempered, and historically this was not used in AML remission induction therapy, consolidation, or in salvage. However, the use of L-asparaginase in AML has recently garnered modest attention again and may be revisited going forward, particularly with developing idea that glutaminase activity may play an increasing role in L-asparaginase anti-neoplastic effect.[14] Despite some use in various non-Hodgkin lymphomas, ALL has been the predominant disease setting for L-asparaginase therapy. The majority of data is found in ALL, and this is where the scope of this review will lie.

MECHANISM OF ACTION

L-asparaginase is an enzyme that catalyzes the hydrolysis of asparagine to aspartic acid and ammonia. To a lesser degree, it catalyzes the hydrolysis of glutamine to glutamic acid and ammonia.[1] As above, both of these reactions occur via deamidation and not deamination, with ammonia being liberated by the amide group. Thus, for asparagine, ammonia is liberated from the amide group off of the beta carbon in this alpha amino acid, not the amino group of the alpha carbon. Similarly, with glutamine, the liberated ammonia in this hydrolytic reaction is via deamidation from the amide group attached to the gamma carbon of the alpha amino acid and not the alpha amino group.[2,3]

Bacterial type L-asparaginases (referred to henceforth as "asparaginases") come in two subtypes defined by where they are localized.[15] Type I localizes to the cytosol and displays less affinity to L-asparagine (referred to henceforth as "asparagine"), while type II localizes to the periplasmic space and exhibits much higher substrate affinity.[16] Depletion of asparagine (and glutamine) in the plasma theoretically deprives ALL lymphoblasts of this amino acid, as these malignant lymphoblasts cannot effectively resynthesize asparagine since they lack asparagine synthetase.[17,18] In actual practice, ALL lymphoblasts do upregulate and produce asparagine synthetase, under conditions of asparagine depletion with asparaginase, *in vitro*, rendering asparaginase ineffective in vitro at killing ALL lymphoblasts.[19] In practicum, there is also some in vivo ALL lymphoblast upregulation and production of asparagine synthetase in the setting of asparagine depletion, but this does not seem to compromise blast killing or clinical outcome.[20]

Acute lymphoblastic leukemia lymphoblasts cannot produce sufficient asparagine for growth (since they lack asparagine synthetase) and rely upon on plasma levels of this amino acid for protein synthesis.[17,18] Thus, asparagine is an essential amino acid for ALL lymphoblasts, and plasma asparagine depletion inhibits protein synthesis. This ultimately leads to, among other effects, inhibition of ribonucleic acid (RNA) and deoxyribonucleic acid (DNA) synthesis, causing subsequent apoptotic cell death of the leukemic blasts.[21] The effects of protein depletion are nonspecific and lead to the various asparaginase toxicities, which are further discussed below.

Although serum asparagine depletion is the goal of the treatment, asparagine depletion is not only dependent on the pool of asparagine deamidated by the drug, but also by the amount of this amino acid to the diet, synthesis by the liver, as well as induction of asparagine synthetase in the leukemia cells. Thus, serum asparagine levels can vary between individual patients being treated with the same dose and schedule of asparaginase, resulting in differing responses to asparaginase.

CHARACTERISTICS OF ASPARAGINASE

Asparaginase has no cross resistance, no known late effects, and has central nervous system (CNS) anti-leukemia activity, even though the drug does not penetrate the brain, given that cerebrospinal fluid asparagine levels are thought to equilibrate with plasma levels. Asparaginase is not myelosuppressive, yet it exhibits a unique toxicity profile that includes hypersensitivity, pancreatitis, and venous thrombosis, all of which can potentially be life-threatening. Among other side effects are hepatotoxicity, hyperglycemia, neuropathy, and a bleeding diathesis (see Toxicity section below).

ASPARAGINASE PREPARATIONS

Three asparaginase preparations are commercially available for use in treatment of ALL. The first developed was *E. coli* asparaginase, on which most of the historical data is based. Another preparation, the pegylated form of *E. coli* asparaginase, PEG-asparaginase, involves polyethylene glycol attached covalently to the native enzyme; thus rendering PEG-asparaginase potentially less immunogenetic and longer-lasting. *Erwinia chrysanthemi* asparaginase is the third preparation and has been FDA approved for use in patients with hypersensitivity to the *E. coli* preparations. Each asparaginase form may be given intravenously (IV) or intramuscularly (IM), and all exhibit half-lives ($t_{1/2}$) that impact dosing schedule. The $t_{1/2}$ of *E. coli* asparaginase is 1.24 days; while PEG-asparaginase's $t_{1/2}$ is much longer, at approximately 6 days, thus rendering an approximate equivalency of 6–9 doses of *E. coli* asparaginase given over 2–3 weeks with one PEG-asparaginase dose. *E. chrysanthemi* asparaginase exhibits the shortest $t_{1/2}$, 0.65 days, which may be of clinical benefit due to its short duration since any treatment toxicity is not exacerbated by long-lasting drug levels. While these $t_{1/2}$ values theoretically predict duration of efficacy of treatment or toxicity duration, practically, development of asparaginase antibodies—which can occur with significant frequency—will shorten the duration of effect by (1) pharmacokinetics, with a shortened $t_{1/2}$ and (2) neutralizing the pharmacodynamic effect asparaginase.

TOXICITY

While the various asparaginase toxicities have been well delineated in the pediatric literature—due to the considerable experience with using the drug compared to in adults—a considerable gap in toxicity data and, more specifically, recommendations on management of adult asparaginase toxicity exists. A detailed review of asparaginase toxicity data and management intricacies is beyond the scope of this review, but Stock et al. reported recommendations from an ALL expert panel that serves as an initial guide for adult toxicity.[22] However, since a dialectic exists between asparaginase's varying toxicities that can often be severe and potentially life-threatening and the fact that effective asparaginase ALL therapy depends on prolonged drug administration and prolonged plasma asparagine depletion, practitioners without significant experience using the drug should proceed with caution. Clinical experience in treating with the drug is paramount in balancing treatment efficacy and managing toxicity.

Adult asparaginase toxicity is qualitatively no different than pediatric toxicity, i.e., the toxicity profile is the same. However, the rates of certain toxicities differ between children and adults. Generally, with increasing age, the rates of most toxicities increase, although this is not always the case since grade 3 and 4 allergy/hypersensitivity seems to occur more frequently in children. Several confounding factors, besides increasing age, may also contribute to the general increased frequencies of toxicity in adults. These include, in adults, more comorbidities, alcohol use, and increased use of other medications that may contribute to toxicity.

Among the various toxicities are: allergy/hypersensitivity, pancreatitis, hyperglycemia, hepatotoxicity, thrombosis, coagulopathy, fatigue, nausea/vomiting, and neuropathy. Since asparaginase is a foreign protein, allergy/hypersensitivity may occur. Clinical manifestations range from mild injection site reactions to anaphylaxis. Furthermore, silent hypersensitivity may occur, with neutralizing antibodies being formed. Silent hypersensitivity poses a challenge since, by definition, it happens without a clinical red flag, and therefore, neutralizing antibodies alter asparaginase pharmacokinetics by decreasing the $t_{1/2}$ and may compromise plasma asparaginase depletion also by rendering it pharmacodynamically ineffective. Often, asparaginase is given with corticosteroids, as either part of the ALL treatment regimen or as prophylaxis for possible asparaginase allergy. This may lower the risk of severe reaction and neutralizing antibody formation.

The mechanism of asparaginase-related pancreatitis, which can either be asymptomatic (isolated amylase or lipase elevations) or symptomatic (clinical pancreatitis), is unknown. Clinical pancreatitis remains one of the true contraindications to further asparaginase therapy. Hyperglycemia occurs with increasing frequency with advancing age and is due to asparaginase's effect on the insulin biosynthesis. Concomitant corticosteroid use places a patient at higher risk for hyperglycemia and insulin administration is often temporarily required. Hepatotoxicity occurs in multiple forms and has an unknown etiology. Frequently, elevated transaminases and hyperbilirubinemia are encountered, with hyperbilirubinemia being more problematic since this may delay dosing of other chemotherapy. The true quantitative risk of asparaginase hepatotoxicity is difficult to assess in adults since asparaginase is almost always given concomitantly with other hepatotoxic agents, such as other cytotoxic chemotherapy or supportive medications.

Other liver protein synthesis effects can be seen, including hypoalbuminemia and decreased production of procoagulants and anticoagulants. Venous thrombosis occurs more frequently than hemorrhage, with the majority of thromboses being catheter related, though the most serious occur in the CNS (sinus vein thrombosis). While the synthesis of many such proteins [antithrombin III (AT III), plasminogen, protein C, protein S, coagulation factors, and fibrinogen] declines, the most clinically relevant to thrombosis and hemorrhage seem to be AT III and fibrinogen, respectively. Care must be taken with repleting AT III and fibrinogen, particularly fibrinogen, since overzealous correction may provoke the opposite effect, e.g., cryoprecipitate may provoke thrombosis, due to repleting fibrinogen but also due to cryoprecipitate containing Factor VIII and von Willebrand factor. If AT III concentrate is not available, fresh frozen plasma (FFP) may be used to replete AT III stores in the setting of thrombosis, but FFP is best avoided if possible since it will replete plasma asparagine stores. While acute thromboembolic events and hemorrhages are treated, there is very little prospective trial data to support general guidelines regarding prophylactic repletion of AT III or fibrinogen in adults. However, consideration may be given to prophylactic administration of these products, especially during induction since the majority of events will occur during that cycle.

Lastly, CNS effects other than thrombosis/hemorrhage may occur during asparaginase therapy; these include the "asparaginase blues", which occur when ammonia is liberated via asparaginase and glutaminase activity. Besides CNS depression via increased plasma ammonia, other rare CNS disturbances can occur, such as coma, seizures, and posterior reversible leukoencephalopathy syndrome.[22]

ADULT ALL PROTOCOL ARCHETYPES

The treatment regimen of ALL in all age groups is very complex, and no standard of care regimen for adults has been established. Despite many regimens being previously developed, almost all regimens are adopted from the German Berlin-Frankfurt-Münster (BFM) or hyperfractionated cyclophosphamide, vincristine, doxorubicin, and dexamethasone (HyperCVAD) regimens.[23,24] All of these regimens provide CNS prophylaxis and maintenance therapy. The German BFM pediatric group developed the BFM-based regimen, while subsequent groups later adopted and modified it.[25-27]

Berlin-Frankfurt-Münster-based Regimens

All BFM-based regimens usually utilize a two-phase induction. The first induction phase involves daunorubicin, vincristine, prednisone, and asparaginase, while the second phase includes cyclophosphamide, cytarabine, and 6-mercaptopurine (6-MP). Notably, asparaginase is used in all BFM-based inductions. Other modifications to the BFM-based regimen, including other agents, have been tried. Following the two-phase induction, multiple successive, intensive multiagent chemotherapy consolidation cycles are administered; this also often involves a delayed reinduction phase.[23]

HyperCVAD

The second major ALL regimen archetype, called the HyperCVAD regimen, was formulated at the MD Anderson Cancer Center.[24] It consists of a cycle A and cycle B, which are alternated four times to provide at total of eight cycles. Cycle A consists of HyperCVAD. Cycle B incorporates high-dose methotrexate plus high-dose cytarabine. Notably, HyperCVAD does not include asparaginase in either of its cycles. To this point, HyperCVAD has been studied only in adults.

Overall, it remains extremely difficult to compare and contrast trials that have different designs, patient populations, risk factors, and age limits. Furthermore, comparisons are difficult to make since these protocols involve many agents provided on a complex schedule; therefore, firm statements about a specific agent's utility are difficult to make. Previously, it had been noted that while the complete remission rates seemed to have improved over time, it was striking that not much difference in outcome if asparaginase was used in induction, in consolidation, in both induction and consolidation (as it is used in most BFM-based regimens), or is not used at all. This was noted despite the variability in the trials. However, more recent review of the existing trial data has yielded optimism of improved outcomes with increasing total asparaginase dose, as well as increasing total doses of noncytotoxic chemotherapy, such as vincristine and corticosteroids.

THE CASE FOR ASPARAGINASE

Landmark Pediatric Trials

Given the impressive initial data from the 1960s and 1970s involving asparaginase in treating ALL, the drug was used in both pediatric and adult regimens. However, it was soon discovered that adults suffered high rates of significant toxicities, which, in retrospect, was probably due to multiple factors including: (1) impurities in the early asparaginase preparations, such as contamination with other *E. coli* proteins and (2) inexperience with supportive care for the multitude of asparaginase-associated toxicities. Nonetheless, these early harsh lessons in adults chastened investigators and practitioners, rendering the use of asparaginase in adults to very infrequent for many years due to what was deemed prohibitive toxicity. And this reticence in using asparaginase in adult ALL was commonly practiced until very recently. However, pediatric protocols continued to make use of this highly active agent over successive decades up until the present. A couple of the landmark trials that particularly serve as evidence buttressing the argument of asparaginase's role in pediatric ALL therapy will be discussed. These trials also served as strong historical evidence providing the impetus to re-explore asparaginase's role in adult ALL.

Dana Farber Cancer Institute's 77-01 Trial

The Dana Farber Cancer Institute's (DFCI's) trial number 77-01 represents a landmark pediatric ALL trial, supporting intensive asparaginase dosing.[28] Pediatric patients with Precursor B-cell ALL were randomized to either receive or not receive intensification with L-asparaginase (25,000 U/m^2 once per week for ages greater than or equal to 6 years; 50,000 U/m^2 once per week for ages less than 6 years) for 20 weeks. This intensification was given after an induction of vincristine, prednisone, and doxorubicin (VPD), which was followed by a brief five-dose asparaginase consolidation given every other day. This schedule attempted to sustain the depletion of asparagine for a long duration of 5 months. Disease free survival (DFS) and event free survival (EFS) were both significantly improved with L-asparaginase-intensification, and EFS between the groups after a median followup of 9.4 years was 71% ± 9% versus 31% ± 11%, respectively, for the asparaginase intensification and non-asparaginase intensification groups.[29] Furthermore, the results were similar when comparing high and low-risk disease.

Dana Farber Consortium Protocol 91-01

Building upon the previous DFCI Consortium ALL protocols, Dana Farber Consortium Protocol 91-01 was conducted between 1991 and 1995.[30] The 377 pediatric patients on protocol were subjected to five randomizations, including (1) a preinduction investigational window, assessing leukemic kill of different corticosteroids/doses given for 3 days prior to induction; (2) high-dose infusional 6-MP versus conventional oral 6-MP dosing during intensification; (3) 48-hour infusional versus standard IV bolus doxorubicin for high risk patients (to determine any differences in late echocardiographic abnormalities) during intensification; (4) hyperfractionated versus conventional cranial radiation to determine any difference in neuropsychologic sequelae, and (5) PEG-asparaginase versus L-asparaginase during intensification.

Patients were randomized to either PEG-asparaginase 2,500 IU/m^2 IM every other week for 15 doses or L-asparaginase 25,000 IU/m^2 weekly for 30 doses during intensification. Patients could be converted to the other asparaginase preparation after a mild clinical allergic reaction, and they were switched to E. chrysanthemi asparaginase if they experienced a second allergic event.

The 5-year EFS for the 377 patients on trial was 83% ± 2%, and no significant difference was found between the standard and high risk groups. No significant difference was found between any of the randomized groups, most notably the

PEG-asparaginase versus L-asparaginase randomization. Overall, 29% of patients experienced asparaginase-related toxicity, but there was no significant difference in the frequency of dose-limiting toxicity between the two preparations. Of all the patients who achieved a CR and survived beyond completion of intensification (n = 352), 15% of patients experienced at least one asparaginase allergic event, but no significant difference in 5-year EFS was noted between patients who experienced an allergy compared to those who did not. More importantly, however, 12% of evaluable patients completed less than 25 weeks (of a possible total of 30 weeks) of asparaginase treatments. These patients who received less asparaginase did display significantly worse 5-year EFS compared with those who received at least 26 weeks of asparaginase therapy (73% ± 7% versus 90% ± 2%). Going further, a multivariate Cox-proportional hazard model that included covariates for asparaginase intolerance, age, initial white blood cell (WBC) count, and immunophenotype showed that asparaginase intolerance was the only prognostically significant variable predicting 5-year EFS.

More evidence of the benefit of increased asparaginase dosing was found when reviewing the most recent preceding DFCI protocols with less asparaginase: 81-01, 85-01, and 87-01. Baseline demographics were similar in all of the trials, as well as remission death rates, but EFS and leukemia free survival was significantly better in 91-01 versus the 81-01, 85-01, and 87-01 conglomerate of patients. Although another major difference between 91-01 and the other trials was 91-01's substitution of dexamethasone, in lieu of prednisone, in post-remission therapy (and dexamethasone has repeatedly shown greater *in vitro* antileukemic activity and better CNS penetration), there still remains strong evidence for asparaginase's role in the improved outcomes.[30]

Retrospective Analyses of Adolescents and Young Adults Comparing Pediatric versus Adult Protocols Outcomes

Children's Cancer Group versus Cancer and Leukemia Group B Retrospective Analysis

One major retrospective analysis was performed by Stock et al.[31] This retrospective comparison of adolescents and young adults (AYAs) aged 16–20 years with newly diagnosed ALL who were treated on consecutive "pediatric" protocols by the Children's Cancer Group (CCG) or "adult" protocols by the Cancer and Leukemia Group B (CALGB) attempted to investigate the outcome gap in long-term survival between pediatric and adult patients.

It had previously been noted that the AYA patient population exhibited much worse long-term outcomes compared to younger children. Furthermore, the AYA ALL population remains an intriguing demographic since AYA ALL is relatively much less common compared to children. Furthermore, historically, this small population of patients has been difficult to analyze since their treatment—either with a pediatric or adult regimen—was often solely determined by referral pattern, i.e., to a pediatric or adult oncologist. Moreover, this relatively small AYA population has been difficult to analyze since their trial results often were included in pediatric or adult reports, thus making heterogeneous study populations that truly may not reflect the true AYA population.

A total of 197 AYA patients, aged 16–20 years, were enrolled by the CCG between 1989 and 1995. The two analyzed trials were CCG 1882 (175 patients) and CCG 1901 (22 patients). During these years, the CCG used a risk-stratified treatment approach, where the 175 patients enrolled on CCG 1882 all received a standard induction. A day 7 bone marrow examination was used to define rapid early responders (RERs), who had 25% or less marrow lymphoblasts (M1 or M2 marrow status), and slow early responders (SERs), who had greater than 25% marrow blasts (M3 marrow status). The RERs proceeded to be treated with a standard, CCG-modified BFM post-remission regimen, which had previously been reported, plus or minus prophylactic cranial irradiation (PCI). The SERs, after the standard induction, proceeded to receive post-remission therapy with either the same standard, CCG-modified BFM regimen plus PCI, or a CCG-augmented BFM post-remission regimen plus PCI. Twenty-two patients with newly diagnosed ALL exhibiting "lymphomatous features" were enrolled on CCG 1901 using the "New York" regimen, which is similar to the five-drug CALGB induction regimen.

For comparison, 124 AYAs, aged 16–20 years, were enrolled on sequential CALGB studies from 1988 to 2001. These sequential trials were CALGB 8811, CALGB 9111, CALGB 9311, CALGB 9511, and CALGB 19802. Except for CALGB 19802, all of the other previous trials, starting with CALGB 8811, used a five-drug induction of cyclophosphamide, daunorubicin, vincristine, prednisone, and L-asparaginase, followed by intensive post-remission therapy modeled after the BFM regimen. Therapy also included intrathecal (IT) chemotherapy and PCI. The subsequent CALGB trials were slight variations of CALGB 8811, with granulocyte colony stimulating factor being tested versus placebo during induction and early intensification in CALGB 9111. An additional drug treatment was included between the two early intensification cycles in CALGB 9311, with monoclonal antibody anti-B4/blocked ricin administered on a 7-day continuous infusion for B-cell disease and high-dose cytarabine administered for T-cell disease. For CALGB 9511, during induction and consolidation, PEG-asparaginase was substituted for L-asparaginase. Lastly, CALGB 19802 had the most treatment distinctions compared to CALGB 8811, as high-dose systemic methotrexate and IT methotrexate were given in lieu of PCI. Also, CALGB 19802 involved higher doses of daunorubicin and cytarabine.

The patient demographics and characteristics were similar between the CCG and CALGB patients, aside from a significant difference in age distribution, with the median ages of the CCG and CALGB trials being 16 and 19 years, respectively. Otherwise, there were no significant differences in other risk factors, including presenting WBC count and cytogenetics. Notably, complete remission rates were 90% for both the CCG and CALGB set of trials; however, a significant difference in long-term outcomes was noted between the two groups. The EFS and overall survival (OS) for the CCG AYA were 63% and 67%, respectively, while the CALGB AYA had EFS and OS of 34% and 46%, respectively. Furthermore, a significant difference in the pattern of relapse was noted, with 7-year CNS relapse rates of 1% and 11%, respectively, for the CCG and CALGB. This difference in long-term CNS relapses may be attributed to earlier and increased doses of CNS prophylaxis, including IT therapy for the CCG.

Looking at Surveillance, Epidemiology and End Results data and other historical studies, it has been well established that age is a risk factor in ALL, with younger patients, aside from the youngest of infants, doing better—even within the pediatric and AYA populations. Thus, it was investigated whether the significant differences in median age between the two groups contributed to the stark difference in outcomes. Overall, within the CCG, no statistical difference in long-term outcomes could be appreciated between the 16–17 and 18–20 years old subgroups. Yet the CALGB did manifest interesting age distribution outcome disparities, as the 7-year EFS for CALGB 16–17 year olds was 55% versus 29% for 18–20 year olds. More interestingly, inter-group comparisons revealed no significant difference between 7-year EFS between 16 and 17 year olds between the CCG and CALGB, which were 64% and 55%, respectively. A significant difference existed, however, between the 18–20 years old subgroups' 7-year EFS, with the CCG being 57% and the CALGB being 29%.

Since ALL is the most common pediatric malignancy, the majority of new ALL diagnoses are in children and pediatric oncologists treat ALL more frequently than their adult oncologist counterparts. It has been repeatedly hypothesized that the relative respective difference in the experience of treating ALL, between pediatric and adult oncologists, leads to differences in outcomes. The hypothesized mechanism for this is protocol adherence, i.e., keeping the appropriate schedule and dosing of drugs in the treatment regimen. However, in Stock's review, this did not seem to be the case. Of all the patients moving on to the maintenance phase of therapy, no significant difference in the 7-year EFS existed between the CCG 1882 patients who initiated maintenance within 30 days of the original treatment schedule compared with those CCG 1882 patients starting maintenance greater than 30 days late. The same lack of difference between "on-time" and late maintenance delivery was appreciated in the CALGB group. Therefore, protocol adherence, at least by these parameters, did not seem to alter long-term outcomes.

No significant differences in EFS and OS between the different intragroup trials within both the CCG and CALGB were noted. However, interesting intergroup differences between the dosing of agents exist. Overall, the CCG used higher doses of non-myelosuppressive drugs, such as corticosteroids, vincristine, and L-asparaginase in the induction remission and post-remission induction phases (Table 8-1).[31] To enable an easier analysis, CCG 1901 patients were not included in this analysis since they represented a small proportion of the total CCG patients (10%), and there were no significant differences between CCG 1882 and 1901 in 7-year EFS and OS.

Table 8-1	Comparison of Myelosuppressive and Non-myelosuppressive Drugs in the Children's Cancer Group and Cancer and Leukemia Group B Retrospective Trial in Adolescents and Young Adult			
	CCG 1882- Standard Post- Remission	CCG 1882- Augmented Post- Remission	CALGB 8811 9111 9311 9511	CALGB 19802
Induction				
Drug				
Prednisone	1,680 mg/m²	1,680 mg/m²	1,260 mg/m²	1,260 mg/m²
Vincristine	8 mg	8 mg	8 mg	8 mg
L-Asparaginase[1]	54,000 units/m²	54,000 units/m²	36,000 units/m²	36,000 units/m²
Daunorubicin	100 mg/m²	100 mg/m²	135 mg/m²	240 mg/m²
Cyclophos-phamide	0	0	1,200 mg/m²	1,200 mg/m²
Post-remission				
Drug				
Dexamethasone	210 mg/m²	420 mg/m²	140 mg/m²	140 mg/m²
Vincristine	22.5 mg/m²	45 mg/m²	14 mg (total)	14 mg (total)
L-Asparaginase[1]	90,000 units/m²	318,000 units/m²	48,000 units/m²	48,000 units/m²
Doxorubicin	75 mg/m²	150 mg/m²	90 mg/m²	90 mg/m²
Cytarabine	1,800 mg/m²	2,400 mg/m²	1,200 mg/m²	12,000 mg/m²
Cyclophos-phamide	3,000 mg/m²	4,000 mg/m²	3,000 mg/m²	3,000 mg/m²
6-Thioguanine	840 mg/m²	1,680 mg/m²	840 mg/m²	840 mg/m²
6-Mercaptopurine	4,080 mg/m²	4,080 mg/m²	5,040 mg/m²	5,040 mg/m²
Methotrexate (IV or Oral)	90 mg/m²	1,000 mg/m²	100 mg/m²	6,600 mg/m²

CCG, Children's Cancer Group; CALGB, Cancer and Leukemia Group B; IV, intravenously.

Source: Adapted from Stock W, La M, Sanford B, et al. What determines the outcomes for adolescents and young adults with acute lymphoblastic leukemia treated on cooperative group protocols? A comparison of Children's Cancer Group and Cancer and Leukemia Group B studies. *Blood.* 2008;112(5):1646-54.

Because of the improved long-term outcomes in the CCG cohort and the other similarities between the CCG and CALGB groups, a strong case may be made for the more intensive use of non-myelosuppressive agents as the basis for the CCG's improved outcomes. Underscored with this is the role of L-asparaginase since the CCG 1882 induction L-asparaginase dose was 150% the CALGB induction dose, while the standard and augmented CCG 1882 post-remission L-asparaginase doses were 187.5% and 662.5% the CALGB post-remission dose, respectively. Furthermore, CALGB 19802 provided much greater doses of cytotoxic chemotherapy—both in induction and post-remission therapy—compared with both the CCG and other CALGB treatment regimens, and this more cytotoxic chemotherapy intensive regimen failed to result in improved long-term outcomes compared with CCG and the previous CALGB trials. This lack of improvement further buttressed the argument that more intensive treatment with noncytotoxic agents improved outcomes.[31]

Pediatric DCOG versus Adult HOVON Trial Outcomes

Other European pediatric and adult cooperative group trials have also explored the differing outcomes of AYA. A retrospective review of outcomes between AYA aged 15–18 years treated on a series of trials by the Dutch Childhood Oncology Group (DCOG) and the Dutch-Belgian Hemato-Oncology Cooperative Study Group (HOVON) showed evidence for significantly superior outcomes in 5-year OS, DFS, and EFS for the DCOG studies.[32] Several variables may have contributed to the outcome differences, including the absence of high-dose systemic methotrexate in the HOVON studies; omitted or shortened maintenance therapy in HOVON studies, and therefore, a shorter duration of therapy; the more frequent use of allogeneic hematopoietic stem cell transplant (HSCT) in the HOVON studies; and the utilization of reinduction/intensification cycles in the DCOG trials, with a previous meta-analysis showing EFS benefit to this approach.[33] However, as with the CCG and CALGB studies, a significant difference between the pediatric and adult cooperative group trials was the pediatric trials' increased usage of noncytotoxic chemotherapy. While the amount of vincristine and corticosteroids (and particularly dexamethasone, which has better CNS penetration than prednisone and may improve both CNS and isolated bone marrow relapse rate) were increased in the DCOG trials, L-asparaginase total dosage was also higher in the DCOG trials. The mean cumulative doses were 101,000 and 70,000 units/m^2 in the DCOG and HOVON trials, respectively.

The French FRALLE-93 and LALA-94 Trials

Similarly, Boissel et al. asked the same question, retrospectively comparing long-term outcomes from the pediatric French Acute Lymphoblastic Leukemia Group

(FRALLE)-93 and adult leucémie Aiguë Lymphoblastique de l'Adulte (LALA)-94 trials. They looked at AYAs aged 15–20 years. They found that, although there was a significant difference in median age between the trials, age did not factor into outcome. Overall, a univariate analysis found that factors influencing the 5-year EFS were: WBC count, cytogenetics, phenotype, and trial, with the FRALLE-93 being favored. Significant differences favoring the pediatric trial were noted in induction CR rate and 5-year OS, DFS, relapse free survival, and EFS. Between the two trials, many of the same differences between pediatric and adult ALL protocols were seen, e.g., higher cumulative doses of corticosteroids, vinca alkaloids, and L-asparaginase in the pediatric FRALLE-93 trial. In fact, LALA-94 did not use L-asparaginase in induction, and the total L-asparaginase doses were 180,000 and 9,000 U/m^2 in FRALLE-93 and LALA-94, respectively.[34]

MRC ALL97/Revised 99 and UKALLXII/ECOG2993 Trials

Ramanujachar et al. reported another comparative retrospective analysis between the pediatric-inspired Medical Research Council (MRC) ALL97/revised 99 trials and the adult UKALLXII/Eastern Cooperative Oncology Group (ECOG) 2993 trial for AYAs aged 15–17 years. Although these trials had multiple variations, including increased allogeneic HSCT in the adult trial, the pediatric protocols trended to perform better than the adult trials, with a significantly improved 5-year OS and EFS, as well as decreased deaths in remission. Once again, the pediatric trials used increased doses of noncytotoxic corticosteroids, vincristine, and L-asparaginase, although the discrepancy in L-asparaginase cumulative dosing was not as striking as in some of the other pediatric and adult retrospective comparisons.[35]

Swedish Pediatric NOPHO-92 versus Adult Protocol

Another retrospective comparison between pediatric and adult ALL protocols in Sweden was undertaken for patients treated in the 1990s.[36] Although this study looked at many different age groups, from 10 years to 40 years, a subset of 59 AYAs aged 15–20 years old were reviewed. Despite the smaller numbers for the AYA subset, a significantly improved 5-year EFS was seen for AYAs treated on the pediatric trial. Furthermore, despite differences in known risk factors between the groups, it should be noted that, among many differences between the trials, the pediatric protocol total L-asparaginase dose was 420,000 IE/m^2, while the adult protocol did not involve any L-asparaginase.

THE ROLE OF ASPARAGINASE—FACTORS TO CONSIDER

Asparaginase's importance in the treatment of ALL is complex since many variables that have not been or cannot be adequately studied exists. Questioning that asparaginase is an active drug in ALL is untenable, however. Its efficacy has been proven in old pediatric phase I/II trials, where single agent asparaginase in the salvage arena induced responses of 30–65% in relapsed patients, although the response duration was short.[37] However, in adults, the exact dose and duration has not yet been fully established. It is possible that the critical factor for efficacy is not the actual dose of asparaginase, but rather the level asparagine depletion, which is dependent on other factors and not only the drug. Theoretically, this view seems sound. However, it remains unclear how long asparagine should be depleted and whether the depletion is required to be sustained or may be intermittent/stuttering. Asparaginase should also be considered in the context of other drugs given in a particular regimen. Other factors to consider are the increased toxicity with age, especially after 55–60 years, and the various mechanisms of resistance, such as anti-asparaginase antibodies or the induction of asparagine synthetase expression in malignant lymphoblasts. The mode of administration, either IV or IM, should also be considered. Formerly, in the United States asparaginase was usually given IM due to concerns associated with IV administration, although IV asparaginase is now being studied and used more frequently in the United States.[38,39] Furthermore there are also three forms of asparaginase: *E. coli*, pegylated *E. coli* (PEG-asparaginase), and *E. chrysanthemi*, each with different benefits and half-lives (see Asparaginase Preparations section).

ASPARAGINASE ENZYMATIC ACTIVITY, ASPARAGINE DEPLETION, AND CLINICAL OUTCOME

A few studies have suggested a relationship between serum enzymatic activity, asparagine depletion, and clinical outcome. A relapsed pediatric ALL study using PEG-asparaginase demonstrated that patients failing to achieve a CR had lower serum asparaginase enzymatic activity.[40] Similarly, CALGB 9511, which used PEG-asparaginase in newly diagnosed adult ALL, showed improved survival in patients achieving asparagine depletion.[41] In another study, asparaginase concentration was measured.[42] Per day 14 assessment, if serum asparagine concentration was depleted below a certain threshold, the relapse rate was 9%, compared to a 55% relapse rate in patients who had higher serum asparagine concentration levels on day 14. Interestingly, differences in the enzymatic activity were not critical to outcome. This lends credence to the hypothesis that asparagine depletion, not asparaginase dose, is the ultimate determinant of treatment efficacy, i.e., asparaginase dose is only a surrogate for plasma asparagine depletion.

Another indirect assessment of efficacy is assaying the development of antibodies that may compromise asparaginase therapy. These antibodies may alter the pharmacokinetics by increasing asparaginase clearance, or they may alter asparaginase pharamcodynamics via neutralizing antibodies. Antibodies develop after an allergic reaction to asparaginase, although these antibodies can also develop without clinical manifestation of allergy, i.e., silent hypersensitivity. Early studies reported that hypersensitivity and antibody formation to *E. coli* asparaginase did not impact clinical outcome. Patients who experienced severe hypersensitivity reactions to *E. coli* asparaginase and were thus switched to the *E. chrysanthemi* formulation did not have shortened response.[43,44] Alternatively, more recently, it was reported that children with silent hypersensitivity had a higher relapse rate than those with clinical or no hypersensitivity.[45] This result is more in keeping with the known risk of decreased efficacy of asparaginase due to antibody formation.

ASPARAGINASE IN PEDIATRIC NEWLY DIAGNOSED ALL
DFCI 77-01 and 91-01

All pediatric protocols use asparaginase. Asparaginase's role in combination therapy has most extensively been studied in randomized trials in children. Please see DFCI 77-01 section above for more details of this trial, suggesting that the improved outcome was due to more prolonged asparaginase treatment and asparagine depletion.[28,29] Please also see DFCI 91-01 section above for more details regarding this trials' results, suggesting improved outcome was due to longer asparagine depletion.[30]

IDH-ALL-91 Trial

In a BFM-based Italian/Dutch/Hungarian (IDH) trial, IDH-ALL-91, L-asparaginase was used in induction and reinduction.[46] Patients subsequently were randomized to an additional 30 weekly doses of L-asparaginase during continuation (n = 178) or not receive L-asparaginase (n = 177) during continuation. Those who received L-asparaginase during continuation had a significantly better DFS when compared to the children who were randomized not to receive an additional L-asparaginase (87.5% vs 78.7%, respectively). A multivariate analysis showed that not receiving additional L-asparaginase during continuation, along with being male, and being older than 10 years all significantly adversely affected outcome.

CCG 1882 Trial

The Children's Cancer Group conducted another study using a BFM backbone in high-risk patients, CCG 1882 (see CCG vs CALGB Retrospective Analysis section), randomizing patients to either standard or augmented intensity chemotherapy.[47] In the augmented arm, although several other drugs were intensified, the doses of vincristine, asparaginase, and methotrexate were increased much more, i.e., incommensurate with the dose increases of the other agents. For the standard regimen, six doses of asparaginase were given in only one consolidation, while, in the augmented arm, multiple doses of asparaginase were administered over five cycles, yielding a total dose of 366,000 U/m^2. The 5-year EFS in the augmented group was 75.0% ± 3.8%, compared to 55.0% ± 4.5% in the standard treatment group. Similarly, a non-randomized pilot study with augmented therapy displayed a 4-year EFS of 70.8% ± 4.6%; the 6-year EFS of the pilot was 65.4% ± 4.9%; all these results being similar to the randomized CCG 1882 data.[48]

ALL-BFM 90 Trial

The pediatric ALL-BFM group performed their own study, ALL-BFM 90, which studied three risk groups: standard risk group (SRG), medium risk group (MRG), and high risk group (HRG); and four treatment modifications, including: (1) dose intensification during induction, with more rapid sequence of drugs; (2) enforced "intense reconsolidation" (as compared to the consolidation that the SRG and MRG received) by rotational elements in the HRG; (3) decreased dose of anthracyclines and decreased dose of prophylactic cranial radiation (12 Gy) in MRG/HRG; and (4) randomization of the MRG to receive consolidation with or without L-asparaginase.[49]

Regarding asparaginase, the SRG and MRG both received the same L-asparaginase dose in the 28-day induction (eight doses of 10,000 U/m^2 = 80,000 U/m^2). HRG patients received only 60,000 U/m^2 during their truncated induction (six doses of 10,000 U/m^2), but were given additional asparaginase during consolidation (termed "intensive reconsolidation"), which consisted of three rotational elements (HR1, HR2, and HR3), each of which contained one dose of L-asparaginase at 25,000 U/m^2. These three rotational elements comprised a set, with three sets comprising the intensive consolidation. Thus the HRG received a total of 285,000 Units/m^2 of L-asparaginase (60,000 Units/m^2 in induction; and 225,000 Units/m^2 in intensive reconsolidation).

The SRG received only a total of 120,000 U/m^2 (80,000 U/m^2 in induction; none in consolidation, and 40,000 U/m^2 in reinduction). The MRG received the same induction and reinduction doses of L-asparaginase as the SRG, but the MRG included a randomization to either receive or not receive additional L-asparaginase during consolidation with 6-MP, high-dose IV methotrexate, and IT methotrexate. If randomized to receive L-asparaginase in consolidation, four doses of 25,000 U/m^2 were given every 2 weeks for a total of 220,000 U/m^2 (80,000 U/m^2 in induction; 100,000 U/m^2 in consolidation, and 40,000 U/m^2 in reinduction), while the MRG that was randomized to not receive L-asparaginase in consolidation had the same total asparaginase dose as the SRG (120,000 U/m^2).

This increased consolidation/total dose of L-asparaginase in the randomized MRG failed to improve the outcome of the MRG. In the MRG, the EFS was 83% ± 2% with additional asparaginase, compared to 81% ± 2% without it. In the HRG, the EFS was 34%, with the total greater L-asparaginase dose due to intensive reconsolidation, compared to an EFS of 48% in high-risk patients in their previous trial (ALL-BFM 86).[50]

CCG 1961 Trial

Children's Cancer Group 1961 investigated augmented post-induction intensification (PII) regimens, augmenting therapy either via increased intensity or via increased duration of therapy (2 × 2 randomization). To summarize, high-risk ALL children who were RERs to a standard induction (standard four-drug induction that included *E. coli* asparaginase) were randomized either to (1) increased PII therapy with PEG-asparaginase or to (2) standard PII regimen of *E. coli* asparaginase. Within each intensification arm (increased vs standard), patients were further randomized to receive their respective therapies for standard or longer duration. Thus, for standard intensity PII, patients received either 5 months of *E. coli* asparaginase (standard duration) or eight months of *E. coli* asparaginase (longer duration). For increased intensity PII, patients received either 6 months of PEG-asparaginase (standard duration) or 10 months of PEG-asparaginase (longer duration). Both the 5-year EFS and OS were significantly higher in the increased intensity PII arm compared to the standard PII arm: 81.2% versus 71.7% (EFS) and 88.7% versus 83.4% (OS), respectively. The duration of therapy randomization failed to show a significant difference between standard or longer duration of therapy.[51]

Other Trials

Comparisons of *E. coli* asparaginase with the shorter acting *E. chrysanthemi* asparaginase form have demonstrated the advantage of longer asparagine depletion. In two studies, patients were randomized to an identical schedule and dose of either *E. coli* or *E. chrysanthemi* asparaginase, and all other chemotherapy drugs in the regimens remained identical.[52,53] One study from the European Organization for Research and Treatment of Cancer used a BFM backbone (Duval), while the other used the DFCI model with multiple doses of asparaginase (Moghrabi).[52,53] In both studies, those treated with *E. coli* asparaginase experienced a better outcome than those treated with the *E. chrysanthemi* form, and significantly more patients randomized to *E. chrysanthemi* experienced a relapse.[53] It is possible that the more continuous serum asparagine depletion with *E. coli* asparaginase may be associated with better outcome than the intermittent asparagine depletion by *E. chrysanthemi* asparaginase.

ASPARAGINASE IN LARGE ADULT ALL TRIALS

The use of asparaginase in adults varies between individual trials, both in terms of total dose and duration. During induction, the drug is mostly given in similar doses, as it is in children. However, it appears that, even if the drug is used in the post-remission phase, it is usually given for one or two early consolidation cycles with a smaller total dose and a shorter duration of time, compared to the doses given in the randomized pediatric studies, which resulted in better outcomes in children. It is possible that asparaginase is not always administered in the post-remission setting in adults because of apparent or perceived toxicity concerns, although this is not well documented. For those who are using asparaginase in adult clinical trials, it would be useful to document, even retrospectively, asparaginase-specific toxicities, the rate of inability of patients to complete the treatment schedule, and the reasons for that inability.

If sustained and prolonged asparagine depletion is an important factor in the effectiveness of asparaginase treatment in adults, as is probably the case in children, this depletion is generally neither attempted nor achieved in the clinical trials that have been previously performed until now. For example, in a very large international ALL trial, MRC UKALL XII/ECOG E2993, which compared standard chemotherapy to allogeneic transplantation, the short-acting *E. coli* asparaginase was given for only three doses on days 2, 9, and 23 and only in one cycle of consolidation.[27] One might speculate that if more asparaginase would have been given, the outcomes of standard chemotherapy may have improved in comparison to allogeneic transplantation. When planning future randomized trials in adult ALL to test the role of asparaginase in a combination regimen, the importance of considering ways to prolong and perhaps even sustain asparagine depletion cannot be over emphasized.

IS ASPARAGINASE A CRITICAL COMPONENT IN THE TREATMENT OF ALL?

Several factors are salient in determining whether asparaginase is a critical component in the treatment of ALL. First, it has been well established that asparaginase is an active drug in ALL. Second, a relationship theoretically exists between serum enzymatic activity, asparagine depletion, and clinical outcome. This also appears to be true based on a small amount of clinical data. Third, in several pediatric randomized controlled trials (which used two asparaginase-containing regimens: the BFM- or the DFCI-based models), modification of the dose and schedules of asparaginase alone resulted in improved outcome and contributed to the overall benefit. Fourth, it also appears that better outcome in pediatric ALL is associated with longer asparaginase treatment and theoretically more sustained asparagine depletion. Finally, in the previous historical adult protocols, asparaginase was used much less in the post-remission phase and for a much shorter duration of time when compared to pediatric protocols.

Without a randomized clinical trial in adult ALL, the role of each component of multi-agent regimens that include asparaginase cannot be clearly defined. However, based on the summary points above and the pediatric data and AYA comparison data between pediatric and adult regimens, it is very possible that asparaginase has a role, especially in the combination regimens based on the BFM model, where it is already included. It is possible that an alternative combination with drugs other than those used in the BFM model without asparaginase (e.g., hyperCVAD) would produce a similar or even better outcome in adult ALL patients. However, the results of the hyperCVAD regimen should be confirmed by multi-institutional studies, similar to what has already been performed in ALL studies that have included asparaginase. Also, based on what we already know about asparagine depletion, it is unclear if combining asparaginase with HyperCVAD would augment results. However, this may not be pharmacokinetically compatible.[54]

Should we abandon such an active drug in front-line therapy of ALL or should we continue optimizing its use, as has been done in several pediatric protocols which emphasize longer duration over several consolidation cycles, resulting in improved outcome? Certainly, asparaginase has not been as well-studies in adults. Because of the toxicity concerns, studies should continue to look at the risk-benefit ratio and feasibility of intensified asparaginase programs in adults, applying multiple doses of asparaginase (or a few doses of long-acting PEG-asparaginase) post-remission. If indeed, asparaginase continues to be considered a critical component, asparaginase's unique toxicities should be accepted in the same manner that the more common risks of profound and prolonged myelosuppression are accepted in patients treated with cytotoxic chemotherapy.

TREATMENT OF ADULT ALL WITH "PEDIATRIC" PROTOCOLS AND INTENSIFIED ASPARAGINASE AND FUTURE DIRECTIONS

Adult studies using intensified pediatric protocols that include more asparaginase have initiated over the last several years. Although the follow-up times are short and much of the data has yet to mature, the preliminary results are promising. Furthermore, rational dosing and timing of asparaginase and other chemotherapeutic agents has been explored. Douer et al. reported pharmacokinetic, pharmacodynamic, and safety data of PEG-asparaginase, which was given IV during induction.[54] In this study, 25 adults aged 17–55 years or younger with newly diagnosed ALL received a single intravenous dose of PEG-asparaginase ($2,000 \text{ IU}/m^2$) on day 16 of a standard BFM induction regimen, instead of the usual 14 doses of *E. coli* asparaginase in the original BFM protocol. Only one patient developed a neutralizing antibody. In the other patients, serum asparagine was found to be completely depleted in all patients 14 days after IV PEG-asparaginase administration (day 30 of Induction protocol), in 81% of patients 21 days after PEG-asparaginase (day 37 of Induction protocol), and in 44% of patients 28 days after PEG-asparaginase dosing (day 44 of induction protocol). Sufficient serum concentrations of the enzymatic activity and asparagine depletion were seen for 21 days, and for even longer in some individuals. The pharmacokinetic/pharmacodynamic (PK/PD) correlation demonstrated that a minimal PEG-asparaginase level (activity) was required for optimal plasma asparagine depletion of 90%. The volume of distribution was 2.43 L/m^2 (equivalent to adult plasma volume), and the $t_{1/2}$ was 7 days. The CR rate was 96%, and Peg-asparaginase was well tolerated, with few grade 3 or 4 side effects. This study demonstrated that, in adults, PEG-asparaginase produces a long duration of sustained asparagine depletion and enzymatic activity for up to 4 weeks and may be administered IV, with a safety profile similar to equivalent multiple doses of intramuscular *E. coli* asparaginase.[54]

Building upon this PK and PD data, a rationally constructed BFM-modeled regimen (USC II) was formulated based on the previous PK/PD data. In this follow-up study, preliminary feasibility results were reported on an intensive pediatric regimen containing multiple doses of PEG-asparaginase (whereas the previous study only evaluated one PEG-asparaginase dose in induction) in 51 adults with newly diagnosed ALL.[55] The backbone of the protocol was an augmented-BFM pediatric ALL regimen that consisted of eight cycles of multi-agent chemotherapy followed by maintenance. PEG-asparaginase (2,000 IU/m^2/dose) was given IV once in six of the eight pre-maintenance cycles: induction phase I (cycle 1; on day 15), induction phase II (cycle 2; on day 15), two cycles of intensification (cycles 3 and 6; on day 16, respectively), and two cycles of delayed reinduction (cycles 5 and 8; on day 15, respectively). The timing of PEG-asparaginase was planned based on previous data. Corticosteroids were given during and around the time of PEG-asparaginase dosing, while certain cytotoxic chemotherapy agents were administered temporally removed from PEG-asparaginase, in order to avoid potentiating adverse effects. In total, 192 PEG-asaparaginase doses were administered, and only three patients experienced an allergic reaction. Of the 51 patients, 28 could not complete all six scheduled doses (Allogeneic HSCT = 7; pancreatitis = 6; Allogeneic HSCT in a patient who had pancreatitis = 1; patient refusal = 1; induction failure = 2; anaphylaxis = 2; allergy other than anaphylaxis = 1; DVT = 1; died in CR = 3; relapse = 4). Only one patient developed a neutralizing antibody, and this occurred after the first dose of PEG-asparaginase. The percentage of patients with grade 3/4 toxicities during the PEG-asparaginase cycles were as follows: anaphylaxis = 4%, pancreatitis = 14%, thrombosis = 16%, elevated liver enzymes = 65%, hyperbilirubinemia = 43%, hyperglycemia = 33%, hypertriglyceridemia = 16%, and fatigue = 8%. All toxicities were reversible, and no asparaginase-related deaths were seen. Overall, 7-year OS and DFS was 51% and 58%, respectively.

The DFCI applied their pediatric ALL approach, based on the high-risk arm of DFCI Childhood ALL Consortium 00-01. After an induction that included L-asparaginase, patients received intensification that involved 30 weekly doses of L-asparaginase (dosed to asparagine depletion) to treat newly diagnosed ALL patients aged 50 years or younger.[56] The median dose for depletion was $16,582 \, U/m^2$. Of 39 patients who could have completed 30 weeks of L-asparaginase intensification, 27 were able to do so. With a short follow-up of 24 months, the EFS was 72.5%, and the OS was 77.1%. The preliminary results suggest that this approach is feasible, with acceptable toxicity.

The CALGB led intergroup trial with the Southwest Oncology Group (SWOG), ECOG, and Children's Oncology Group (COG) are collaborating on a clinical trial in AYA up to age 39 with newly diagnosed ALL. Patients are being treated with a fully augmented BFM pediatric therapeutic regimen, and one of the arms of this pediatric protocol is being applied in adults. This study will examine if outcomes for AYA ALL will be similar when treated using an identical therapeutic program by either adult or pediatric hematologist/oncologists. Among the issues that will be assessed in this study are outcomes of patients treated on the CALGB/SWOG study compared with those treated on the COG AALL0232 study, toxicities of a pediatric therapeutic regimen when it is applied to young adults up to age 39, and protocol adherence by patients and their caregivers.

SUMMARY

In adults, although asparaginase is included in most protocols, its use has been more limited and less thoroughly studied, mainly due to concerns related to toxicity. Several large randomized pediatric studies show that asparaginase has an important role in the treatment of newly diagnosed pediatric ALL, suggesting that it should probably also be included in adult protocols, especially in those based on the BFM model. Greater efficacy may be achieved with approaches that have a longer duration of asparaginase during post-remission therapy, producing more sustained asparagine depletion, rather than giving higher doses of the drug, i.e., dose density over dose intensity. This may be accomplished by using multiple doses of the long-acting PEG-asparaginase. Overall, asparaginase-related toxicities might be reduced by lowering the rate of hypersensitivity reaction by using PEG-asparaginase and/or adding moderate doses of steroids (at the risk of worsened hyperglycemia); reducing risk of clotting of large veins by allowing the fibrinogen to drop when the platelet counts are adequate; carefully monitoring patients and early treatment of pancreatitis; and limiting the upper age limit to 55–60 years, above which, the risk to benefit ratio of asparaginase may be too skewed. The preliminary results of studies using multiple doses of *E. coli* and PEG-asparaginase suggest this approach is feasible.

The outcome of pediatric ALL has improved dramatically over the last 40 years through a systematic approach of well-designed large trials, making specific and assessable inquiries, and without adding new drugs. Based on these studies' results, as well as the CALGB-SWOG-CCG clinical trial, well designed randomized trials are needed to define the role of asparaginase in adult ALL, as has been already done in childhood ALL. In a more general sense, the treatment of ALL in adults should be studied in the same systematic fashion, including studying the role of asparaginase and comparing the different models of treatment. Since ALL is less common in adults, this may be a challenge that is best delegated to the large cooperative groups.

REFERENCES

1. Kurtzberg J. Asparaginase. In: Holland JF, Blast RJC, Morton DL, editors. Cancer Medicine, 4th ed. Baltimore, MD: Williams and Wilkins; 1997. p. 1027.
2. Available from: http://www.worthington-biochem.com/aspr/images/reaction.jpg. [Accessed August 2013].
3. Available from: http://chemwiki.ucdavis.edu/@api/deki/files/11401/=image048.png. [Accessed August 2013].
4. Furth O, Friedmann M. Uber die verbreitung asparaginsspaltender organfermente. Biochem Z. 1910;26:435-40.
5. Clementi A. Desaminidation enzymatique de l'asparagine. Arch Int Physiol. 1922;19:369-73.
6. Kidd JG. Regression of transplanted lymphomas induced in vivo by means of normal guinea pig serum. I. Course of transplanted cancers of various kinds in mice and rats given guinea pig serum, horse serum, or rabbit serum. J Exp Med. 1953;98(6):565-82.
7. Broome JD. Evidence that the L-asparaginase of guinea pig serum is responsible for its antilymphoma effects. I. Properties of the L-asparaginase of guinea pig serum in relation to those of the antilymphoma substance. J Exp Med. 1963;118:99-120.
8. Old LJ, Boyse EA, Campbell HA, et al. Leukaemia-inhibiting properties and L-asparaginase activity of sera from certain South American rodents. Nature. 1963;198:801.
9. Mashburn LT, Wriston JC. Tumor inhibitory effect of l-asparaginase from escherichia coli. Arch Biochem Biophys. 1964;105:450-2.
10. Oettgen HF, Old LJ, Boyse EA, et al. Inhibition of leukemias in man by L-asparaginase. Cancer Res. 1967;27(12):2619-31.
11. Hill MJ, Roberts J, Loeb E, et al. L-asparaginase therapy for leukemia and other malignant neoplasms. Remission in human leukemia. JAMA. 1967;202(9):882-8.
12. Ohnuma T, Holland JF, Nagel G, et al. Effects of L-asparaginase in acute myelocytic leukemia. JAMA. 1969;210(10):1919-21.
13. Beard ME, Crowther D, Galton DA, et al. L-asparaginase in treatment of acute leukaemia and lymphosarcoma. Br Med J.1970;1:191-5.
14. Wise DR, Thompson CB. Glutamine addiction: a new therapeutic target in cancer. Trends Biochem Sci. 2010;35(8):427-33.
15. Worthington Enzyme Manual. Available from: www.worthington-biochem.com/aspr/default. html. [Accessed August 2013].
16. Available from: http://www.bio.davidson.edu/Courses/Molbio/MolStudents/spring2005/ Champaloux/total_membrane.gif. [Accessed August 2013].
17. Haskell CM, Canellos GP. l-asparaginase resistance in human leukemia—asparagine synthetase. Biochem Pharmacol. 1969;18(10):2578-80.
18. Cooney DA, Handschumacher RE. L-asparaginase and L-asparagine metabolism. Annu Rev Pharmacol. 1970;10:421-40.
19. Alslanian AM, Kilberg MS. Multiple adaptive mechanisms affect asparagine synthetase substrate availability in asparaginase-resistant MOLT-4 human leukaemia cells. Biochem J. 2001;358:59-67.
20. Appel IM, den Boer M, Meijerink JP, et al. Up-regulation of asparagine synthetase expression is not linked to the clinical response L-asparaginase in pediatric acute lymphoblastic leukemia. Blood. 2006;107(11):4244-9.

21. Nandy P, Periclou AP, Avramis VI. The synergism of 6-mercaptopurine plus cytosine arabinoside followed by PEG-asparaginase in human leukemia cell lines (CCRF/CEM/0 and (CCRF/CEM/ara-C/7A) is due to increased cellular apoptosis. *Anticancer Res.* 1998; 18(2A):727-37.

22. Stock W, Douer D, DeAngelo DJ, et al. Prevention and management of asparaginase/pegasparaginase-associated toxicities in adults and older adolescents: recommendations of an expert panel. *Leuk Lymphoma.* 2011;52(12):2237-53.

23. Hoelzer D, Thiel E, Loffler H, et al. Prognostic factors in a multicenter study for treatment of acute lymphoblastic leukemia in adults. *Blood.* 1988;71(1):123-31.

24. Kantarjian H, Thomas D, O'Brien S, et al. Long-term follow-up results of hyperfractionated cyclophosphamide, vincristine, doxorubicin, and dexamethasone (Hyper-CVAD), a dose-intensive regimen, in adult acute lymphocytic leukemia. *Cancer.* 2004;101(12):2788-801.

25. Goekbuget N, Arnold R, Buechner T, et al. Intensification of induction and consolidation improves only subgroups of adult ALL: analysis of 1200 patients in GMALL study 05/03. *Blood.* 2001;98:802 [Abstract].

26. Larson RA, Dodge RK, Burns CP, et al. A five-drug remission induction regimen with intensive consolidation for adults with acute lymphoblastic leukemia: cancer and leukemia group B study 8811. *Blood.* 1995;85(8):2025-37.

27. Goldstone AH, Richards SM, Lazarus HM. In adults with standard-risk acute lymphoblastic leukemia, the greatest benefit is achieved from a matched sibling allogeneic transplantation in first complete remission, and an autologous transplantation is less effective than conventional consolidation/maintenance chemotherapy in all patients: final results of the International ALL Trial (MRC UKALL XII/ECOG E2993). *Blood.* 2008;111(4):1827-33.

28. Sallan SE, Hitchcock-Bryan S, Gelber R. Influence of intensive asparaginase in the treatment of childhood non-T-cell acute lymphoblastic leukemia. *Cancer Res.* 1983;43(11):5601-7.

29. Sallan SE, Gelber RD, Kimball V, et al. More is better! Update of Dana-Farber Cancer Institute/Children's Hospital childhood acute lymphoblastic leukemia trials. *Haemotol Blood Transfus.* 1990;33:459-66.

30. Silverman LB, Gelber RD, Dalton VK, et al. Improved outcome for children with acute lymphoblastic leukemia: results of Dana-Farber Consortium Protocol 91-01. *Blood.* 2001; 97(5):1211-8.

31. Stock W, La M, Sanford B, et al. What determines the outcomes for adolescents and young adults with acute lymphoblastic leukemia treated on cooperative group protocols? A comparison of Children's Cancer Group and Cancer and Leukemia Group B studies. *Blood.* 2008;112(5):1646-54.

32. de Bont JM, Holt Bv, Dekker AW, et al. Significant difference in outcome for adolescents with acute lymphoblastic leukemia treated on pediatric vs adult protocols in the Netherlands. *Leukemia.* 2004;18(12):2032-35.

33. Childhood ALL Collaborative Group. Duration and intensity of maintenance chemotherapy in acute lymphoblastic leukaemia: overview of 42 trials involving 12,000 randomised children. *Lancet.* 1996;347(9018):1783-8.

34. Boissel N, Auclerc MF, Lhéritier V, et al. Should adolescents with acute lymphoblastic leukemia be treated as old children or young adults? Comparison of the French FRALLE-93 and LALA-94 trials. *J Clin Oncol.* 2003;21(5):774-80.

35. Ramanujachar R, Richards S, Hann I, et al. Adolescents with acute lymphoblastic leukaemia: outcome on UK national paediatric (ALL97) and adult (UKALLXII/E2993) trials. *Pediatr Blood Cancer.* 2007;48(3):254-61.

36. Hallböök H, Gustafsson G, Smedmyr B, et al. Treatment outcome in young adults and children > 10 years of age with acute lymphoblastic leukemia in Sweden: a comparison between a pediatric protocol and an adult protocol. *Cancer.* 2006;107(7):1551-61.

37. Ertel IJ, Nesbit ME, Hammond D, et al. Effective dose of L-asparaginase for induction of remission in previously treated children with acute lymphocytic leukemia: a report from Childrens Cancer Study Group. *Cancer Res.* 1979;39(10):3893-6.

38. Nesbit M, Chard R, Evans A, et al. Evaluation of intramuscular versus intravenous administration of L-asparaginase in childhood leukemia. *Am J Pediatr Hematol/Oncol.* 1979;1(1):9-13.

39. Evans WE, Tsiatis A, Rivera G, et al. Anaphylactoid reactions to *Escherichia coli* and *Erwinia asparaginase* in children with leukemia and lymphoma. *Cancer.* 1982;49(7):1378-83.

40. Abshire TC, Pollock BH, Billett AL, et al. Weekly polyethylene glycol conjugated L-asparaginase compared with biweekly dosing produces superior induction remission rates in childhood relapsed acute lymphoblastic leukemia: a Pediatric Oncology Group Study. *Blood.* 2000;96(5):1709-15.

41. Wetzler M, Sanford BL, Kurtzberg J, et al. Effective asparagine depletion with pegylated asparaginase results in improved outcomes in adult acute lymphoblastic leukemia: Cancer and Leukemia Group B Study 9511. *Blood.* 2007;109(10):4164-67.

42. Avramis VI, Holcenberg JS, Ettinger AG, et al. Failure of asparagine (ASN) depletion, not in adequate asparaginase (ASNase) activity, predicts relapse in standard risk (SR) chilldhood acute lymphoblastic leukemia (ALL): A Children's Oncology Group (COG) report. *Blood.* 2007;110:588 [Abstract].

43. Larson RA, Fretzin MH, Dodge RK, et al. Hypersensitivity reactions to L-asparaginase do not impact on the remission duration of adults with acute lymphoblastic leukemia. *Leukemia.* 1998;12(5):660-5.

44. Woo MH, Hak LJ, Storm MC, et al. Hypersensitivity or development of antibodies to asparaginase does not impact treatment outcome of childhood acute lymphoblastic leukemia. *J Clin Oncol.* 2000;18(7):1525-32.

45. Panosyan EH, Seibel NL, Martin-Aragon S, et al. Asparaginase antibody and asparaginase activity in children with higher-risk acute lymphoblastic leukemia: Children's Cancer Group Study CCG-1961. *J Pediatr Hematol/Oncol.* 2004;26(4):217-26.

46. Pession A, Valsecchi MG, Masera G, et al. Long-term results of a randomized trial on extended use of high dose L-asparaginase for standard risk childhood acute lymphoblastic leukemia. *J Clin Oncol.* 2005;23(28):7161-7.

47. Nachman JB, Sather HN, Sensel MG, et al. Augmented post-induction therapy for children with high-risk acute lymphoblastic leukemia and a slow response to initial therapy. *N Engl J Med.* 1998;338(23):1663-71.

48. Nachman JB, Sather HN, Gaynon PS, et al. Augmented Berlin-Frankfurt-Munster therapy abrogates the adverse prognostic significance of slow early response to induction chemo-therapy for children and adolescents with acute lymphoblastic leukemia and unfavorable presenting features: a report from the Children's Cancer Group. *J Clin Oncol.* 1997;15(6):2222-30.

49. Schrappe M, Reiter A, Ludwig WD, et al. Improved outcome in childhood acute lymphoblastic leukemia despite reduced use of anthracyclines and cranial radiotherapy: results of trial ALL-BFM 90. German-Austrian-Swiss ALL-BFM Study Group. *Blood.* 2000;95(11):3310-22.

50. Reiter A, Schrappe M, Ludwig WD, et al. Chemotherapy in 998 unselected childhood acute lymphoblastic leukemia patients. Results and conclusions of the multicenter trial ALL-BFM 86. *Blood.* 1994;84(9):3122-33.

51. Seibel NL, Steinherz PG, Sather HN, et al. Early postinduction intensification therapy improves survival for children and adolescents with high-risk acute lymphoblastic leukemia: a report from the Children's Oncology Group. *Blood.* 2008;111(5):2548-55.

52. Duval M, Suciu S, Ferster A, et al. Comparison of Escherichia coli-asparaginase with Erwinia-asparaginase in the treatment of childhood lymphoid malignancies: results of a randomized

European Organisation for Research and Treatment of Cancer-Children's Leukemia Group phase 3 trial. *Blood.* 2002;99(8):2734-9.

53. Moghrabi A, Levy DE, Asselin B, et al. Results of the Dana-Farber Cancer Institute ALL Consortium Protocol 95-01 for children with acute lymphoblastic leukemia. *Blood.* 2007; 109(3):896-904.

54. Douer D, Yampolsky H, Cohen LJ, et al. Pharmacodynamics and safety of intravenous pegaspargase during remission induction in adults aged 55 years or younger with newly diagnosed acute lymphoblastic leukemia. *Blood.* 2007;109(7):2744-50.

55. Douer D, Aldoss I, Lunning M, et al. Pharmacokinetics-based modifications of intravenous pegylated asparaginase dosing in the context of a "pediatric-inpired" protocol in adults with newly diagnosed acute lymphoblastic leukemia (ALL). *Blood.* 2012;120:1495 [Abstract].

56. DeAngelo DJ, Dahlberg S, Silverman LB, et al. A multicenter phase II study using a dose intensified pediatric regimen in adults with untreated acute lymphoblastic leukemia. *Blood.* 2007;110:587 [Abstract].

CHAPTER 9 — Monitoring of Minimal Residual Disease to Guide Therapy of Acute Lymphoblastic Leukemia

Allen EJ Yeoh, Dario Campana

INTRODUCTION

In patients with acute lymphoblastic leukemia (ALL), risk of relapse is closely related to the degree of resistance to initial treatment. This relationship was already noted during the initial efforts to treat childhood ALL with a curative, rather than a palliative intent.[1] Subsequent studies found that relapse occurred more frequently among patients with a higher number of residual lymphoblasts in peripheral blood after 7 days of prednisone (PRED)[2] or multiagent remission-induction therapy,[3] or residual lymphoblasts in bone marrow after 1 or 2 weeks of therapy.[4,5] However, a considerable number of relapses occurred in patients believed to be good responders by the above morphologic criteria, suggesting that a better risk discrimination might be achievable with the application of more sensitive and reliable methods to measure residual disease. Moreover, detecting relapse before it becomes clinically apparent may allow a more timely switch to more intensive therapy or allogeneic hematopoietic stem cell transplant, which intuitively might be more effective when the residual tumor burden is low.

The above considerations provided the rational framework for the development of methods to monitor minimal residual disease (MRD), a terminology that indicates leukemic cells not detectable by conventional morphology. The expectation was that a proportion of patients considered to be in remission by morphology would have MRD, and that MRD should be prognostically important. During the early days of MRD studies, the latter prediction was not embraced by many who believed that leukemia distribution during treatment was very heterogeneous and that this would lead to variable and ultimately uninformative MRD estimates. Others thought that low levels of leukemia might persist during remission but remain under immunosurveillance, rendering prognostication based on MRD measurements unreliable. Despite these apprehensions, some investigators went ahead and took advantage of new technologies, such as cell marker analysis or polymerase chain reaction (PCR), to explore the remission status of patients with ALL and demonstrated that the initial predictions were correct.

The history of MRD in ALL starts in the late 1970s to early 1980s. Thus, its development extends over three decades and parallels the evolution of technologies for cellular and genetic analyses. The first original article that reported detection of "MRD" in ALL was published by George Janossy, Ken Bradstock, and their colleagues working at the Royal Free Hospital in London.[6] These authors had noticed that a feature of T-lineage ALL lymphoblasts was the simultaneous expression of terminal deoxynucleotidyl transferase (TdT) and T-cell antigens and that this immunophenotype was absent in the bone marrow of healthy donors. With great insight, they applied these markers (using polyclonal antisera and fluorescence microscopy) to search for MRD in 18 patients with T-lineage ALL and detected it in 6 patients. Immunologic analysis of MRD evolved from this pioneering finding through the development of monoclonal antibodies and flow cytometry,[7,8] to the current state-of-the-art which relies on analyzing a multiplicity of cell markers with extremely sophisticated instruments. Another momentous event in the history of MRD was the development of PCR, which was swiftly applied to detect genetic abnormalities,[9,10] and clonal rearrangements of T-cell receptor (TCR) and immunoglobulin (Ig) genes.[11-13] Collectively, studies of MRD in patients with ALL have shown that (1) post-treatment samples considered to be in morphologic remission can conceal a variable amount of leukemic cells, and (2) levels of MRD predict the risk of relapse. In this chapter, we discuss MRD methodologies and their clinical application in childhood and adult ALL.

MONITORING MRD BY FLOW CYTOMETRY

Methodologic Notes

Acute lymphoblastic leukemia cells express cell marker profiles which are different from those expressed by normal hematopoietic cells, and therefore, can be used to identify MRD. In T-lineage ALL, leukemic lymphoblasts can be distinguished by the expression of a T-cell precursor immunophenotype characterized by terminal TdT and/or cluster of differentiation (CD) 34 together with T-cell markers, such as CD3 and/or CD5.[14,15] This T-cell precursor immunophenotype is not expressed by normal peripheral blood and bone marrow cells. To this basic marker combination, one can add other T-cell markers, e.g., CD99.[16]

In cases of B-lineage ALL, the main task is to distinguish leukemic cells from normal B-cell progenitors, which are normally present in the bone marrow, and can be particularly abundant in children and in samples recovering after chemotherapy.[17-19] Indeed, B-lineage ALL cells express such distinctive profiles in the majority of cases.[14,20,21] Among the 422 children and adolescents with newly diagnosed ALL enrolled in the St Jude Total XV study, 418 (99.1%) had a leukemia expressing immunophenotypes that allowed monitoring MRD with a sensitivity of 1 leukemic cell among 10,000 normal mononucleated cells.[22] New markers, which are potentially useful for MRD monitoring in B-lineage ALL, have been reported.[23,24] Using gene expression arrays to identify differences between normal and leukemic cells, an early study pointed to CD58 as a useful marker for MRD studies in B-lineage ALL,[25] a finding that was confirmed by others leading to its wide adoption as MRD marker.[26-28] In a more recent study, the genome-wide gene expression of lymphoblasts from 270 patients with newly diagnosed B-lineage ALL was compared to that of normal CD19+CD10+ B-cell progenitors.[29] Expression of 30 genes differentially expressed by greater than or equal to threefold was then tested by flow cytometry in 200 B-lineage ALL and 61 nonleukemic bone marrow samples, including bone marrow samples recovering from chemotherapy. Twenty two of the thirty markers were differentially expressed in up to 81.4% of ALL cases.[29] Results of MRD detection by flow cytometry with these markers correlated with those of PCR testing, and sequential studies during treatment and diagnosis-relapse comparisons documented their stability.[29] The availability of these new markers, which are now incorporated into our routine panels for MRD monitoring, allows us to take full advantage of modern flow cytometers which can detect eight or more markers simultaneously, producing a better discrimination between normal and leukemic cells, and consequently a more reliable and sensitive assay.

After the first 2–3 weeks of remission-induction therapy, bone marrow samples typically become devoid of B-cell precursors.[30] This situation can be exploited to monitor MRD with a simplified panel of markers, consisting only of CD19, CD34, and CD10. This idea was tested by comparing the results obtained with the simplified panel with those obtained by flow cytometric detection of aberrant immunophenotypes selected according to the immunophenotype of leukemic cells at diagnosis. Discordant results were seen in only 4 (1.1%) of the 376 samples, in which the simplified panel detected CD19+ cells expressing CD10 and/or CD34 (0.35%; range, 0.04–0.47%), while the full panel showed that these were normal B-cell progenitors.[30] This basic assay, which has low cost and yields results that are relatively simple to analyze, is now used by several laboratories worldwide to measure early treatment response. However, it must be emphasized that the assay should not be used at other times during or after treatments because normal B-cell progenitors will be present invalidating the rationale for the test.

The process for MRD monitoring by flow cytometry starts at diagnosis when leukemia-associated immunophenotypes are identified in each patient. Although MRD studies can be done by applying a universal panel of markers with no information about the immunophenotype of the leukemic cells at diagnosis,[31] negative MRD results are difficult to interpret under these circumstances. Nevertheless, with the plethora of markers currently available to distinguish ALL cells, further studies are warranted as diagnostic material may not always be available. The sensitivity of MRD detection by flow cytometry is dictated by the degree of immunophenotypic differences between leukemic and normal cells in each case, and by the number of cells available for analysis. The typical sensitivity achievable routinely is 1 leukemic cell in 10,000 normal cells.[14] However, with the availability of large antibody panels, the sensitivity can potentially increase to 1 in 100,000 in many cases.

Correlations with Treatment Outcome

During the last 15 years, there have been numerous studies that demonstrated the prognostic significance of measuring MRD by flow cytometry in childhood ALL. These studies included patients with newly diagnosed[32-39] or relapsed ALL,[40,41] as well as recipients of allogeneic hematopoietic stem cell transplant.[42,43]

To determine the prognostic significance of MRD in children with newly diagnosed ALL, a prospective study collected MRD results, which were not communicated to treating physicians, and hence were not used to guide treatment intensity. Among the 195 patients enrolled in the St Jude Total XIII study, MRD levels greater than or equal to 0.01% in bone marrow on days 19, 46, or later intervals were strongly associated with a higher risk of relapse.[32-34] MRD remained a significant prognostic factor after adjusting for presenting features and for levels of peripheral blood lymphoblasts after the first week of remission-induction therapy.[33] In a subsequent trial (St Jude Total XV), MRD was used to guide intensity of therapy. Nevertheless, detection of MRD greater than or equal to 0.01% on day 19 and at the end of remission-induction therapy remained significant adverse prognostic factors, and MRD greater than or equal to 1% at the end of remission induction was a major independent adverse prognosticator.[22]

A large correlative study between MRD and outcome analyzed bone marrow samples collected at the end of remission induction (day 29) from 1,971 patients with newly diagnosed B-lineage ALL enrolled in the 9,900 series trials of the Children's Oncology Group (COG).[36] Levels of MRD correlated with adverse outcome. Thus, 5-year event-free survival was 59% ± 5% for patients with MRD 0.01–0.1% (n = 175), 49% ± 6% for those with 0.1–1% MRD (n = 141) and 30% ± 8% for those with greater than or equal to 1% (n = 67), in contrast to 88% ± 1% for patients with undetectable MRD (n = 1,588).[36] In another large study, MRD was analyzed on day 15 of treatment in 830 patients enrolled in the Associazione Italiana Ematologia Oncologia Pediatrica (AIEOP)-Berlin-Frankfurt-Münster (BFM) ALL 2000 study.[37] The preceding treatment consisted of 14 days of steroids, and one dose of vincristine, daunorubicin, asparaginase, as well as intrathecal methotrexate. Three MRD-based risk groups were identified: (1) standard risk (SR) (<0.1% MRD; 42%); (2) intermediate risk (IR) (0.1% ≤10% MRD; 47%); and (3) high risk (HR) (≥10%; 11%) with a 5-year cumulative incidence of relapse of 8%, 18% and 47%, respectively.[37]

Correlative studies between MRD detected by flow cytometry and treatment outcome have also been performed in adult patients, indicating the clinical importance of monitoring MRD in this setting.[20,44-48] Thus, Vidriales et al.[45] found that MRD on day 35 of treatment independently predicted relapse-free survival among 102 adolescents and adults with ALL. Among 53 patients with T-lineage ALL enrolled in the Italian cooperative GIMEMA (Gruppo Italiano Malattie Ematologiche dell'Adulto) LAL0496 protocol, probability of relapse was significantly related to MRD measured at different TP during treatment.[46] Among 116 patients with Philadelphia-negative ALL enrolled in the Polish Adult Leukemia Group ALL 4-2002 study, MRD greater than or equal to 0.1% after remission-induction therapy was an independent predictor for relapse.[47] Giebel et al.[48] analyzed the results of autologous hematopoietic stem cell transplant according to MRD as measured by flow cytometry at the time of transplant in 79 adult patients with ALL. They found that among Philadelphia-negative ALL, the 5-year probability of leukemia-free survival at 5 years was 58% for MRD less than 0.1% patients versus 17% for patients with higher MRD levels.

MONITORING MRD BY PCR
Methodologic Notes

Gene translocations are distinguishing traits of leukemic cells and can be amplified by PCR. The most common abnormalities that are targeted for MRD monitoring are transcript of gene fusions, including BCR-ABL1, MLL-AFF1, TCF3-PBX1, and ETV6-RUNX1.[49] Such aberrant transcripts are suitable targets for MRD monitoring in approximately 40% of children and 50% of adults with ALL, although this percentages may increase if less frequent transcripts are also targeted. More recently, identified gene fusions, such as immunoglobulin heavy chain locus (IGH@) to cytokine receptor-like factor 2 (CRLF2) and P2RY8-CRLF2, which are found in about half of ALL patients with Down syndrome, and in approximately 15% of adult ALL and of high-risk childhood B-lineage ALL cases lacking other fusion transcripts,[50-53] could also be included in the panels. The transcripts are typically amplified using "real-time" quantitative PCR (RQ-PCR) and the sensitivity of the assay is assessed by running mixtures of diagnostic leukemic and normal ribonucleic acid (RNA).[54,55] The sensitivity of detection that can be achieved with this method is around 1 leukemia cell in 10,000–100,000. A downside of using fusion transcripts as a target in MRD studies is that it is difficult to determine the level of MRD precisely due to the fact that the number of transcript copies per cell is unknown, and may vary from patient to patient and at different stages of the disease.

A hallmark of lymphoid cells, including leukemic lymphoblasts, is the rearrangement of Ig and TCR genes which can be used as a genetic fingerprint for MRD studies; RQ-PCR is widely used for their detection. The BIOMED-2 concerted action BMH4-CT98-3936 project optimized primers and methods, and issued guidelines for interpretation, thus setting standards for the use of these assays for MRD detection.[54,55] The junctional regions of these genes form a molecular sequence, which is unique to each clone, and can, therefore, be used as a target to monitor MRD. Typically, the identity of the clonal rearrangements in each leukemia is identified at diagnosis by sequencing the PCR product obtained with primers matched to the V and J regions of the Ig and TCR genes.[56] Then, matching junctional region-specific oligonucleotides, also called allele-specific oligonucleotides, are synthesized and used as primers for RQ-PCR in follow-up samples where MRD is quantified by comparing the signal to those of serial dilutions of leukemic and normal deoxyribonucleic acid (DNA).[56] The sensitivity of detection that can be achieved with RQ-PCR amplification of Ig and TCR genes is 1 leukemia cell in 10,000–100,000. In general, MRD quantification of Ig and TCR rearrangements is precise as DNA is stable and the target genes are represented in 1 copy per cell.[56]

The majority of B-lineage ALL cases have Ig gene rearrangements as well as cross-lineage TCR gene rearrangements.[57] The latter are rearranged in most cases of T-lineage ALL, while cross-lineage Ig gene rearrangements occur in approximately 20% of T-cell acute lymphocytic leukemia (T-ALL).[56] Among 3,341 diagnostic samples studied in the AIEOP-BFM ALL 2000 trial, only 88 (3%) did not have rearrangements and another 7% had sequences which were not sufficiently distinct to reach a sensitivity of at least 0.01%.[58] In a study performed in patients enrolled in St Jude Total Studies 13–15, 475 of 539 (88%) samples from patients with newly diagnosed B-lineage ALL had gene rearrangements suitable for PCR monitoring with a sensitivity of at least 0.001%.[59] Investigators had previously recommended to use at least two rearrangements with a potential sensitivity of 1 in 10,000 or more as a target to avoid the risk of false-negative results due to oligoclonality and clonal evolution.[58,60] However, this is rather a restrictive approach; it may limit the applicability of the assay and, ultimately, may not be necessary. To this end, BFM investigators showed that the prognosis of patients classified according to MRD results obtained by a 2-marker analysis was similar to those who had only one marker available.[61] In fact, the recently reported Ma-Spore (Malaysia-Singapore) 2003 trial, targeted a single rearrangement in each patient, and achieved effective risk-stratification and excellent clinical results with this simpler and less expensive approach.[62]

Correlations with Treatment Outcome

In ALL, systematic studies of MRD targeting fusion transcripts have been reported infrequently. Among 42 adult patients with Philadelphia-chromosome positive ALL, the 28 with greater than 2 log reduction of residual disease after induction and greater than 3 log reductions after consolidation therapy had a 2-year relapse-free survival 38% versus 0% for the 14 poor responders.[63] In a study of 100 patients with Philadelphia-positive ALL treated with imatinib-containing chemotherapy, MRD was monitored using RQ-PCR for BCR-ABL1 transcripts.[64] Although MRD levels at the end of induction therapy did not significantly correlate with relapse, increasing MRD levels at subsequent time points preceded relapse in 12 of the 13 patients who did not receive allogeneic hematopoietic stem cell transplant, while relapse occurred in 6 of the 16 who underwent transplant.[64] Wassmann et al.[65] studied 27 patients with Philadelphia chromosome-positive ALL who received imatinib upon detection of MRD after transplant. MRD became undetectable in 14 patients after 0.9–3.7 (median, 1.5) months, and remained in remission for the duration of imatinib treatment. By contrast, 12 of the 13 patients who failed to achieve MRD negativity relapsed. Madzo et al.[66] targeted ETV6-RUNX1 fusion transcripts in patients with this leukemia subtype at the end of remission-induction therapy: among the 55 patients studied, 41 were MRD negative and none developed a relapse, as compared to 4 relapses among the 14 patients who were MRD positive.

The experience of MRD monitoring targeting Ig and TCR receptor gene rearrangements is considerably wider, with numerous studies demonstrating its clinical significance in patients with newly diagnosed ALL,[58,59,61,62,67-82] as well as in patients who relapse and then achieve a second remission,[83,84] and in those receiving hematopoietic stem cell transplantation.[85-88] The largest study using this approach in childhood B-lineage ALL was reported by Conter et al.[61] who studied MRD in 3,184 patients with newly diagnosed ALL on days 33 and 78 of treatment and derived an MRD-based risk classification based on the results. Patients with MRD less than 0.01% at both time points (42%) had a 5-year event-free survival of 92%; this was 50% for those with MRD greater than or equal to 0.1% on day 78 (6%) and 78% for the remaining patients (52%). In a parallel study performed in 464 patients with T-lineage ALL, 16% were MRD less than 0.01% at both time points and had 7-year event-free survival of 91%; this was 50% and 81% for the other two groups (representing 21% and 63% of patients, respectively).[77] The Ma-Spore 2003 study used a similar criteria to build an MRD risk classification in 420 with newly diagnosed childhood ALL: 202 (36%) were good responders, 28 (5%) poor responders, and 190 (34%) had an intermediate MRD response; the 6-year event-free survival was 93%, 32%, and 84%, respectively.[62] In 455 patients with B-lineage ALL enrolled in St Jude Total 13–15 studies, MRD as detected by targeting Ig and TCR genes was an adverse prognostic factor. Moreover, patients with low levels of MRD (0.001% $\leq$ 0.01%; n = 63) had a significantly higher 5-year cumulative incidence of relapse (13%) than those with findings below 0.001% (n = 319) (5%).[59]

Studies in adult patients also demonstrated the informative potential of monitoring MRD by PCR amplification of antigen-receptor genes.[48,78,79,82] Bassan et al.[81] targeted either fusion transcripts or antigen-receptor gene rearrangements to monitor MRD at the end of consolidation in 112 adult patients with ALL, of whom 58 were MRD-negative and 54 MRD-positive. Five-year disease-free survival was 72% and 14%, respectively and MRD was the most significant risk factor for relapse.

This group of investigators used a similar approach to monitor MRD in patients undergoing transplantation: 3-year overall for the 12 patients transplanted while PCR-negative was 80% versus 49% for the 25 who were PCR-positive, and cumulative incidence of relapse was 0% and 46%, respectively.[80]

CLINICAL APPLICATION OF MRD MONITORING

Methodology

Each method for MRD monitoring has different characteristics, and hence different advantages and disadvantages (Table 9-1). Results of flow cytometry are usually in good concordance with those of PCR amplification of Ig/TCR genes when a

Table 9-1	Main Characteristics of Different Methods to Measure Minimal Residual Disease in ALL		
Characteristics	*Flow cytometry*	*PCR on fusion transcripts*	*PCR on Ig/TCR genes*
Sensitivity	0.01%	0.01–0.001%	0.01–0.001%
Percentage of patients	>98%	~40%	*B-lineage ALL:* • 1 target: >90% • 2 targets: ~74% *T-lineage ALL:* • 1 target: ~85% • 2 targets: ~65%
Sample stability	Cells viability decreases over time; samples must be processed within 24–48 hours	RNA highly unstable; needs to be processed within 6–12 hours of collection	DNA stable; samples must be processed transported within 3–4 days
Clonal evolution	Possible, hence the use of multiple markers	No	Possible, hence the use of >1 target
Standardization	Significant differences in sample preparation, markers and analysis by different groups	• Clinically meaningful cutoffs uncertain • BCR-ABL1 p210 standards for CML	Yes
Advantages	Precise quantification of MRD and information on sample composition and quality	Standard primer and PCR conditions for each fusion transcript	High sensitivity and precise quantification of MRD
Disadvantages	Requires high expertise to analyze results	• Plasmid contamination leading to false-positive results • Standard curve using cell line dilution is cumbersome • mRNA degradation leading to false-negative results	Time-consuming to sequence and construct patient-specific markers

ALL, acute lymphoblastic leukemia; PCR, polymerase chain reaction; Ig, immunoglobulin; TCR, T-cell receptor; RNA, ribonucleic acid; DNA, deoxyribonucleic acid; CML, chronic myeloid leukemia; MRD, minimal residual disease; mRNA, messenger RNA.

threshold of 0.01% to define MRD positivity is used.[89-91] Thus, in a study in which MRD was measured by both assays in 227 children with B-lineage ALL, MRD was less than 0.01% in 1,200 of 1,375 samples, and greater than or equal to 0.01% in 129 by both assays; MRD levels measured by the two methods were highly correlated.[89] Among the 46 samples with discordant results, 28 were MRD-positive by flow cytometry and less than 0.01% by PCR but PCR was nevertheless positive at lower levels in 26 of these samples. In the remaining 18 samples, MRD was greater than or equal to 0.01% by PCR but negative by flow cytometry, although in 8 samples (of the 9 in which markers allowed a sensitivity higher than 1 in 10,000), cells with aberrant immunophenotypes were detectable at level lower than 0.01%.[89]

Definitive comparisons between results of MRD studies targeting fusion transcripts and other techniques have not been performed. Metzler et al.[92] compared MRD results of ETV6-RUNX1 fusion transcripts and antigen-receptor gene rearrangements in 12 patients with t(12;21)-positive ALL. In 10 patients, there was concordance of results, while in 2 had persistence of ETV6-RUNX1 with MRD negative Ig/TCR and remaining in complete remission (CR). Zaliova et al.[93] compared results of MRD targeting BCR-ABL1 transcripts Ig/TCR PCR method in 218 samples from 17 children with Philadelphia chromosome-positive ALL and found a rather poor correlation between the two methods; 20% of the sample studies were negative by Ig/TCR gene rearrangements but positive for the fusion transcript.

While flow cytometry is broadly available, only a minority of laboratories has the necessary expertise to perform MRD studies correctly. To this end, there are efforts to improve the currently available software to facilitate the discrimination between normal and leukemic cells. For example, pattern classification algorithms have been applied to automatically discriminate leukemic cells from normal peripheral blood B-cells,[94] and hierarchical clustering analysis has been used in to measure MRD in ALL.[95] There are much fewer laboratories that can perform MRD studies based on PCR amplification of Ig/TCR genes. Because specific PCR primers need to be developed for each patient and PCR assay conditions need to be individually optimized, the process is generally laborious and precludes timely measurements of MRD at early time intervals, such as day 15. However, it is now possible to use consensus primers to amplify all rearranged Ig or TCR segments at diagnosis, subject the amplified product to high-throughput parallel sequencing, and then track the leukemic clones during follow-up by applying the same method.[96-98] The early results obtained with this technology indicate great reliability and potential for outstanding sensitivity.

Tailoring Treatment According to MRD

The time intervals at which MRD is measured vary according to protocol. For childhood ALL, protocols at St Jude Children's Research Hospital typically measure MRD in bone marrow after 2 and 6 weeks of treatment;[22] protocols of the COGs measure MRD in peripheral blood on day 8 and in bone marrow on day 29;[36] those of the AIEOP-BFM group traditionally measure MRD in bone marrow on days 33 and 78.[61,77] The usefulness of measuring MRD beyond the initial phases of treatment is somewhat less well established. In general, MRD positive patients at the end of remission should be closely monitored as conversion to MRD negativity is associated with a favorable outcome while persistence of MRD almost invariably predicts relapse.[33] In patients with T-lineage ALL, subsequent monitoring can be performed in peripheral blood instead of bone marrow as levels are typically equivalent in either tissue in this subtype of ALL.[99,100]

Although MRD is often used to select candidates for more intensive therapy and/ or transplant, it can also be used to identify patients who can be treated with less intensive therapy thus reducing treatment toxicity. For example, in the Ma-Spore ALL 2003 study, 30% of patients who cleared their MRD below 0.01%, had reduced high-dose methotrexate from 5 g/m^2 to 2 g/m^2 for all the four courses, and had two instead of three blocks of chemotherapy during reinduction (Figure 9-1).[62]

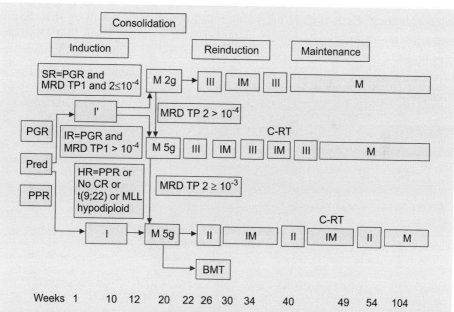

SR, standard risk; PGR, prednisone good responder; MRD, minimal residual disease; TP, time points; IM, interim maintenance; IR, intermediate risk; PRED, prednisone; HR, high risk; CR, complete remission; PPR, prednisone poor responder; MLL, mixed-lineage leukemia; C-RT, cranial radiation therapy; BMT, bone marrow transplantation.

Figure 9-1 Schematic representation of the Ma-Spore (Malaysia-Singapore) 2003 treatment protocol which incorporated minimal residual disease (MRD) for risk stratification. *Reproduced from:* Yeoh AE, Ariffin H, Chai EL, et al. Minimal residual disease-guided treatment deintensification for children with acute lymphoblastic leukemia: results from the Malaysia-Singapore acute lymphoblastic leukemia 2003 study. *J Clin Oncol.* 2012;30(19):2384-92, *with permission.*

These patients had an excellent 6-year event-free survival of 93%. MRD is the most important prognostic factor in childhood ALL but presenting clinical features, such as age, leukocyte count, and cytogenetics can help refine risk assignment strategies. In our current Ma-Spore ALL 2010 study, patients older than 9 years of age or younger than 1 year, do not receive further deintensification of therapy despite rapid clearance of MRD to less than 0.01% at week 5.

SUMMARY

Minimal residual disease testing is now widely used for risk assignment in ALL. Table 9-2 shows an example of how MRD can be applied to the treatment of childhood ALL. It should be noted, however, that the clinical significance of an MRD test depends on the treatment context and it is difficult to directly extrapolate MRD applications from one protocol to another. Moreover, for a group of patients who retain high levels of MRD after initial therapy, current treatment is inadequate and relapse rates are high. For example, children who failed to clear MRD by week 12 in the Ma-Spore 2003 study, 6-year event-free survival was only 32% despite treatment intensification.[62] Nevertheless, early identification of these patients by MRD testing and subsequent allogeneic hematopoietic stem cell transplant in first remission may improve outcome.[22,43] Regardless, these patients are candidates for innovative therapies that can either eradicate MRD or reduce leukemia cell load prior to transplant.

Table 9-2	An Example of Risk Classification for Childhood ALL Incorporating Minimal Residual Disease and Treatment Action		
	Standard risk (SR)	*High risk (HR)*	*Intermediate risk (IR)*
Presenting features	B-lineage with: • Age 1 years to <10 years • WBC <50 × 10⁹/L • No unfavorable genetics	Unfavorable genetics (BCR-ABL1, hypodiploidy <45 chromosomes, MLL gene rearrangements, or IKZF1 deletions)	All others
MRD (depending on protocol type)	<0.01% on weeks 2 and 6 (St Jude), day 29 (COG), weeks 5 and 12 (AIEOP-BFM, Ma-Spore)	≥1% on week 6 (St Jude), on day 29 (COG); ≥0.1% on week 12 (AIEOP-BFM, Ma-Spore)	All others
Treatment action	Possible treatment deintensification (e.g. reduced anthracyclines, lower methotrexate dose)	Treatment intensification, allogeneic hematopoietic stem cell transplant, novel agents to reduce leukemia burden	Standard treatment

ALL, acute lymphoblastic leukemia; WBC, white blood count; MLL, mixed-lineage leukemia; IKZF1, Ikaros family zinc finger 1; MRD, minimal residual disease; COG, Children's Oncology Group; AIEOP, Associazione Italiana Ematologia Oncologia Pediatrica; BFM, Berlin-Frankfurt-Münster; Ma-Spore, Malaysia-Singapore.

A less used but probably equally important role of MRD risk assignment is to accurately identify low-risk patients who could be offered reduced intensity of therapy. Although improvement of supportive care and availability of new antifungal agents in developed countries can handle treatment, related complications of contemporary high-intensity therapy, the costs and risk of late effects are increasing. For countries with more limited resources, treatment-related morbidity and mortality eliminates any improvement in overall survival seen in developed countries. MRD monitoring including simplified flow cytometric testing,[30] or single PCR-based marker targeting Ig/TCR rearrangements[62] should be sufficient to identify candidates for reduced intensity therapy.

In conclusion, MRD studies have transformed prognostication and protocol design in childhood ALL, and are being progressively introduced in treatment schemas for adult ALL.[101] They can also refine eligibility criteria for novel agents, and provide surrogate end-points for activity.[102] They are a key step toward a highly customized, and hence more effective, treatment for patients with ALL.

REFERENCES

1. Jacquillat C, Weil M, Gemon MF, et al. Combination therapy in 130 patients with acute lymphoblastic leukemia (protocol 06 LA 66-Paris). *Cancer Res.* 1973;33(12):3278-84.
2. Möricke A, Zimmermann M, Reiter A, et al. Long-term results of five consecutive trials in childhood acute lymphoblastic leukemia performed by the ALL-BFM study group from 1981 to 2000. *Leukemia.* 2010;24(2):265-84.
3. Gajjar A, Ribeiro R, Hancock ML, et al. Persistence of circulating blasts after 1 week of multiagent chemotherapy confers a poor prognosis in childhood acute lymphoblastic leukemia. *Blood.* 1995;86(4):1292-5.
4. Steinherz PG, Gaynon PS, Breneman JC, et al. Cytoreduction and prognosis in acute lymphoblastic leukemia—the importance of early marrow response: report from the Children's Cancer Group. *J Clin Oncol.* 1996;14(2):389-98.
5. Schultz KR, Massing B, Spinelli JJ, et al. Importance of the day 7 bone marrow biopsy as a prognostic measure of the outcome in children with acute lymphoblastic leukemia. *Med Pediatr Oncol.* 1997;29(1):16-22.
6. Bradstock KF, Janossy G, Tidman N, et al. Immunological monitoring of residual disease in treated thymic acute lymphoblastic leukaemia. *Leuk Res.* 1981;5(4-5):301-9.
7. Hurwitz CA, Loken MR, Graham ML, et al. Asynchronous antigen expression in B lineage acute lymphoblastic leukemia. *Blood.* 1988;72(1):299-307.
8. Campana D, Coustan-Smith E, Janossy G. The immunologic detection of minimal residual disease in acute leukemia. *Blood.* 1990;76(1):163-71.
9. Kawasaki ES, Clark SS, Coyne MY, et al. Diagnosis of chronic myeloid and acute lymphocytic leukemias by detection of leukemia-specific mRNA sequences amplified in vitro. *Proc Natl Acad Sci U S A.* 1988;85(15):5698-702.
10. Hermans A, Gow J, Selleri L, et al. BCR-ABL oncogene activation in Philadelphia chromosome-positive acute lymphoblastic leukemia. *Leukemia.* 1988;2(10):628-33.
11. d'Auriol L, Macintyre E, Galibert F, et al. In vitro amplification of T cell gamma gene rearrangements: a new tool for the assessment of minimal residual disease in acute lymphoblastic leukemias. *Leukemia.* 1989;3(2):155-8.
12. Hansen-Hagge TE, Yokota S, Bartram CR. Detection of minimal residual disease in acute lymphoblastic leukemia by in vitro amplification of rearranged T-cell receptor delta chain sequences. *Blood.* 1989;74(5):1762-7.

13. Yamada M, Hudson S, Tournay O, et al. Detection of minimal disease in hematopoietic malignancies of the B-cell lineage by using third-complementarity-determining region (CDR-III)-specific probes. *Proc Natl Acad Sci U S A*. 1989;86(13):5123-7.

14. Campana D, Coustan-Smith E. Detection of minimal residual disease in acute leukemia by flow cytometry. *Cytometry*. 1999;38(4):139-52.

15. Campana D. Minimal residual disease monitoring in childhood acute lymphoblastic leukemia. *Curr Opin Hematol*. 2012;19(4):313-8.

16. Dworzak MN, Fröschl G, Printz D, et al. CD99 expression in T-lineage ALL: implications for flow cytometric detection of minimal residual disease. *Leukemia*. 2004;18(4):703-8.

17. Rimsza LM, Larson RS, Winter SS, et al. Benign hematogone-rich lymphoid proliferations can be distinguished from B-lineage acute lymphoblastic leukemia by integration of morphology, immunophenotype, adhesion molecule expression, and architectural features. *Am J Clin Pathol*. 2000;114(1):66-75.

18. van Wering ER, van der Linden-Schrever BE, Szczepański T, et al. Regenerating normal B-cell precursors during and after treatment of acute lymphoblastic leukaemia: implications for monitoring of minimal residual disease. *Br J Haematol*. 2000;110(1):139-46.

19. McKenna RW, Washington LT, Aquino DB, et al. Immunophenotypic analysis of hematogones (B-lymphocyte precursors) in 662 consecutive bone marrow specimens by 4-color flow cytometry. *Blood*. 2001;98(8):2498-507.

20. Ciudad J, San Miguel JF, López-Berges MC, et al. Prognostic value of immunophenotypic detection of minimal residual disease in acute lymphoblastic leukemia. *J Clin Oncol*. 1998;16(12):3774-81.

21. Lucio P, Gaipa G, van Lochem EG, et al. BIOMED-I concerted action report: flow cytometric immunophenotyping of precursor B-ALL with standardized triple-stainings. BIOMED-1 Concerted Action Investigation of Minimal Residual Disease in Acute Leukemia: International Standardization and Clinical Evaluation. *Leukemia*. 2001;15(8):1185-92.

22. Pui CH, Campana D, Pei D, et al. Treating childhood acute lymphoblastic leukemia without cranial irradiation. *N Engl J Med*. 2009;360(26):2730-41.

23. Muzzafar T, Medeiros LJ, Wang SA, et al. Aberrant underexpression of CD81 in precursor B-cell acute lymphoblastic leukemia: utility in detection of minimal residual disease by flow cytometry. *Am J Clin Pathol*. 2009;132(5):692-8.

24. DiGiuseppe JA, Fuller SG, Borowitz MJ. Overexpression of CD49f in precursor B-cell acute lymphoblastic leukemia: potential usefulness in minimal residual disease detection. *Cytometry B Clin Cytom*. 2009;76(2):150-5.

25. Chen JS, Coustan-Smith E, Suzuki T, et al. Identification of novel markers for monitoring minimal residual disease in acute lymphoblastic leukemia. *Blood*. 2001;97(7):2115-20.

26. Veltroni M, De Zen L, Sanzari MC, et al. Expression of CD58 in normal, regenerating and leukemic bone marrow B cells: implications for the detection of minimal residual disease in acute lymphocytic leukemia. *Haematologica*. 2003;88(11):1245-52.

27. Lee RV, Braylan RC, Rimsza LM. CD58 expression decreases as nonmalignant B cells mature in bone marrow and is frequently overexpressed in adult and pediatric precursor B-cell acute lymphoblastic leukemia. *Am J Clin Pathol*. 2005;123(1):119-24.

28. Mejstríková E, Fronková E, Kalina T, et al. Detection of residual B precursor lymphoblastic leukemia by uniform gating flow cytometry. *Pediatr Blood Cancer*. 2010;54(1):62-70.

29. Coustan-Smith E, Song G, Clark C, et al. New markers for minimal residual disease detection in acute lymphoblastic leukemia. *Blood*. 2011;117(23):6267-76.

30. Coustan-Smith E, Ribeiro RC, Stow P, et al. A simplified flow cytometric assay identifies children with acute lymphoblastic leukemia who have a superior clinical outcome. *Blood*. 2006;108(1):97-102.

31. Wells DA, Sale GE, Shulman HM, et al. Multidimensional flow cytometry of marrow can differentiate leukemic from normal lymphoblasts and myeloblasts after chemotherapy and bone marrow transplantation. *Am J Clin Pathol*. 1998;110(1):84-94.

32. Coustan-Smith E, Behm FG, Sanchez J, et al. Immunological detection of minimal residual disease in children with acute lymphoblastic leukaemia. *Lancet.* 1998;351(9102):550-4.

33. Coustan-Smith E, Sancho J, Hancock ML, et al. Clinical importance of minimal residual disease in childhood acute lymphoblastic leukemia. *Blood.* 2000;96(8):2691-6.

34. Coustan-Smith E, Sancho J, Behm FG, et al. Prognostic importance of measuring early clearance of leukemic cells by flow cytometry in childhood acute lymphoblastic leukemia. *Blood.* 2002;100(1):52-8.

35. Dworzak MN, Fröschl G, Printz D, et al. Prognostic significance and modalities of flow cytometric minimal residual disease detection in childhood acute lymphoblastic leukemia. *Blood.* 2002;99(6):1952-8.

36. Borowitz MJ, Devidas M, Hunger SP, et al. Clinical significance of minimal residual disease in childhood acute lymphoblastic leukemia and its relationship to other prognostic factors: a Children's Oncology Group study. *Blood.* 2008;111(12):5477-85.

37. Basso G, Veltroni M, Valsecchi MG, et al. Risk of relapse of childhood acute lymphoblastic leukemia is predicted by flow cytometric measurement of residual disease on day 15 bone marrow. *J Clin Oncol.* 2009;27(31):5168-74.

38. Motwani J, Jesson J, Sturch E, et al. Predictive value of flow cytometric minimal residual disease analysis in childhood acute lymphoblastic leukaemia at the end of remission induction therapy: results from a single UK centre. *Br J Haematol.* 2009;144(1):133-5.

39. Bowman WP, Larsen EL, Devidas M, et al. Augmented therapy improves outcome for pediatric high risk acute lymphocytic leukemia: results of Children's Oncology Group trial P9906. *Pediatr Blood Cancer.* 2011;57(4):569-77.

40. Coustan-Smith E, Gajjar A, Hijiya N, et al. Clinical significance of minimal residual disease in childhood acute lymphoblastic leukemia after first relapse. *Leukemia.* 2004;18(3):499-504.

41. Raetz EA, Borowitz MJ, Devidas M, et al. Reinduction platform for children with first marrow relapse in acute lymphoblastic Leukemia: A Children's Oncology Group Study [corrected]. *J Clin Oncol.* 2008;26(24):3971-8.

42. Elorza I, Palacio C, Dapena JL, et al. Relationship between minimal residual disease measured by multiparametric flow cytometry prior to allogeneic hematopoietic stem cell transplantation and outcome in children with acute lymphoblastic leukemia. *Haematologica.* 2010;95(6):936-41.

43. Leung W, Campana D, Yang J, et al. High success rate of hematopoietic cell transplantation regardless of donor source in children with very high-risk leukemia. *Blood.* 2011;118(2):223-30.

44. Sánchez J, Serrano J, Gómez P, et al. Clinical value of immunological monitoring of minimal residual disease in acute lymphoblastic leukaemia after allogeneic transplantation. *Br J Haematol.* 2002;116(3):686-94.

45. Vidriales MB, Pérez JJ, López-Berges MC, et al. Minimal residual disease in adolescent (older than 14 years) and adult acute lymphoblastic leukemias: early immunophenotypic evaluation has high clinical value. *Blood.* 2003;101(12):4695-700.

46. Krampera M, Vitale A, Vincenzi C, et al. Outcome prediction by immunophenotypic minimal residual disease detection in adult T-cell acute lymphoblastic leukaemia. *Br J Haematol.* 2003;120(1):74-9.

47. Holowiecki J, Krawczyk-Kulis M, Giebel S, et al. Status of minimal residual disease after induction predicts outcome in both standard and high-risk Ph-negative adult acute lymphoblastic leukaemia. The Polish Adult Leukemia Group ALL 4-2002 MRD Study. *Br J Haematol.* 2008;142(2):227-37.

48. Giebel S, Stella-Holowiecka B, Krawczyk-Kulis M, et al. Status of minimal residual disease determines outcome of autologous hematopoietic SCT in adult ALL. *Bone Marrow Transplant.* 2010;45(6):1095-101.

49. Gabert J, Beillard E, van der Velden V, et al. Standardization and quality control studies of "real-time" quantitative reverse transcriptase polymerase chain reaction of fusion gene

transcripts for residual disease detection in leukemia—a Europe Against Cancer program. *Leukemia*. 2003;17(12):2318-57.

50. Mullighan CG, Collins-Underwood JR, Phillips LA, et al. Rearrangement of CRLF2 in B-progenitor- and Down syndrome-associated acute lymphoblastic leukemia. *Nat Genet*. 2009;41(11):1243-6.

51. Harvey RC, Mullighan CG, Chen IM, et al. Rearrangement of CRLF2 is associated with mutation of JAK kinases, alteration of IKZF1, Hispanic/Latino ethnicity, and a poor outcome in pediatric B-progenitor acute lymphoblastic leukemia. *Blood*. 2010;115(26):5312-21.

52. Yoda A, Yoda Y, Chiaretti S, et al. Functional screening identifies CRLF2 in precursor B-cell acute lymphoblastic leukemia. *Proc Natl Acad Sci U S A*. 2010;107(1):252-7.

53. Cario G, Zimmermann M, Romey R, et al. Presence of the P2RY8-CRLF2 rearrangement is associated with a poor prognosis in non-high-risk precursor B-cell acute lymphoblastic leukemia in children treated according to the ALL-BFM 2000 protocol. *Blood*. 2010; 115(26):5393-7.

54. van der Velden V, Hochhaus A, Cazzaniga G, et al. Detection of minimal residual disease in hematologic malignancies by real-time quantitative PCR: principles, approaches, and laboratory aspects. *Leukemia*. 2003;17(6):1013-34.

55. Brüggemann M, Schrauder A, Raff T, et al. Standardized MRD quantification in European ALL trials: proceedings of the Second International Symposium on MRD assessment in Kiel, Germany, 18-20 September 2008. *Leukemia*. 2010;24(3):521-35.

56. van der Velden VH, van Dongen JJ. MRD detection in acute lymphoblastic leukemia patients using Ig/TCR gene rearrangements as targets for real-time quantitative PCR. *Methods Mol Biol*. 2009;538:115-50.

57. Szczepanski T, Beishuizen A, Pongers-Willemse MJ, et al. Cross-lineage T cell receptor gene rearrangements occur in more than ninety percent of childhood precursor-B acute lymphoblastic leukemias: alternative PCR targets for detection of minimal residual disease. *Leukemia*. 1999;13(2):196-205.

58. Flohr T, Schrauder A, Cazzaniga G, et al. Minimal residual disease-directed risk stratification using real-time quantitative PCR analysis of immunoglobulin and T-cell receptor gene rearrangements in the international multicenter trial AIEOP-BFM ALL 2000 for childhood acute lymphoblastic leukemia. *Leukemia*. 2008;22(4):771-82.

59. Stow P, Key L, Chen X, et al. Clinical significance of low levels of minimal residual disease at the end of remission induction therapy in childhood acute lymphoblastic leukemia. *Blood*. 2010;115(23):4657-63.

60. Szczepanski T, Willemse MJ, Brinkhof B, et al. Comparative analysis of Ig and TCR gene rearrangements at diagnosis and at relapse of childhood precursor-B-ALL provides improved strategies for selection of stable PCR targets for monitoring of minimal residual disease. *Blood*. 2002;99(7):2315-23.

61. Conter V, Bartram CR, Valsecchi MG, et al. Molecular response to treatment redefines all prognostic factors in children and adolescents with B-cell precursor acute lymphoblastic leukemia: results in 3184 patients of the AIEOP-BFM ALL 2000 study. *Blood*. 2010;115(16): 3206-14.

62. Yeoh AE, Ariffin H, Chai EL, et al. Minimal residual disease-guided treatment deintensification for children with acute lymphoblastic leukemia: results from the Malaysia-Singapore acute lymphoblastic leukemia 2003 study. *J Clin Oncol*. 2012;30(19):2384-92.

63. Pane F, Cimino G, Izzo B, et al. Significant reduction of the hybrid BCR/ABL transcripts after induction and consolidation therapy is a powerful predictor of treatment response in adult Philadelphia-positive acute lymphoblastic leukemia. *Leukemia*. 2005;19(4):628-35.

64. Yanada M, Sugiura I, Takeuchi J, et al. Prospective monitoring of BCR-ABL1 transcript levels in patients with Philadelphia chromosome-positive acute lymphoblastic leukaemia undergoing imatinib-combined chemotherapy. *Br J Haematol*. 2008;143(4):503-10.

65. Wassmann B, Pfeifer H, Stadler M, et al. Early molecular response to posttransplantation imatinib determines outcome in MRD+ Philadelphia-positive acute lymphoblastic leukemia (Ph+ ALL). *Blood.* 2005;106(2):458-63.

66. Madzo J, Zuna J, Muzíková K, et al. Slower molecular response to treatment predicts poor outcome in patients with TEL/AML1 positive acute lymphoblastic leukemia: prospective real-time quantitative reverse transcriptase-polymerase chain reaction study. *Cancer.* 2003; 97(1):105-13.

67. Brisco MJ, Condon J, Hughes E, et al. Outcome prediction in childhood acute lymphoblastic leukaemia by molecular quantification of residual disease at the end of induction. *Lancet.* 1994;343(8891):196-200.

68. Cave H, van der Werff ten Bosch J, Suciu S, et al. Clinical significance of minimal residual disease in childhood acute lymphoblastic leukemia: European Organization for Research and Treatment of Cancer–Childhood Leukemia Cooperative Group. *N Engl J Med.* 1998; 339(9):591-8.

69. van Dongen JJ, Seriu T, Panzer-Grümayer ER, et al. Prognostic value of minimal residual disease in acute lymphoblastic leukaemia in childhood. *Lancet.* 1998;352(9142):1731-8.

70. Goulden NJ, Knechtli CJ, Garland RJ, et al. Minimal residual disease analysis for the prediction of relapse in children with standard-risk acute lymphoblastic leukaemia. *Br J Haematol.* 1998;100(1):235-44.

71. Panzer-Grümayer ER, Schneider M, Panzer S, et al. Rapid molecular response during early induction chemotherapy predicts a good outcome in childhood acute lymphoblastic leukemia. *Blood.* 2000;95(3):790-4.

72. Biondi A, Valsecchi MG, Seriu T, et al. Molecular detection of minimal residual disease is a strong predictive factor of relapse in childhood B-lineage acute lymphoblastic leukemia with medium risk features. A case control study of the International BFM study group. Leukemia. 2000;14(11):1939-43.

73. Zhou J, Goldwasser MA, Li A, et al. Quantitative analysis of minimal residual disease predicts relapse in children with B-lineage acute lymphoblastic leukemia in DFCI ALL Consortium Protocol 95-01. *Blood.* 2007;110(5):1607-11.

74. Attarbaschi A, Mann G, Panzer-Grümayer R, et al. Minimal residual disease values discriminate between low and high relapse risk in children with B-cell precursor acute lymphoblastic leukemia and an intrachromosomal amplification of chromosome 21: the Austrian and German acute lymphoblastic leukemia Berlin-Frankfurt-Münster (ALL-BFM) trials. *J Clin Oncol.* 2008;26(18):3046-50.

75. Van der Velden VH, Corral L, Valsecchi MG, et al. Prognostic significance of minimal residual disease in infants with acute lymphoblastic leukemia treated within the Interfant-99 protocol. *Leukemia.* 2009;23(6):1073-9.

76. Sutton R, Venn NC, Tolisano J, et al. Clinical significance of minimal residual disease at day 15 and at the end of therapy in childhood acute lymphoblastic leukaemia. *Br J Haematol.* 2009;146(3):292-9.

77. Schrappe M, Valsecchi MG, Bartram CR, et al. Late MRD response determines relapse risk overall and in subsets of childhood T-cell ALL: results of the AIEOP-BFM-ALL 2000 study. *Blood.* 2011;118(8):2077-84.

78. Brüggemann M, Raff T, Flohr T, et al. Clinical significance of minimal residual disease quantification in adult patients with standard-risk acute lymphoblastic leukemia. *Blood.* 2006;107(3):1116-23.

79. Raff T, Gökbuget N, Lüschen S, et al. Molecular relapse in adult standard-risk ALL patients detected by prospective MRD monitoring during and after maintenance treatment: data from the GMALL 06/99 and 07/03 trials. *Blood.* 2007;109(3):910-5.

80. Spinelli O, Peruta B, Tosi M, et al. Clearance of minimal residual disease after allogeneic stem cell transplantation and the prediction of the clinical outcome of adult patients with high-risk acute lymphoblastic leukemia. *Haematologica.* 2007;92(5):612-8.

81. Bassan R, Spinelli O, Oldani E, et al. Improved risk classification for risk-specific therapy based on the molecular study of minimal residual disease (MRD) in adult acute lymphoblastic leukemia (ALL). *Blood.* 2009;113(18):4153-62.

82. Patel B, Rai L, Buck G, et al. Minimal residual disease is a significant predictor of treatment failure in non T-lineage adult acute lymphoblastic leukaemia: final results of the international trial UKALL XII/ECOG2993. *Br J Haematol.* 2010;148(1):80-9.

83. Eckert C, Biondi A, Seeger K, et al. Prognostic value of minimal residual disease in relapsed childhood acute lymphoblastic leukaemia. *Lancet.* 2001;358(9289):1239-41.

84. Paganin M, Zecca M, Fabbri G, et al. Minimal residual disease is an important predictive factor of outcome in children with relapsed 'high-risk' acute lymphoblastic leukemia. *Leukemia.* 2008;22(12):2193-200.

85. Knechtli CJ, Goulden NJ, Hancock JP, et al. Minimal residual disease status before allogeneic bone marrow transplantation is an important determinant of successful outcome for children and adolescents with acute lymphoblastic leukemia. *Blood.* 1998;92(11):4072-9.

86. Knechtli CJ, Goulden NJ, Hancock JP, et al. Minimal residual disease status as a predictor of relapse after allogeneic bone marrow transplantation for children with acute lymphoblastic leukaemia. *Br J Haematol.* 1998;102(3):860-71.

87. Krejci O, van der Velden VH, Bader P, et al. Level of minimal residual disease prior to haematopoietic stem cell transplantation predicts prognosis in paediatric patients with acute lymphoblastic leukaemia: a report of the Pre-BMT MRD Study Group. *Bone Marrow Transplantation.* 2003;32(8):849-51.

88. Bader P, Kreyenberg H, Henze GH, et al. Prognostic value of minimal residual disease quantification before allogeneic stem-cell transplantation in relapsed childhood acute lymphoblastic leukemia: the ALL-REZ BFM Study Group. *J Clin Oncol.* 2009;27(3):377-84.

89. Neale GA, Coustan-Smith E, Stow P, et al. Comparative analysis of flow cytometry and polymerase chain reaction for the detection of minimal residual disease in childhood acute lymphoblastic leukemia. *Leukemia.* 2004;18(5):934-8.

90. Kerst G, Kreyenberg H, Roth C, et al. Concurrent detection of minimal residual disease (MRD) in childhood acute lymphoblastic leukaemia by flow cytometry and real-time PCR. *Br J Haematol.* 2005;128(6):774-82.

91. Ryan J, Quinn F, Meunier A, et al. Minimal residual disease detection in childhood acute lymphoblastic leukaemia patients at multiple time-points reveals high levels of concordance between molecular and immunophenotypic approaches. *Br J Haematol.* 2009;144(1):107-15.

92. Metzler M, Mann G, Monschein U, et al. Minimal residual disease analysis in children with t(12;21)-positive acute lymphoblastic leukemia: comparison of Ig/TCR rearrangements and the genomic fusion gene. *Haematologica.* 2006;91(5):683-6.

93. Zaliova M, Fronkova E, Krejcikova K, et al. Quantification of fusion transcript reveals a subgroup with distinct biological properties and predicts relapse in BCR/ABL-positive ALL: implications for residual disease monitoring. *Leukemia.* 2009;23(5):944-51.

94. Pedreira CE, Costa ES, Almeida J, et al. A probabilistic approach for the evaluation of minimal residual disease by multiparameter flow cytometry in leukemic B-cell chronic lymphoproliferative disorders. *Cytometry A.* 2008;73A(12):1141-50.

95. Fišer K, Sieger T, Schumich A, et al. Detection and monitoring of normal and leukemic cell populations with hierarchical clustering of flow cytometry data. *Cytometry A.* 2012;81(1):25-34.

96. Boyd SD, Marshall EL, Merker JD, et al. Measurement and clinical monitoring of human lymphocyte clonality by massively parallel VDJ pyrosequencing. *Sci Transl Med.* 2009;1(12):12-23.

97. Wu D, Sherwood A, Fromm JR, et al. High-throughput sequencing detects minimal residual disease in acute T lymphoblastic leukemia. *Sci Transl Med.* 2012;4(134):134-63.

98. Faham M, Zheng J, Moorhead M, et al. Deep-sequencing approach for minimal residual disease detection in acute lymphoblastic leukemia. *Blood.* 2012;120(26):5173-80.

99. Coustan-Smith E, Sancho J, Hancock ML, et al. Use of peripheral blood instead of bone marrow to monitor residual disease in children with acute lymphoblastic leukemia. *Blood.* 2002;100(7):2399-402.

100. van der Velden VH, Jacobs DC, Wijkhuijs AJ, et al. Minimal residual disease levels in bone marrow and peripheral blood are comparable in children with T cell acute lymphoblastic leukemia (ALL), but not in precursor-B-ALL. *Leukemia.* 2002;16(8):1432-6.

101. Campana D. Should minimal residual disease monitoring in acute lymphoblastic leukemia be standard of care? *Curr Hematol Malig Rep.* 2012;7(2):170-7.

102. Topp MS, Kufer P, Gökbuget N, et al. Targeted therapy with the T-cell-engaging antibody blinatumomab of chemotherapy-refractory minimal residual disease in B-lineage acute lymphoblastic leukemia patients results in high response rate and prolonged leukemia-free survival. *J Clin Oncol.* 2011;29(18):2493-8.

Prophylaxis and Treatment of CNS Involvement in Acute Lymphoblastic Leukemia

10

Rebecca L Olin, Lloyd E Damon

INTRODUCTION

Central nervous system (CNS) involvement by acute lymphoblastic leukemia (ALL) represents a major obstacle in the treatment of this disease. CNS involvement is relatively uncommon at diagnosis, occurring in approximately 3–8% of patients (5% in a recently published large clinical trial).[1-3] However, without specific CNS-directed prophylaxis, greater than 50% of patients will develop CNS relapse.[4] In the 1970s, CNS prophylaxis was introduced into pediatric ALL trials, consisting of cranial radiation in combination with intrathecal (IT) chemotherapy. Because of the long-term toxicity of cranial radiation, recent efforts have focused on the use of high-dose CNS-penetrating systemic chemotherapy in combination with IT treatment, reserving cranial irradiation for active CNS disease or prophylaxis of high-risk patients. Using these strategies, the risk of CNS relapse with appropriate prophylaxis is now 3–5% in children[5,6] and 2–8% in adults.[3,7-9]

Clinically, CNS leukemia is most commonly diagnosed by analysis of cerebrospinal fluid (CSF) obtained via lumbar puncture (LP). CSF involvement is defined as white blood cells (WBC) greater than or equal to $5/\mu L$ with the presence of lymphoblasts; the further classification of CSF results is discussed below. CNS leukemia also can present symptomatically as meningeal infiltration or cranial neuropathies, sometimes in the absence of CSF positivity. In particular, chin numbness (mental nerve involvement, referred to as numb chin syndrome) is associated with the mature B-cell subtype of ALL.[1] Risk factors for CNS involvement at diagnosis and for CNS recurrence, for pediatric and adult patients, are summarized in table 10-1.

In children with ALL, multiple trials have shown that CNS involvement at diagnosis is associated with significantly decreased event-free survival (EFS),[6,13-15] although one recently published study did not support this.[16] In adults, the prognosis of CNS involvement at diagnosis is less clear. In two large trials, CNS involvement at diagnosis did increase the probability of a CNS relapse, but did not seem to impact 5-year EFS.[3,17] Overall survival (OS) at 5 years was decreased in one trial (29% with CNS disease versus 38% without, p = 0.03; Figure 10-1)[3] but not the other [35% with CNS disease versus 31% without, p = NS (non-significant p value)].[17] At present, CNS

Table 10-1	Risk Factors for CNS Involvement at Diagnosis and CNS Recurrence	
CNS disease at diagnosis	*CNS recurrence*	
Adult	*Pediatric*	*Adult*
Immunophenotype (T cell, mature B cell)[3]	Immunophenotype (T cell)[10]	CNS involvement at diagnosis[3]
High WBC[3]	High WBC[10]	
Mediastinal mass[3]	Ph+, t(4;11)[10]	
Elevated LDH[11]	Presence of blasts in CSF at diagnosis (including traumatic LP)[10,12]	

ALL, acute lymphoblastic leukemia; CNS, central nervous system; WBC, white blood cells; Ph+, Philadelphia chromosome-positive; LDH, lactate dehydrogenase; CSF, cerebrospinal fluid.

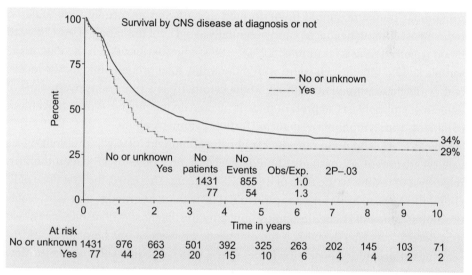

Figure 10-1 Overall survival (OS) by central nervous system (CNS) involvement at diagnosis in the Medical Research Council (MRC) United Kingdom Adult Lymphoblastic Leukemia XII (UKALL XII)/Eastern Cooperative Oncology Group (ECOG) E2993 study. *From* Lazarus HM, Richards SM, Chopra R, et al. Central nervous system involvement in adult acute lymphoblastic leukemia at diagnosis: results from the international ALL trial MRC UKALL XII/ECOG E2993. *Blood.* 2006;108(2):465-72, *with permission.*

involvement at diagnosis is not widely considered to be a sufficiently poor prognostic sign to warrant allogeneic transplant as postremission therapy.

CLINICAL EVALUATION OF CNS INVOLVEMENT

Evaluation for CNS involvement in a patient with newly diagnosed ALL is based predominantly on CSF analysis from a LP. CNS imaging is not routine and is performed if neurologic signs or symptoms are present. Imaging may reveal parenchymal or leptomeningeal involvement by ALL, or may reveal intracranial hemorrhage. If suspicion for intracranial hemorrhage is present clinically, imaging should be performed prior to the LP.

The timing of the initial LP should occur according to the protocol on which therapy will be based, but in general, this assessment should occur either prior to initiating therapy or during the first phase of induction. The rationale behind performing the LP prior to or with administration of systemic therapy is to avoid false-negative results that might occur if systemic therapy was to penetrate and "sterilize" the CNS. Alternatively, the first LP is sometimes delayed until circulating blasts are reduced or eliminated, in order to avoid false-positive results due to contamination of the CSF with peripheral blood.[18]

Lumbar puncture should be performed using a Sprotte˚ needle if possible, to reduce post-lumbar headaches and potentially avoid contamination of the CSF with blood (referred to as a "traumatic LP").[19] CSF studies performed on the diagnostic sample should include cell count with differential, total protein and glucose levels, and cytologic examination. Although flow cytometry is a more sensitive means of detecting lymphoblasts, at present there is no data on the prognosis or management of patients with lymphoblasts detected by flow cytometry alone.

Because IT chemotherapy is a critical component of CNS prophylaxis as well as treatment all patients should receive a first dose of IT chemotherapy, regardless of results, at the time of first of CSF staging. Therefore, the first dose of IT chemotherapy can be given during the initial LP without knowledge of results. Delay of administration of IT chemotherapy until after the diagnostic LP results are known may decrease its effectiveness, if the diagnostic LP itself causes hematoma and/or scarring in the epidural or subarachnoid space, with subsequent changes in the flow of CSF and poor distribution of IT chemotherapy.[12]

Classification of diagnostic CSF results is shown in table 10-2. Patients with CNS-1 status have no CNS disease and receive prophylaxis; patients with CNS-3 have active

Table 10-2	Classification of Cerebrospinal Fluid Resulting from a Diagnostic Lumbar Puncture
Classification	*Definition*
CNS-1	Absence of identifiable lymphoblasts in CSF
CNS-2	Lymphoblasts present with total CSF WBC $< 5/\mu L$
CNS-3	Lymphoblasts present with total CSF WBC $\geq 5/\mu L$ and/or brain parenchymal disease and/or cranial nerve abnormalities
Traumatic LP	CSF erythrocytes $> 10/\mu L$

CNS, central nervous system; CSF, cerebrospinal fluid; WBC, white blood cells; LP, lumbar puncture.

CNS disease and receive additional CNS-directed therapy. However, management of patients with CNS-2 status is less clear. The prognosis of patients with CNS-2 status is controversial; some studies have demonstrated a worse prognosis compared to CNS-1 patients but this has not been confirmed in others (Table 10-3). CNS-2 status does appear to be a risk factor for CNS recurrence in many but not all trials. Treatment of patients with CNS-2 varies by protocol and institution.

Interpretation of CSF results from a traumatic LP may be facilitated using the Steinherz-Bleyer algorithm (unpublished). The algorithm compares the CSF ratio of WBC/red blood cells (RBC) to the blood ratio of WBC/RBC. If the CSF ratio is greater than two times the blood ratio, then the CSF sample is considered as CNS-3 status. If the CSF ratio is less than or equal to two times the blood ratio, then the CSF sample is considered as CNS-2.

Prognosis of patients with traumatic LP is worse than those without a traumatic LP (Table 10-3). It is unclear whether this is a causal relationship or merely an association. It is possible that a traumatic LP causes iatrogenic introduction of lymphoblasts into the CNS; alternatively it may lead to hematoma and/or scarring in the epidural or subarachnoid space and subsequent poor distribution of IT chemotherapy. Conversely, traumatic LPs may simply be associated with more advanced leukemia, or may obscure unrecognized CNS-3 cases. Because of the concern that a traumatic diagnostic LP can cause a worse prognosis, some institutions take specific steps to avoid traumatic LP, including platelet transfusions and having an experienced clinician who performs the LP.[12]

Table 10-3	Event-free Survival and Risk of Any CNS Relapse According to CNS-2 Status or Traumatic Lumbar Puncture			
Study	CNS-2		Traumatic LP	
	EFS	CNS relapse	EFS	CNS relapse
SJCRH XI[20]	p < 0.01	p < 0.01		
POG 8602[21]		p = 0. 002		
CCG 1800/1900[22]	p = 0.0165	p = 0.0018		
BFM 95[23]	NS	p < 0.05	p = 0.003	p < 0.05
EORTC 58881[16]	NS	NS	NS	NS
CCG 105[24]	NS	NS		
DCLSG ALL-7 and 8[25]	NS	NS	p < 0.01	NS
SJCRH XIIIB[26]	NS	NS	NS	NS
SJCRH XI and XII[27]			p = 0.026	NS

SJCRH, St Jude Children's Research Hospital; POG, Pediatric Oncology Group; CCG, Children's Cancer Group; BFM, Berlin-Frankfurt-Münster; EORTC, European Organization for Research and Treatment of Cancer; DCLSG, Dutch Childhood Leukemia Study Group; CNS, central nervous system; LP, lumbar puncture; EFS, event-free survival; NS, non-significant p value.

PRIMARY TREATMENT OF CNS LEUKEMIA

The primary treatments directed at the CNS include cranial radiation, IT/ intraventricular chemotherapy, and systemic chemotherapy (Table 10-4). For simplicity, going forward, "IT" and "intraventricular" will be considered equivalent routes of CSF chemotherapy administration.

Table 10-4	Treatments Directed at the Central Nervous System	
Treatment	*Dose*	*Comments*
Radiation[26,28,29]	• 12–24 Gy cranium in 8–16 1.5 Gy fractions • 6–20 Gy spinal axis (rarely used)	*Late affects:* Secondary neoplasms, neurocognitive defects, endocrinopathies, prolonged growth hormone deficiency[30]
Intrathecal (IT) methotrexate (MTX)[6]	*Children:* • 8 mg (age 1–1.99 year) • 10 mg (age 2–2.99 year) • 12 mg (age ≥3 year) *Adults:* • 12–15 mg	
IT cytarabine (Ara-C)[6]	*Children:* Single agent • 40 mg (age 1–1.99 year) • 50 mg (age 2–2.99 year) • 60 mg (age ≥3 year) *Children:* In triple therapy • 24 mg (age 1–1.99 year) • 30 mg (age 2–2.99 year) • 36 mg (age ≥3 year) *Adults:* • 50–100 mg	
IT liposomal Ara-C[31,32]	50 mg	Dexamethasone (Dex) as arachnoiditis prophylaxis; caution—more neurotoxicity if given in conjunction with IV high-dose Ara-C[33]
IT hydrocortisone (HC)[6]	*Children:* • 16 mg (age 1–1.99 year) • 20 mg (age 2–2.99 year) • 24 mg (age ≥3 year) *Adults:* • 50 mg	Intraventricular HC is highly emetogenic
IT thiotepa[34]	5–11.5 mg/m^2	
Systemic Dex[6]	8–20 mg/m^2/day in 5 day pulses	

Continued

Continued

Treatment	Dose	Comments
Systemic asparaginase	*Children:* • *E. coli* L-asparaginase 25,000 units/m² weekly or 10,000 units/m² thrice weekly; Peg-asparaginase 2,500 units/m² per dose *Adults:* • *E. coli* L-asparaginase 6,000 units/m² per dose; Peg-asparaginase 500–2,500 units/m²	Depletion of CSF glutamine occurs
Systemic thioguanine[35,36]	40–60 mg/m²/day	11–20% VOD (veno-occlusive disease of liver) and 5% portal hypertension[35,37]
Systemic MTX[6]	0.5–8 g/m² over 4–36 hours (regimen-dependent)	In children, titrate the dose to achieve a steady state blood level of 33 µM (low risk) or 65 µM (standard risk)
Systemic Ara-C[38]	0.5–3 g/m² per dose	Doses need to be modified for renal function to avoid neurotoxicity[39,40]
Systemic thiotepa[41]	50–65 mg/m² per dose	
Systemic dasatinib	100 mg daily	Penetrates into the CNS; for patients with t(9;22)[42]

IV, intravenous; CSF, cerebrospinal fluid; *E. coli, Escherichia coli*; CNS, central nervous system.

Radiation Therapy

Historically, radiation has been a mainstay to treat active CNS leukemia but has long-term consequences, which include neurocognitive defects, secondary neoplasms, endocrinopathies (including prolonged growth hormone deficiency), and short stature.[30,43] Neurocognitive defects are less pronounced in adults compared to children, but is still a significant issue, especially in adults over 60 years of age.[44,45] The secondary neoplasms associated with radiation in pediatric ALL patients and their percent cumulative probability at 20 years are: basal cell carcinoma of skin (7.5%), meningioma (3.7%), brain cancer (0.65%), myeloid neoplasm (0.8%), soft tissue sarcoma (1.5%), Hodgkin lymphoma (0.2%), and other carcinomas (5.6%).[30] The cumulative risk of a non-basal cell carcinoma secondary neoplasm at 20 years was 13.3% compared to 0.95% in nonradiated patients and was sixfold higher than expected compared to the general population. As such, efforts to reduce or eliminate the routine use of radiation in patients with CNS positive ALL have been in play. In addition, spinal radiation has been eliminated as a standard treatment due to its toxicity (severe myelosuppression) and the lack of clear benefit in the setting of intense, CNS-directed systemic chemotherapy and IT chemotherapy.

Intrathecal Chemotherapy

Intrathecal chemotherapy plays an important role in both the treatment and prophylaxis of CNS leukemia. The primary agents used are methotrexate (MTX), alone or in combination with Ara-C and hydrocortisone (HC) (triple therapy). Triple therapy is commonly used in children and single-agent MTX is commonly used in adults. The doses of chemotherapy are age-dependent (Table 10-4) to account for the expansion of CSF volume with advancing age. The side effects of IT chemotherapy include non-supine headache, arachnoiditis, and hematoma and/ or scarring in the epidural or subarachnoid space. Maneuvers to reduce these side effects and maximize CSF distribution of the chemotherapeutic agents include the use of a noncutting spinal needle, the use of greater than or equal to 6 mL of diluent per injection, the use of conscious sedation in children, and the maintenance of the supine position for at least 1 hour after the injection. The schedule and total number of IT injections is protocol-dependent and in part determined whether the injections are for prophylaxis or for active CNS treatment of leukemia. Intraventricular chemotherapy is generally reserved for patients with active CNS leukemia, and is performed via an Ommaya reservoir. Intraventricular HC is highly emetogenic.

Intrathecal liposomal Ara-C is Food and Drug Administration (FDA)-approved for the treatment of lymphomatous meningitis. Liposomal Ara-C has a CSF half-life of 130–277 hours (compared to 3–4 hours for conventional Ara-C) and only needs to be given every 2 weeks.[32] The primary side effect from liposomal Ara-C is a sterile arachnoiditis. Dexamethasone (Dex) is given before and after IT injections of liposomal Ara-C to ameliorate this problem. In one study, 16% of patients receiving liposomal Ara-C experienced neurotoxicity, primarily when given during a treatment cycle including high-dose intravenous (IV) MTX and Ara-C.[33] Thus, IT liposomal Ara-C should be avoided when high-dose IV MTX or high-dose IV Ara-C is being administered. In patients with active meningeal non-Hodgkin lymphoma (NHL) or ALL, the cytopathologic response rate to liposomal Ara-C as a single agent ranges from 67% to 100% (57–67% complete).[32,46]

Intrathecal thiotepa has been used to treat active CNS leukemia but is not a common choice.[34] Overall responses (partial in all but one) in ALL patients with CNS leukemia have been reported in 8 of 12 assessable cases.[34,47,48]

Systemic Chemotherapy

Certain systemic chemotherapeutic agents play a role in treating or preventing CNS leukemia. Depending on the drug and its dose and route of administration, penetration of the blood-brain barrier is possible with the achievement of therapeutic

CSF and CNS parenchymal drug levels. Taking advantage of this effect has led to the reduction or elimination of routine cranial radiation in many modern ALL protocols with an acceptably low risk of CNS relapse.

Systemic Dex is one example of a CNS-active agent. Dex penetrates the CNS better than prednisone (Pred)/prednisolone due to its lower protein binding [70% (concentration-independent) versus 60–95% (concentration-dependent), respectively] and its longer CSF half-life (4.1 hours vs 2.9 hours in a nonhuman primate model, respectively), providing improved CNS bioavailability.[49] The exposure to Pred/prednisolone in the CSF is estimated to be only 10–20% that of Dex. The enhanced CSF exposure to Dex is clinically evident based on the effectiveness of Dex as an antiemetic and due to increased CNS side effects compared to Pred/prednisolone. The benefits of high-dose Dex compared to Pred in treating or preventing CNS leukemia need to be weighed against its toxicities, including an increased risk of septic death during induction and an increased risk of osteonecrosis of joints in patients 10 years or older. Children's Oncology Group (COG) AALL0232 randomized 2,575 children and young adults to Dex (10 mg/m^2 per day for 14 days) or to Pred (60 mg/m^2 per day for 28 days) during induction.[50] Overall, Dex was associated with a greater risk of osteonecrosis [11.6% vs 8.7%, p = 0.014; hazard ratio (HR) 1.64]. The increased risk of osteonecrosis was evident in patients greater than or equal to 10 years of age (17.2% vs 12.6%, p = 0.006; HR 1.79) but was not in patients less than 10 years old. The protocol was amended to give all patients greater than or equal to 10 years old Pred during induction.

The relative CNS benefits of Dex also need to be appreciated within the context of Pred/prednisolone and Dex dosing. The accepted bioequivalence ratio of Pred/prednisolone to Dex dosing is 6–7.[51] Randomized studies comparing Pred/prednisolone to Dex at ratios greater than 7 are not making a fair comparison of the two agents. Data regarding the effectiveness of high-dose Dex for active (primary or relapsed) CNS leukemia is notably lacking.

Parenteral asparaginase has CNS activity. Asparaginase has been demonstrated to reduce CSF asparagine and glutamine levels to biologically meaningful levels, although the drug itself does not penetrate into the CNS.[52-54] The clinical expression of this effect has been the demonstration of asparaginase-induced seizures even in the absence of intracranial vascular thrombosis.[55,56] Not all asparaginase products are created equal. The risk of CNS ALL relapse is sixfold higher with Erwinia-derived asparaginase (5-year cumulative risk 6%) compared to *Escherichia coli*-derived asparaginase (5-year cumulative risk 1%; p < 0.1) when the same doses were used (25,000 IU/m^2 weekly for 20 weeks).[57] The standard asparaginase used for ALL patients in the United States has been *E. coli*-derived (native or pegylated), mainly for availability reasons rather than CNS relapse reasons. However, this difference should be kept in mind when asparaginase choices are made since the Erwinia-derived product is now FDA-approved in the United States. Asparaginase is routinely given as part of multiagent induction and postinduction therapy in patients with a new diagnosis of ALL with primary CNS involvement, so its true level of CNS activity in this setting cannot be dissected.

Oral thiopurines, such as 6-mercaptopurine and thioguanine are active in ALL, and appear to have a role in CNS leukemia. There is indirect evidence for this as a study comparing 6-mercaptopurine (n = 1,017; 75 mg/m^2 daily) to thioguanine (n = 1010; 50-60 mg/m^2 daily) in children with ALL found a lower CNS relapse rate in those given thioguanine (3.5%) than those given 6-mercaptopurine (5.5%; p = 0.01).[35] Another study also found a lower isolated CNS relapse risk for thioguanine compared to 6-mercaptopurine [HR 0.53; 95% confidence interval (CI), 0.30–0.92; p = 0.02] in 1,492 randomized patients, while a third study found a CNS relapse rate of zero in 51 patients receiving IV thioguanine at 480 mg/m^2 during consolidation and maintenance.[36,37] All of these studies showed excess hepatotoxicity with thioguanine. The risk of serious veno-occlusive disease (VOD) of liver is thioguanine dose-dependent, and ranges from 11% to 20% with a 5% risk of portal hypertension, substantially higher than with 6-mercaptopurine.[35,37]

A very active agent for CNS leukemia is high-dose IV MTX, certainly at doses 0.5 g/m^2 or greater. Doses up to 8 g/m^2 IV over 4 hours have been shown to be safe in patients with ALL, usually with IV leucovorin rescue beginning 24 hours later. High-dose IV MTX is able to cross the blood-brain barrier and produce therapeutic CSF levels. It has clinical activity for both leptomeningeal disease in ALL and NHL, and for parenchymal disease in primary CNS and intraocular lymphoma.[58-60] The Children's Cancer Group (CCG) (protocols 191P, 139P, and 144P) gave a mega-dose of IV MTX (33.6 g/m^2 over 24 hours with leucovorin rescue beginning 12 hours later) to children with ALL but without cranial radiation as CNS prophylaxis.[61] This dose of MTX produced a median steady state CSF MTX level of 12 mcM (3–122) with levels of greater than or equal to 1 mcM considered therapeutic. Despite this, the survivals of patients receiving mega-dose MTX were no better than patients receiving standard MTX doses combined with cranial radiation, although they had better neurocognitive testing. Further, the CNS relapse rate was 19%, an unexpected finding and perhaps explained by the early use of leucovorin and the relative lack of intensity of the systemic regimen delivered. The long-term consequence of high-dose IV MTX is leukoencephalopathy, usually reversible, and best diagnosed with diffusion-weighted magnetic resonance (MR) imaging.[62,63]

Cytarabine is another antimetabolite that at high IV doses penetrates the CNS and is active in CNS leukemia and NHL. IV Ara-C at 0.5-3 g/m^2 per dose for 4–12 doses produces therapeutic CSF levels.[38] High-dose IV Ara-C is a common salvage regimen for relapsed CNS leukemia and lymphoma and is a consolidation treatment for primary CNS lymphoma.[60,64,65] The primary side effects of high-dose IV Ara-C are CNS toxicity (mainly cerebellum, cerebrum, and cranial nerves, mediated through triggering of apoptosis of neurons), keratoconjunctivitis, and myelo-suppression.[39,66,67] The most important risk factor for Ara-C-induced neurotoxicity is reduced renal function: the rate of neurotoxicity is 8% when the estimated glomerular filtration rate (GFR) is greater than or equal to 60 mL/min compared to 76% when the GFR is less than 60 mL/min.[39] Modifying the IV Ara-C dose when there is reduced renal function virtually eliminates the risk of neurotoxicity.[40] Due to its significant potential toxicities, especially myelosuppression, it is more common to use high-dose IV MTX than Ara-C as a single agent to treat CNS leukemia.

The alkylating agent thiotepa is notable for its CNS penetration.[41] Its dose-limiting toxicity as a single agent is central nervous toxicity, with the maximum tolerated dose 1,125 mg/m^2 (in the setting of hematopoietic stem cell support).[68] One-half of patients with first CNS leukemia relapse cleared their CSF blasts with a single IV dose of thiotepa at 50–60 mg/m^2.[69] Another alkylating agent with high-CNS penetration is ifosfamide, at doses of 2 g/m^2 or greater. Neurotoxicity is also an undesirable side effect of ifosfamide. There is little data on using either agent for active primary CNS leukemia, although high-dose thiotepa has been used as part of conditioning regimens for autologous stem cell transplant in relapsed primary CNS lymphoma.[70,71]

In patients with Philadelphia chromosome-positive (Ph$^+$) ALL [t(9;22)] and active CNS leukemia, the tyrosine-kinase inhibitor of choice is dasatinib. Dasatinib penetrates into the CSF at therapeutic levels (1.4–20.1 nM) and should help control CNS disease.[42] Dasatinib produced tumor responses in a mouse model of CNS leukemia using the human BCR-ABL+ chronic myelogenous leukemia cell line K562.[42] Dasatinib was used to treat CNS ALL in 14 children with chronic myeloid leukemia (CML) lymphoid blast crisis or Ph$^+$ ALL; five children also received IT chemotherapy. Of 11 evaluable patients, 11 responded, 7 completely.[42] Responses lasted more than 6 months in five patients and more than 1 year in two patients.

Overall Approach to Primary Treatment of CNS Leukemia

The historical mainstay of treatment of CNS leukemia has been cranial-spinal radiation with intensified IT (or intraventricular) chemotherapy. Traditional radiation dosing is 24 Gy to the cranium and 12 Gy to the spinal axis. Spinal radiation, mainly due to its myelosuppressive qualities and lack of clear data supporting its importance in active CNS leukemia, has been dropped as a primary therapy for CNS leukemia. As modern therapeutic regimens are risk-adapted and systemically intensified with high-dose IV MTX, high-dose IV Ara-C, and high-dose Pred or Dex, and enriched with asparaginase, the dose of cranial radiation has been dropped to 18 Gy even in CNS-3 disease[13] and in some regimens eliminated altogether in both children and adults (see discussion on primary prophylaxis).[6] Cranial radiation is still recommended in patients presenting with cranial nerve abnormalities and/or brain parenchymal disease.

SECONDARY TREATMENT OF CNS LEUKEMIA

Isolated relapse in the CNS is now an uncommon event (<1–4% in children and 1–11% in adults) with modern treatment protocols.[6,37] Isolated CNS relapse is a harbinger for bone marrow and/or testicular relapse, and is generally treated with CNS-directed therapy and systemic therapy. The prognosis of relapse of ALL in the CNS is relatively poor in both children and adults, worse in patients with high-risk features at diagnosis, shorter first remissions, and the use of cranial radiation during the initial treatment regimen.[72,73] The 4-year EFS was longer in children with an isolated CNS relapse beyond 18 months from first complete remission (CR) (78%) compared to those with a relapse shorter than 18 months (51%).[69] In adults with an isolated CNS relapse, the long-term survival is less than 7%.[9,74,75]

In patients who have not received prior cranial radiation, radiation in conjunction with IT chemotherapy and systemic chemotherapy may be considered. One trial gave 18 Gy cranial radiation to pediatric ALL patients with first remissions over 18 months and 24 Gy cranial radiation and 15 Gy spinal radiation for those with first remission under 18 months (the outcomes were described above).[69] However, the additional value of cranial radiation in this setting is unclear, especially considering its toxicities, and particularly in adults where the prognosis is so dismal. Complicating this cranial radiation decision-making is the general intention, certainly in adults, to try and get the patient into a second CR, find a suitable hematopoietic stem cell donor, and culminate in allogeneic stem cell transplant, which often involves total body irradiation (TBI). Adding TBI to a patient who has previously received cranial radiation will likely adversely affect that individual's long-term neurocognitive function.

Most CNS leukemia salvage treatment approaches will use aggressive IT chemotherapy, initially two to three times weekly until the CSF clears, and then a weekly to monthly schedule for a protracted period of time as tolerated.[74] This will typically be triple drug therapy in children and young adults and single drug therapy in older adults (above age 30 years). As a single agent, IT liposomal Ara-C achieves a CSF cytopathologic response in 67–100% of patients (57–67% complete) in patients with ALL or NHL.[32,46] The use of IT liposomal Ara-C must be scheduled carefully as it is associated with an increased risk of central neurotoxicity when administered just before or just after high-dose IV MTX or Ara-C.[33,76] Further, the risk of central neurotoxicity is likely substantial when liposomal Ara-C is administered soon before, or later after, the conditioning regimen for hematopoietic stem cell transplantation (HSCT). In one report, central neurotoxicity occurred in 2 of 6 patients who received liposomal Ara-C following HSCT.[77]

The general use of high-dose IV MTX and/or Ara-C for relapsed CNS leukemia is a common approach. The outcomes following these agents are difficult to define as these patients are often getting other systemic drugs as well and treatment goals differ (curative vs palliative) based on age, time to relapse, and comorbidities. It is safe to conclude that there is no established standard of care for isolated CNS relapse of ALL.

Dasatinib has been used to successfully treat a patient with CNS relapse of Ph^+ ALL that was refractory to cranial radiation and imatinib.[78]

PRIMARY CNS PROPHYLAXIS

Trials examining the role of various CNS prophylactic therapies have not routinely distinguished patients with CNS-1 or CNS-2 disease from those with CNS-3 disease or traumatic LPs. Rather, the trials have lumped all such patients together in order to examine CNS-directed therapies, referred to as "CNS prophylaxis", aimed at preventing CNS relapse in the combined cohort. Thus, CNS prophylaxis is really the initial CNS-directed therapy for anyone with the first diagnosis of ALL, regardless of whether CNS leukemia is present or absent.

Cranial Radiation

In the recent past, primary CNS prophylaxis included cranial radiation (18–24 Gy) in conjunction with IT chemotherapy and systemic chemotherapy in all children with ALL. Two sequential trials in children with medium- or high-risk ALL compared cranial radiation doses of 18 Gy (n = 259) to 12 Gy (n = 570).[13] The 6-year cumulative incidence of CNS relapse was not different, 4% with 18 Gy and 6.7% with 12 Gy (p = 0.19). Further, then 6-year EFSs were 68% and 77%, respectively (p = 0.003). Thus, in the setting of intense systemic chemotherapy, the dose of cranial radiation could be safely dropped to 12 Gy.

This observation led to the question of eliminating prophylactic cranial radiation altogether. A meta-analysis was performed of eight trials (1,448 patients) in which cranial radiation plus IT chemotherapy was randomly compared to prolonged IT chemotherapy as CNS prophylaxis.[79] There was a trend toward less CNS relapse with radiation (HR 0.78; 95% CI, 0.59–1.03) but no differences in EFS (HR 0.96; 95% CI, 0.85–1.08) or OS (10-year OS 64% vs 63%) (Figure 10-2). This led to the elimination of routine cranial radiation for children with low risk for CNS recurrence but the retention of cranial radiation for children at high risk. High-risk patients included: pre-B cell ALL with a WBC greater than 100,000/μL; T-cell ALL with a WBC greater than 50,000/μL; high-risk karyotypes [t(9;22), mixed-lineage leukemia (MLL) rearrangement, or hypodiploidy], CNS-2 or CNS-3 disease, or a traumatic LP with CSF blasts[72,73] (Table 10-1). In high-risk patients with CNS-1 disease and in those with CNS-2 disease, the cranial radiation dose was 12 Gy; in those with CNS-3

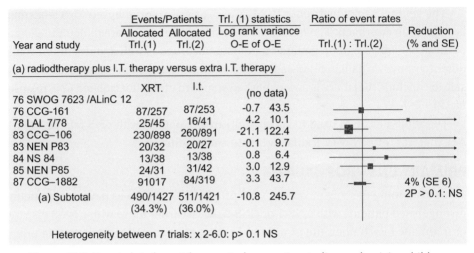

Year and study	Events/Patients Allocated Trl.(1)	Allocated Trl.(2)	Trl. (1) statistics Log rank variance O-E of O-E	Ratio of event rates Trl.(1) : Trl.(2)	Reduction (% and SE)
(a) radiodtherapy plus I.T. therapy versus extra I.T. therapy					
	XRT.	I.t.	(no data)		
76 SWOG 7623 /ALinC 12					
76 CCG-161	87/257	87/253	-0.7 43.5		
78 LAL 7/78	25/45	16/41	4.2 10.1		
83 CCG-106	230/898	260/891	-21.1 122.4		
83 NEN P83	20/32	20/27	-0.1 9.7		
84 NS 84	13/38	13/38	0.8 6.4		
85 NEN P85	24/31	31/42	3.0 12.9		
87 CCG-1882	91017	84/319	3.3 43.7		4% (SE 6)
(a) Subtotal	490/1427 (34.3%)	511/1421 (36.0%)	-10.8 245.7		2P > 0.1: NS

Heterogeneity between 7 trials: x 2-6.0: p> 0.1 NS

Figure 10-2 Forest plot of event-free survival comparing studies randomizing children with acute lymphoblastic leukemia to cranial radiation or no cranial radiation. *From* Clarke M, Gaynon P, Hann I, et al. CNS-directed therapy for childhood acute lymphoblastic leukemia: Childhood ALL Collaborative Group overview of 43 randomized trials. *J Clin Oncol.* 2003;21(9):1798-809, *with permission.*

disease, the cranial radiation dose was 18 Gy.[73] With this approach, only 2–20% of children required cranial radiation and the CNS relapse rate was 1–2%.[13,80] Several randomized and nonrandomized studies suggested that cranial radiation could be eliminated in the setting of aggressive IT chemotherapy in children with medium- to high-risk ALL without an obvious increase in CNS relapse.[81,82] The exception appeared to still be T-cell patients with a WBC greater than 100,000/μL where cranial radiation still seemed important.[82]

This led to the St Jude Total Therapy XV (TT-XV) trial that eliminated cranial radiation in all children with newly diagnosed ALL, even in those considered high risk for CNS relapse.[6] In that trial, patients received triple-drug IT chemotherapy and intensified systemic therapy. The 5-year cumulative CNS relapse risk was 2.7% (95% CI, 1.1–4.3%) (Figure 10-3). The continued CR duration of 71 patients at high risk for CNS relapse treated on TT-XV who would have previously received cranial radiation was longer than the 56 similar patients who received cranial radiation while on St Jude Total Therapy XIII (TT-XIII) [5-year probability of continued first CR, 91% (95% CI, 76–100%) vs 73% (61–85%), p = 0.04] (Figuer 10-4). In TT-XV, only 11 patients had an isolated CNS relapse—the risk factors for CNS relapse were: t(1;19)(TCF3-PBX1), CNS-3 disease at diagnosis, and T-cell disease. The conclusion from TT-XV was that cranial radiation and its attendant long-term morbidities could be safely eliminated in children with newly diagnosed ALL provided the treatment regimen included triple-drug IT chemotherapy and intense systemic chemotherapy. This successful

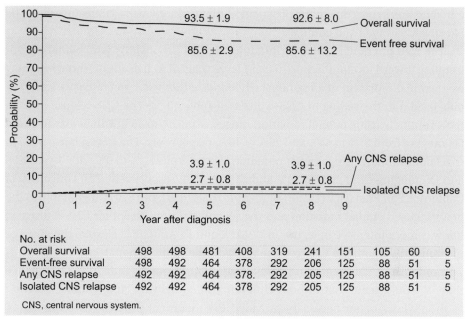

Figure 10-3 Outcomes of children with acute lymphoblastic leukemia (ALL) treated on St Jude Total Therapy XV (TT-XV) protocol without the use of prophylactic cranial radiation. *From* Pui CH, Campana D, Pei D, et al. Treating childhood acute lymphoblastic leukemia without cranial irradiation. *N Engl J Med.* 2009;360(26):2730-41, *with permission.*

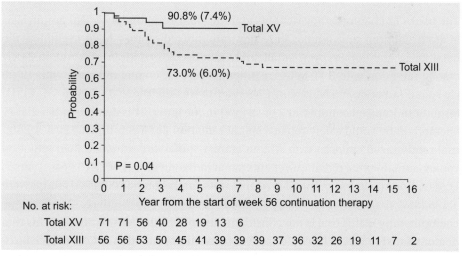

Figure 10-4 Continuous complete remission durations in 71 patients at high risk for central nervous system relapse treated on St Jude Total Therapy XV protocol without cranial radiation compared to 56 similar patients treated on St Jude Total Therapy XIII protocol with cranial radiation. *From* Pui CH, Campana D, Pei D, et al. Treating childhood acute lymphoblastic leukemia without cranial irradiation. *N Engl J Med.* 2009;360(26):2730-41, *with permission.*

outcome was in part due to the observation that children with CNS relapse could be effectively salvaged and cured.

The role of cranial radiation in adults as CNS prophylaxis is in evolution but trending toward its elimination. In eight large trials of ALL in adults, three routinely used cranial radiation of all patients while four either used no cranial radiation or only used it in the setting of CNS-3 disease (Table 10-5). The CNS relapse rates in trials routinely using cranial radiation ranged from 1% to 15% with 5-year EFS and OS ranging from 27% to 44% and 29% to 48%, respectively. The CNS relapse rates in trials not routinely using cranial radiation ranged from 1.2% to 9% with 5-year EFS and OS ranging from 25% to 52% and 31% to 40%, respectively. The University of California, San Francisco (UCSF) sequential trials (8001 and 8707) are notable as the first trial used cranial radiation and the second did not (except for CNS-3 disease) but was more intensive in its use of IV MTX and IV Ara-C.[83,84] Despite the absence of cranial radiation, the CNS relapse rate was the same in both trials, 1%. There is no randomized data regarding cranial radiation in adults with ALL. On balance then, it would seem that in both children and adults with ALL, cranial radiation as prophylaxis is not necessary provided the treatment protocol uses intense IT chemotherapy and intense systemic chemotherapy generally including high doses of MTX and high doses of Ara-C. In adults, a consensus is lacking on whether to use cranial radiation at diagnosis for CNS-3 disease.

Intrathecal Chemotherapy

The use of IT chemotherapy remains an important component of CNS prophylaxis in both children and adults. Very few randomized studies have examined the need for IT chemotherapy. A small study randomized children with ALL to 24 Gy cranial radiation with 5 IT MTX treatments or 24 Gy cranial radiation with 15–20 Gy spinal radiation.[28] The rate of CNS relapse was the same: 3 of 45 (6.6%) in the former randomized cohort and 2 of 49 (4%) in the latter. This demonstrated that IT chemotherapy could safely replace spinal radiation as CNS prophylaxis. A second trial randomized children with ALL to cranial-spinal and extended field radiation versus cranial-spinal radiation versus cranial radiation plus IT MTX (6 doses) versus IT MTX alone (6 doses).[29] The CNS relapse rates for the four randomized groups were 4/135 (3%), 6/152 (4%), 11/159 (7%), and 54/178 (30%), respectively. The systemic chemotherapy in this trial is not considered intense by modern standards. This trial demonstrated that IT MTX could safely replace spinal radiation as CNS prophylaxis, but that 6 IT MTX doses was inadequate CNS prophylaxis in the absence of cranial radiation and intense systemic chemotherapy.

As systemic chemotherapy has intensified, IT chemotherapy has remained as the basic platform for CNS prophylaxis. Depending on the age group, disease features and treatment protocol, the actual IT chemotherapy regimen varies enormously in

Table 10-5 Central Nervous System Relapses in Adult ALL Trials with or without Cranial Radiation

Protocol	Number of patients enrolled	CNS involvement at diagnosis	Cranial radiation?	CR	CNS relapse	5-year EFS	5-year OS
UCSF 8001[83]	109	6%	Yes, 18 Gy (28 Gy if CNS-3)	96 (88%)	1/96 (1%)	35%	40%
UK ALLXII/ECOG E2993[3]	1,508	5%	Yes, 24 Gy cranium and 12 Gy spinal axis (only if no HSCT planned)	1,356 (90%)	85/1356 (6.3%)	27% if CSF+ 34% if CSF- (p = 0.06)	29% if CSF + 38% if CSF- (p = 0.03)
CALGB 8811[85]	197	NS	Yes, 24 Gy	167 (85%)	25/167 (15%)	44%	48%
UCSF 8707[84]	84	6.7%	No, only for CNS-3 (18 Gy)	78 (93%)	1/78 (1.3%)	52%	NS
PETHEMA ALL-89, -93, -96, -97[9]	467	4%	No	381 (82%)	22/381 (6%)	NS	NS
LALA-87 and -94[17]	1,493	6.5%	No, only for CNS-3 (18 Gy)	1,227 (82%)	109/1227 (9%)	37% CSF+ 29% CSF- p = NS	35% CSF + 31% CSF- p = NS
Hyper-CVAD[8]	288	7%	No, only if CNS-2 or -3 (24–30 Gy)	264 (92%)	7/264 (2.7%)	38% (CR duration)	40%
CALGB 1980[86]	161	NS	No	128 (80%)	9/128 (7%)	25% (DFS)	39%

CNS, central nervous system; ALL, acute lymphoblastic leukemia; CR, complete remission; EFS, event-free survival; OS, overall survival; UCSF, University of California, San Francisco; UK, United Kingdom; ECOG, Eastern Cooperative Oncology Group; CSF, cerebrospinal fluid; HSCT, hematopoietic stem cell transplantation; CALGB, Cancer and Leukemia Group B; NS, not stated; PETHEMA, Programa para el Estudio y Tratamiento de Hemopatías Malignas; LALA, Leucemies Aigues Lymphoblastiques de L'Adulte; Hyper-CVAD, hyperfractionated cyclophosphamide, vincristine, doxorubicin and dexamethasone; DFS, disease-free survival.

terms of the number of agents, doses of the agents, the schedule of administration, and the total number of administrations. In adults, MTX is often used alone. Ara-C is sometimes added to MTX for additional anti-leukemia effect. HC is usually added to MTX and Ara-C, so-called "triple therapy", initially to reduce arachnoiditis from Ara-C and MTX, but it may have antileukemic effects in its own right.[73] The Children's Cancer Study Group protocol 1952 randomized 2,037 standard-risk children with ALL to IT triple therapy or to IT MTX within the context of intense systemic therapy.[87] Twenty-four Gy cranial and six Gy spinal radiations were given to everyone with CNS-3 disease, a traumatic LP, or cranial nerve abnormality. The 6-year cumulative incidence of CNS relapse was 3.4% ± 1.0% and 5.9% ± 1.2% for IT triple therapy and IT MTX, respectively (p = 0.004). There were more bone marrow and testicular relapses with IT triple therapy. The 5-year EFS for the two regimens was 80.7% versus 82.5%, respectively (p = 0.3); the 5-year OS for the two regimens was 90.3% versus 94.4%, respectively (p = 0.01), favoring IT MTX. Since IT triple therapy provided better CNS control, it remains the preferred treatment in children with ALL in the setting of systemic therapy that is intensified to reduce bone marrow and testicular relapse.

Another trial in children with standard-risk ALL randomized 164 patients to extended IT triple therapy or to 18 Gy cranial radiation and a shortened course of IT MTX plus Ara-C.[57] The CNS relapse rates were similar [5 of 83 (6%) and 0 of 81 (0%), respectively], as were the 5-year EFS-pairing IT triple agent to double agent therapy.

To date, only two trials have examined the safety of liposomal Ara-C as CNS prophylaxis in adult ALL.[33,88] Liposomal Ara-C was given intrathecally throughout the Hyper-CVAD (hyperfractionated cyclophosphamide, vincristine, doxorubicin, and dexamethasone) regimen.[33] There were no recorded CNS relapses in 31 patients. Symptomatic neurotoxicity developed in 16% of patients, but only when liposomal Ara-C was given during the IV MTX/Ara-C cycles of therapy.

Dexamethasone

Six prospective, randomized trials comparing Dex to Pred/prednisolone during induction therapy (and continuing the randomized therapy during some postinduction treatment phases in four trials) have been reported (Table 10-6).[89] All six trials demonstrated a significant decrease in CNS relapse with Dex (HR 0.53; 95% CI, 0.44–0.65) without a reduction in bone marrow relapses (HR 0.90; 95% CI, 0.69–1.18). In the four trials where the Pred to Dex ratio was less than 7, Dex reduced the EFS (HR, 0.73; 95% CI, 0.66–0.81) and the CNS relapse risk (HR 0.52; 95% CI, 0.45–0.64) compared to Pred. In contrast, in the two trials where the Pred to Dex ratio was greater than 7, Dex had no effect on EFS (HR 1.01; 95% CI, 0.84–1.22) while still reducing the CNS relapse risk (HR 0.59; 95% CI, 0.37–0.95) compared to Pred. Toxicity with Dex was greater, especially death during induction [risk ratio (RR) 2.31;

Table 10-6	Randomized Trials Comparing Dexamethasone to Prednisone During Induction Chemotherapy in Children with ALL					
Trial	Number of patients enrolled	Pred/ Dex ratio	Courses involving corticosteroid randomization	High-risk patients included	HR*, EFS	HR*, CNS relapse
CALGB 7111[90]	493	6.6	I, M	Yes	NS	0.58 (0.38, 0.81)
CCG-1922[91]	1,060	6.6	I, C, M	No	0.67 (0.52, 0.87)	0.54 (0.32, 0.92)
MRC ALL 97/99[92]	1,603	6.2	I, IM, M	Yes	0.7 (0.57, 0.87)	0.49 (0.32, 0.74)
AIEOP-BFM ALL 2000[93]	3,655	6	I	Yes	0.78 (0.66, 0.87)	0.51 (0.34, 0.75)
TCCSG L95-14[94]	359	7.5	I, In	No	1.01 (0.64, 1.58)	0.67 (0.11, 3.96)
EORTC 58951[95]	1,703	10	I	Yes	1.02 (0.83, 1.25)	0.59 (0.36, 0.96)

*Hazard ratios significantly less than 1 favoring Dex over Pred.

ALL, acute lymphoblastic leukemia; Pred, prednisone; Dex, dexamethasone; HR, hazard ratio (95% CI); EFS, event-free survival; CNS, central nervous system; CALGB, Cancer and Leukemia Group B; I, induction; M, maintenance; NS, not stated; CCG, Children's Cancer Group; C, consolidation; MRC, Medical Research Council; ALL, acute lymphoblastic leukemia; IM, intensified maintenance; AIEOP, Associazione Italiana Ematologia Oncologia Pediatrica; BFM, Berlin-Frankfurt-Münster; TCCSG, Tokyo Children's Cancer Study Group; In, intensification; EORTC, European Organization for Research and Treatment of Cancer.

95% CI, 1.46–3.66]. There was also a trend toward a greater risk of osteonecrosis with Dex (RR 1.11; 95% CI, 0.82–1.50) in patients greater than or equal to 10 years old, as discussed previously.

The large COG AALL0232 trial compared Dex to Pred (Pred to Dex ratio 6) during induction in 2,575 pediatric and young adolescent high-risk patients with ALL. The unblinded outcomes have not yet been published, but the composite blinded outcomes have been reported in abstract form.[96] In patients less than 16 years compared to patients greater than or equal to 16 years, the 5-year cumulative incidence of any relapse is 13.4% versus 21.3% (p = 0.0018) and the 5-year cumulative incidence of CNS relapse was 3.7% versus 5.2% (p = 0.58). Whether Dex was associated with a reduced risk of CNS relapse relative to Pred remains to be seen. In any event, the CNS relapse rate is very low in this intensive trial of high-risk patients with ALL where no CNS radiation is administered but high-dose systemic MTX is given (see below).

Intravenous Methotrexate

Intravenous MTX has been developed within ALL treatment protocols as a component of CNS prophylaxis due to its ability to cross the blood-brain barrier.

A recent meta-analysis explored the outcomes of IV MTX in children with ALL randomized to IV MTX versus long-term IT MTX or to cranial radiation with short-term IT MTX (eight clinical trials).[79] In that analysis, which included IV MTX doses of 0.5–8 g/m^2, there was a trend toward reducing the incidence of CNS relapse with IV MTX (HR 0.81; 95% CI, 0.63–1.03; p = 0.08). Patients randomized to IV MTX had a 17% reduction in all ALL events (p = 0.02) and had a better 10-year EFS, 68.1% versus 61.9% (p = 0.003), but no improvement in OS (80.1% vs 76.8%, p = 0.09). The advantage in IV MTX appeared to be more weighted toward better systemic control of disease than to CNS control, which was unexpected. The meta-analysis was admittedly tainted by different MTX doses, schedules, and number of doses delivered across the eight trials. Perhaps IV MTX doses at the higher end of the spectrum would be better to prevent CNS relapse.

The previously described St Jude TT-XV trial gave IV MTX doses such that a steady state blood level of 33 µM (mean MTX dose, 2.5 g/m^2) was achieved for low-risk children with ALL or 65 µM (mean MTX dose, 5 g/m^2) was achieved for standard- or high-risk children with ALL.[6] This IV MTX was delivered four times during the consolidation phase of therapy. This led to a low 8-year cumulative CNS relapse rate of 2.7% without cranial radiation. This suggests, but does not prove, that intensified doses of IV MTX are effective in preventing CNS leukemia relapse in childhood ALL, and help permit the elimination of cranial radiation as CNS prophylaxis.

The AALL0232 trial took another approach to IV MTX to reduce CNS relapse in children and young adults with ALL.[97] This trial randomized children and young adults (up to age 30 years) to four doses of IV MTX (5 g/m^2 per dose) during interim maintenance-1 to "Capizzi MTX" (IV MTX 100 mg/m^2 days 1, 11, 21, 31, and 41 with pegylated-asparaginase 2,500 units/m^2 IV days 2 and 22). In 2,426 randomized patients, the 5-year incidence of CNS relapse was 1.8% in patients receiving 5 g/m^2 IV MTX and 2.6% in patients receiving Capizzi MTX (p value not stated) with the 5-year EFS favoring high-dose MTX (82% vs 75%, respectively; p = 0.006). Due to the long half-life of pegylated-asparaginase and hence its prevention of leukemic cells reentering the S-phase of the cell cycle (MTX is only active during the S-phase), perhaps the Capizzi MTX arm was destined to fail on its MTX every 10 day schedule.

Interpreting the outcomes of IV MTX dose administered as CNS prophylaxis must also be tempered by the schedule of leucovorin administration and the different metabolisms of leucovorin in the malignancy being treated. There is concern that some protocols have started leucovorin rescue too early (between 12 hours and 24 hours after the MTX dose) and/or at too high of a dose such that the leucovorin in part protected leukemic cells from MTX cytotoxicity.[61] There is also evidence that the ALL lineage of origin also plays a role: patients with low-risk pre-B-cell ALL seem to do equally as well with IV MTX doses of 1–2 g/m^2 as T-cell patients receiving 5 g/m^2 per dose.[61]

Intermediate- and high-doses of IV MTX have become common in adult ALL regimens as a component of CNS prophylaxis.[98] At least seven adult trials have utilized IV MTX, in part, as a replacement for cranial radiation (Table 10-7). These trials used MTX doses of 0.5–3 g/m^2 given over 2–36 hours for 2–12 cycles. All trials also required IT chemotherapy. The CNS relapse rates ranged from 1.3% to 11%, with the lower relapse rates tending to be in protocols using higher MTX doses and more intense systemic regimens. Of note, the Hyper-CVAD regimen had a low (2.7%) relapse rate yet does not incorporate L-asparaginase, suggesting L-asparaginase is not critical for CNS prophylaxis in the setting of an otherwise very intense systemic regimen.

Intravenous Cytarabine

High doses of IV Ara-C ($\geq$2 g/m^2 per dose) have been used to provide prophylaxis against CNS relapse in patients with ALL and in the setting of eliminating cranial radiation.[8,84,101] Proof that high-doses of IV Ara-C are effective in reducing the risk of CNS relapse is lacking. The fact that therapeutic levels of Ara-C are present in the

Table 10-7	Central Nervous System Relapse in Adult Acute Lymphoblastic Leukemia Trials Using High-dose Intravenous Methotrexate and Intrathecal Chemotherapy Without Cranial Radiation					
Protocol	Number of patients enrolled	No. with CSF (+) at diagnosis	CR	IV MTX dosing	IT chemo-therapy	CNS relapse
MOAD[99]	55	NS	42 (76%)	100 mg/kg × 12		4/42 (10%)
Norway[100]	79	NS	65 (82%)	0.5 g/m^2 × 2	MTX	7/65 (11%)
UCSF 8707[84]	84	6 (7%)	78 (93%)	2.38 g/m^2 over 36 hour × 6	MTX × 6	1/78 (1.3%)
GIMEMA ALL/0288[7]	778	3 (0.4%)	627 (82%)	1 g/m^2 × 3	MTX/MPD × 16	50/627 (8%)
Hyper-CVAD[8]	288	20 (7%)	264 (92%)	1 g/m^2 over 26 hour × 4	MTX or Ara-C × 4–16	7/264 (2.7%)
PETHEMA ALL-89, -93, -96, -97[9]	467	18 (4%)	381 (81%)	3 g/m^2 × 2–6	MTX/Ara-C/ HC × 12–14	22/381 (6%)
CALGB 19802[86]	161	NS	128 (80%)	1 g/m^2 over 3 hour × 6	MTX × 6	9/128 (7%)

ALL, acute lymphoblastic leukemia; CSF, cerebrospinal fluid; CR, complete remission; IV, intravenous; IT, intrathecal; CNS, central nervous system; MOAD, methotrexate, vincristine, asparaginase and dexamethasone; NS, not stated; MTX, methotrexate; UCSF, University of California, San Francisco; GIMEMA, Gruppo Italiano Malattie Ematologiche dell'Adulto; MPD, methylprednisolone; Hyper-CVAD, hyperfractionated cyclophosphamide, vincristine, doxorubicin and dexamethasone; Ara-C, cytarabine; PETHEMA, Programa para el Estudio y Tratamiento de Hemopatias Maligns; LALA, Leucemies Aigues Lymphoblastiques de L'Adulte; HC, hydrocortisone; CALGB, Cancer and Leukemia Group B.

CSF after IV Ara-C doses of greater than or equal to 0.5 g/m^2 per dose promotes the concept that high-doses of systemic Ara-C might prevent CNS relapse of ALL.[38] High-dose Ara-C is an integral piece of three adult ALL regimens, the UCSF 8707 protocol ($2 \text{ g/m}^2 \times 4$ done twice), the Hyper-CVAD regimen ($3 \text{ g/m}^2 \times 4$ done four times), and Cancer and Leukemia Group B (CALGB) 19802 ($2 \text{ g/m}^2 \times 3$ done twice).[8,84,86] These regimens had low CNS relapse rates 1.3%, 2.7%, and 6%, respectively. CNS neurotoxicity as a complication of high-dose IV Ara-C likely tempers enthusiasm using this agent routinely in children and adults with ALL.[39,40]

Tyrosine-Kinase Inhibitors

As the tyrosine-kinase inhibitor dasatinib penetrates into the CSF at therapeutic levels, it has the potential to act as CNS prophylaxis in patients with Ph+ ALL when combined with systemic chemotherapy and routine CNS prophylaxis.[42] To date, there is no prospective data to support its role in CNS prophylaxis.

SECONDARY CNS PROPHYLAXIS

A common question arises in the setting of systemic relapse of ALL: how to again address the CNS? Certainly these patients are again at risk for CNS relapse. There is no answer to this question based on evidence. The adult UCSF hematologic malignancies program policy is to restart CNS prophylaxis as if this were the primary diagnosis of ALL. Since most of our adult patients have received UCSF 8707 protocol therapy, we again give six IT MTX administrations to patients at ALL relapse with CNS-1 or CNS-2 disease in the setting of aggressive systemic chemotherapy. For those with CNS-3 disease or a traumatic LP, the CNS treatment prescription is physician dependent.

TREATMENT OF THE CNS BEFORE OR AFTER ALLOGENEIC TRANSPLANT

The major risk factor for development of CNS relapse after allogeneic transplant is the presence of CNS involvement prior to transplant. Otherwise, the risk of CNS relapse after allogeneic transplant is low (2–3% in patients with no prior CNS involvement).[102-104] This may be attributable to an effective "graft-versus-leukemia" (GVL) effect in the CNS. Evidence to support this includes documentation of donor cells within the CSF[105] and long-term leukemia-free survival when allogeneic transplant is used to treat isolated CNS relapse in children.[106] However, in one report, donor lymphocyte infusion given for systemic relapse after allogeneic transplant resulted in systemic remission but with subsequent isolated CNS relapse, arguing against a GVL effect in the CNS.[107]

Little data exists to guide the use of CNS prophylactic therapy in the setting of planned allogeneic transplant [reviewed by the European Group for Blood and

Marrow Transplant (EBMT)].[108] In a survey of 90 EBMT centers, 53% administer CNS prophylaxis to ALL patients pretransplant and 23% do so post-transplant. However, no studies exist to evaluate the benefit of IT prophylaxis prior to transplant. With regard to IT prophylaxis given after transplant, one study has shown a decreased risk of CNS relapse,[109] but others have suggested that this is not necessary in patients with no history of CNS disease.[102,103] One study has even shown an increased risk of CNS relapse with post-transplant IT chemotherapy, even when adjusting for a history of CNS disease prior to transplant.[104] Based on the available data, the EBMT does not recommend CNS prophylaxis for patients with ALL undergoing allogeneic transplant who have no history of CNS involvement.

SUMMARY

It seems clear from the literature that CNS "prophylaxis" in ALL overlaps with CNS "treatment" in ALL, as the goal of both is to reduce the risk of future CNS relapse. That said, the evidence supports the elimination of both cranial and spinal radiations in patients with CNS-1, CNS-2, and CNS-3 disease at primary diagnosis, in both children and adults, provided the systemic chemotherapy administered is sufficiently intensive and IT chemotherapy is administered as well. Cranial radiation should still be considered early for cranial nerve and/or brain parenchymal abnormalities from ALL. The role of Dex versus Pred in the prevention of CNS relapse remains unclear, especially in the context of increased osteonecrosis with Dex in children with ALL over age 10 years. Intensive dosing and scheduling of IV MTX and parenteral asparaginase seems important in minimizing CNS relapse in ALL patients not receiving cranial radiation therapy. High-dose IV Ara-C plays a role in modern ALL regimens in adults as CNS prophylaxis. Thioguanine may be more effective than 6-mercaptopurine in preventing a CNS relapse in children, but is discouraged based on an unacceptably high incidence of VOD of liver.

Intrathecal MTX, triple therapy, thiotepa, or liposomal Ara-C should be considered when a CNS relapse occurs as well as cranial radiation (with particular attention to the morbidities of cranial radiation, especially if a salvage allogeneic stem cell transplant with TBI is planned). The role of secondary CNS prophylaxis at the time of systemic ALL relapse is undefined. It is critical that clinicians use a uniform published treatment protocol for their ALL patients, including the systemic and CNS-directed therapies, to maximize the best outcome for their patients not enrolled on a clinical trial.

REFERENCES

1. Jabbour EJ, Faderl S, Kantarjian HM. Adult acute lymphoblastic leukemia. *Mayo Clin Proc.* 2005;80(11):1517-27.
2. Seibel NL. Treatment of acute lymphoblastic leukemia in children and adolescents: peaks and pitfalls. *Hematology Am Soc Hematol Educ Program.* 2008:374-80.

3. Lazarus HM, Richards SM, Chopra R, et al. Central nervous system involvement in adult acute lymphoblastic leukemia at diagnosis: results from the international ALL trial MRC UKALL XII/ECOG E2993. *Blood.* 2006;108(2):465-72.

4. Laningham FH, Kun LE, Reddick WE, et al. Childhood central nervous system leukemia: historical perspectives, current therapy, and acute neurological sequelae. *Neuroradiology.* 2007;49(11):873-88.

5. Kamps WA, Bökkerink JP, Hakvoort-Cammel FG, et al. BFM-oriented treatment for children with acute lymphoblastic leukemia without cranial irradiation and treatment reduction for standard risk patients: results of DCLSG protocol ALL-8 (1991-1996). *Leukemia.* 2002; 16(6):1099-111.

6. Pui CH, Campana D, Pei D, et al. Treating childhood acute lymphoblastic leukemia without cranial irradiation. *N Engl J Med.* 2009;360(26):2730-41.

7. Annino L, Vegna ML, Camera A, et al. Treatment of adult acute lymphoblastic leukemia (ALL): long-term follow-up of the GIMEMA ALL 0288 randomized study. *Blood.* 2002;99(3):863-71.

8. Kantarjian H, Thomas D, O'Brien S, et al. Long-term follow-up results of hyperfractionated cyclophosphamide, vincristine, doxorubicin, and dexamethasone (Hyper-CVAD), a dose-intensive regimen, in adult acute lymphocytic leukemia. *Cancer.* 2004;101(12):2788-801.

9. Sancho JM, Ribera JM, Oriol A, et al. Central nervous system recurrence in adult patients with acute lymphoblastic leukemia: frequency and prognosis in 467 patients without cranial irradiation for prophylaxis. *Cancer.* 2006;106(12):2540-6.

10. Pui CH. Central nervous system disease in acute lymphoblastic leukemia: prophylaxis and treatment. *Hematology Am Soc Hematol Educ Program.* 2006:142-6.

11. Kantarjian HM, Walters RS, Smith TL, et al. Identification of risk groups for development of central nervous system leukemia in adults with acute lymphocytic leukemia. *Blood.* 1988; 72(5):1784-9.

12. Pui CH. Toward optimal central nervous system-directed treatment in childhood acute lymphoblastic leukemia. *J Clin Oncol.* 2003;21(2):179-81.

13. Schrappe M, Reiter A, Ludwig WD, et al. Improved outcome in childhood acute lymphoblastic leukemia despite reduced use of anthracyclines and cranial radiotherapy: results of trial ALL-BFM 90. German-Austrian-Swiss ALL-BFM Study Group. *Blood.* 2000;95(11):3310-22.

14. Silverman LB, Declerck L, Gelber RD, et al. Results of Dana-Farber Cancer Institute Consortium protocols for children with newly diagnosed acute lymphoblastic leukemia (1981-1995). *Leukemia.* 2000;14(12):2247-56.

15. Pui CH, Boyett JM, Rivera GK, et al. Long-term results of Total Therapy studies 11, 12 and 13A for childhood acute lymphoblastic leukemia at St Jude Children's Research Hospital. *Leukemia.* 2000;14(12):2286-94.

16. Sirvent N, Suciu S, Rialland X, et al. Prognostic significance of the initial cerebro-spinal fluid (CSF) involvement of children with acute lymphoblastic leukaemia (ALL) treated without cranial irradiation: results of European Organization for Research and Treatment of Cancer (EORTC) Children Leukemia Group study 58881. *Eur J Cancer.* 2011;47(2):239-47.

17. Reman O, Pigneux A, Huguet F, et al. Central nervous system involvement in adult acute lymphoblastic leukemia at diagnosis and/or at first relapse: results from the GET-LALA group. *Leuk Res.* 2008;32(11):1741-50.

18. Manabe A, Tsuchida M, Hanada R, et al. Delay of the diagnostic lumbar puncture and intrathecal chemotherapy in children with acute lymphoblastic leukemia who undergo routine corticosteroid testing: Tokyo Children's Cancer Study Group study L89-12. *J Clin Oncol.* 2001;19(13):3182-7.

19. Strupp M, Schueler O, Straube A, et al. "Atraumatic" Sprotte needle reduces the incidence of post-lumbar puncture headaches. *Neurology.* 2001;57(12):2310-2.

20. Mahmoud HH, Rivera GK, Hancock ML, et al. Low leukocyte counts with blast cells in cerebrospinal fluid of children with newly diagnosed acute lymphoblastic leukemia. *N Engl J Med.* 1993;329(5):314-9.

21. Lauer S, Shuster J, Kirchner P, et al. Prognostic significance of cerebrospinal fluid (CSF) lymphoblasts (LB) at diagnosis (dx) in children with acute lymphoblastic leukemia (ALL). *Proc Am Soc Clin Oncol.* 1994;13:317.

22. Nachman J, Cherlow J, Sather HN, et al. Effect of initial central nervous system (CNS) status on event-free survival (EFS) in children and adolescents with acute lymphoblastic leukemia (ALL). *Med Pediatr Oncol.* 2002;39:277.

23. Burger B, Zimmermann M, Mann G, et al. Diagnostic cerebrospinal fluid examination in children with acute lymphoblastic leukemia: significance of low leukocyte counts with blasts or traumatic lumbar puncture. *J Clin Oncol.* 2003;21(2):184-8.

24. Gilchrist GS, Tubergen DG, Sather HN, et al. Low numbers of CSF blasts at diagnosis do not predict for the development of CNS leukemia in children with intermediate-risk acute lymphoblastic leukemia: a Children's Cancer Group report. *J Clin Oncol.* 1994;12(12):2594-600.

25. Dutch Childhood Oncology Group, te Loo DM, Kamps WA, et al. Prognostic significance of blasts in the cerebrospinal fluid without pleiocytosis or a traumatic lumbar puncture in children with acute lymphoblastic leukemia: experience of the Dutch Childhood Oncology Group. *J Clin Oncol.* 2006;24(15):2332-6.

26. Pui CH, Sandlund JT, Pei D, et al. Improved outcome for children with acute lymphoblastic leukemia: results of Total Therapy Study XIIIB at St Jude Children's Research Hospital. *Blood.* 2004;104(9):2690-6.

27. Gajjar A, Harrison PL, Sandlund JT, et al. Traumatic lumbar puncture at diagnosis adversely affects outcome in childhood acute lymphoblastic leukemia. *Blood.* 2000;96(10):3381-4.

28. Aur RJ, Hustu HO, Verzosa MS, et al. Comparison of two methods of preventing central nervous system leukemia. *Blood.* 1973;42(3):349-57.

29. Ortega JA, Nesbit ME, Sather HN, et al. Long-term evaluation of a CNS prophylaxis trial—treatment comparisons and outcome after CNS relapse in childhood ALL: a report from the Children's Cancer Study Group. *J Clin Oncol.* 1987;5(10):1646-54.

30. Pui CH, Cheng C, Leung W, et al. Extended follow-up of long-term survivors of childhood acute lymphoblastic leukemia. *N Engl J Med.* 2003;349(7):640-9.

31. Kim S, Khatibi S, Howell SB, et al. Prolongation of drug exposure in cerebrospinal fluid by encapsulation into DepoFoam. *Cancer Res.* 1993;53(7):1596-8.

32. Bomgaars L, Geyer JR, Franklin J, et al. Phase I trial of intrathecal liposomal cytarabine in children with neoplastic meningitis. *J Clin Oncol.* 2004;22(19):3916-21.

33. Jabbour E, O'Brien S, Kantarjian H, et al. Neurologic complications associated with intrathecal liposomal cytarabine given prophylactically in combination with high-dose methotrexate and cytarabine to patients with acute lymphocytic leukemia. *Blood.* 2007;109(8):3214-8.

34. Fisher PG, Kadan-Lottick NS, Korones DN. Intrathecal thiotepa: reappraisal of an established therapy. *J Pediatr Hematol Oncol.* 2002;24(4):274-8.

35. Stork LC, Matloub Y, Broxson E, et al. Oral 6-mercaptopurine versus oral 6-thioguanine and veno-occlusive disease in children with standard-risk acute lymphoblastic leukemia: report of the Children's Oncology Group CCG-1952 clinical trial. *Blood.* 2010;115(14):2740-8.

36. Vora A, Mitchell CD, Lennard L, et al. Toxicity and efficacy of 6-thioguanine versus 6-mercaptopurine in childhood lymphoblastic leukaemia: a randomised trial. *Lancet.* 2006;368(9544):1339-48.

37. Jacobs SS, Stork LC, Bostrom BC, et al. Substitution of oral and intravenous thioguanine for mercaptopurine in a treatment regimen for children with standard risk acute lymphoblastic leukemia: a collaborative Children's Oncology Group/National Cancer Institute pilot trial (CCG-1942). *Pediatr Blood Cancer.* 2007;49(3):250-5.

38. Damon LE, Plunkett W, Linker CA. Plasma and cerebrospinal fluid pharmacokinetics of 1-beta-D-arabinofuranosylcytosine and 1-beta-D-arabinofuranosyluracil following the repeated intravenous administration of high- and intermediate-dose 1-beta-D-arabinofuranosylcytosine. *Cancer Res.* 1991;51(16):4141-5.

39. Damon LE, Mass R, Linker CA. The association between high-dose cytarabine neurotoxicity and renal insufficiency. *J Clin Oncol.* 1989;7(10):1563-8.

40. Smith GA, Damon LE, Rugo HS, et al. High-dose cytarabine dose modification reduces the incidence of neurotoxicity in patients with renal insufficiency. *J Clin Oncol.* 1997;15(2):833-9.

41. Heideman RL, Cole DE, Balis F, et al. Phase I and pharmacokinetic evaluation of thiotepa in the cerebrospinal fluid and plasma of pediatric patients: evidence for dose-dependent plasma clearance of thiotepa. *Cancer Res.* 1989;49(3):736-41.

42. Porkka K, Koskenvesa P, Lundán T, et al. Dasatinib crosses the blood-brain barrier and is an efficient therapy for central nervous system Philadelphia chromosome-positive leukemia. *Blood.* 2008;112(4):1005-12.

43. Haupt R, Fears TR, Robison LL, et al. Educational attainment in long-term survivors of childhood acute lymphoblastic leukemia. *JAMA.* 1994;272(18):1427-32.

44. Tucker J, Prior PF, Green CR, et al. Minimal neuropsychological sequelae following prophylactic treatment of the central nervous system in adult leukaemia and lymphoma. *Br J Cancer.* 1989;60(5):775-80.

45. Laack NN, Brown PD. Cognitive sequelae of brain radiation in adults. *Semin Oncol.* 2004; 31(5):702-13.

46. Glantz MJ, LaFollette S, Jaeckle KA, et al. Randomized trial of a slow-release versus a standard formulation of cytarabine for the intrathecal treatment of lymphomatous meningitis. *J Clin Oncol.* 1999;17(10):3110-6.

47. Gutin PH, Weiss HD, Wiernik PH, et al. Intrathecal N, N′, N″-triethylenethiophosphoramide [thio-TEPA (NSC 6396)] in the treatment of malignant meningeal disease: phase I-II study. *Cancer.* 1976;38(4):1471-5.

48. Ochocka M, Barancewicz M, Ciepielewska D. [Thiotepa in the treatment of central nervous system leukemia in children]. *Acta Haematol Pol.* 1978;9(4):263-7.

49. Balis FM, Lester CM, Chrousos GP, et al. Differences in cerebrospinal fluid penetration of corticosteroids: possible relationship to the prevention of meningeal leukemia. *J Clin Oncol.* 1987;5(2):202-7.

50. Mattano LA, Nachman JB, Devidas M, et al. (2008). Increased incidence of osteonecrosis (ON) with a dexamethasone (DEX) induction for high risk acute lymphoblastic leukemia (HR-ALL): a report from the Children's Oncology Group (COG). [online] Available from ash. confex.com/ash/2008/webprogram/Paper2380.html. [Accessed August, 2013].

51. Inaba H, Pui CH. Glucocorticoid use in acute lymphoblastic leukaemia. *Lancet Oncol.* 2010;11(11):1096-106.

52. Woo MH, Hak LJ, Storm MC, et al. Cerebrospinal fluid asparagine concentrations after Escherichia coli asparaginase in children with acute lymphoblastic leukemia. *J Clin Oncol.* 1999;17(5):1568-73.

53. Rizzari C, Zucchetti M, Conter V, et al. L-asparagine depletion and L-asparaginase activity in children with acute lymphoblastic leukemia receiving i.m. or i.v. Erwinia C. or E. coli L-asparaginase as first exposure. *Ann Oncol.* 2000;11(2):189-93.

54. Avramis VI, Sencer S, Periclou AP, et al. A randomized comparison of native Escherichia coli asparaginase and polyethylene glycol conjugated asparaginase for treatment of children with newly diagnosed standard-risk acute lymphoblastic leukemia: a Children's Cancer Group study. *Blood.* 2002;99(6):1986-94.

55. Hamdan MY, Frenkel EP, Bick R. L-asparaginase-provoked seizures as singular expression of central nervous toxicity. *Clin Appl Thromb Hemost.* 2000;6(4):234-8.

56. Maytal J, Grossman R, Yusuf FH, et al. Prognosis and treatment of seizures in children with acute lymphoblastic leukemia. *Epilepsia.* 1995;36(8):831-6.

57. Moghrabi A, Levy DE, Asselin B, et al. Results of the Dana-Farber Cancer Institute ALL Consortium Protocol 95-01 for children with acute lymphoblastic leukemia. *Blood.* 2007; 109(3):896-904.

58. Bokstein F, Lossos A, Lossos IS, et al. Central nervous system relapse of systemic non-Hodgkin's lymphoma: results of treatment based on high-dose methotrexate combination chemotherapy. *Leuk Lymphoma.* 2002;43(3):587-93.
59. Wieduwilt MJ, Valles F, Issa S, et al. Immunochemotherapy with intensive consolidation for primary CNS lymphoma: a pilot study and prognostic assessment by diffusion-weighted MRI. *Clin Cancer Res.* 2012;18(4):1146-55.
60. Rubenstein J, Hsi ED, Johnson JL, et al. Intensive chemotherapy and immunotherapy in patient with newly diagnosed primary CNS lymphoma: CALGB 50202 (Alliance 50202). *J Clin Oncol.* 2013;31:3061-8.
61. Pui CH, Relling MV, Evans WE. Is mega dose of methotrexate beneficial to patients with acute lymphoblastic leukemia? *Leuk Lymphoma.* 2006;47(12):2431-2.
62. Aradillas E, Arora R, Gasperino J. Methotrexate-induced posterior reversible encephalopathy syndrome. *J Clin Pharm Ther.* 2011;36(4):529-36.
63. Salkade PR, Lim TA. Methotrexate-induced acute toxic leukoencephalopathy. *J Cancer Res Ther.* 2012;8(2):292-6.
64. Witzig TE, Geyer SM, Kurtin PJ, et al. Salvage chemotherapy with rituximab DHAP for relapsed non-Hodgkin lymphoma: a phase II trial in the North Central Cancer Treatment Group. *Leuk Lymphoma.* 2008;49(6):1074-80.
65. Soussain C, Suzan F, Hoang-Xuan K, et al. Results of intensive chemotherapy followed by hematopoietic stem-cell rescue in 22 patients with refractory or recurrent primary CNS lymphoma or intraocular lymphoma. *J Clin Oncol.* 2001;19(3):742-9.
66. Enokido Y, Araki T, Aizawa S, et al. p53 involves cytosine arabinoside-induced apoptosis in cultured cerebellar granule neurons. *Neurosci Lett.* 1996;203(1):1-4.
67. Besirli CG, Deckwerth TL, Crowder RJ, et al. Cytosine arabinoside rapidly activates Bax-dependent apoptosis and a delayed Bax-independent death pathway in sympathetic neurons. *Cell Death Differ.* 2003;10(9):1045-58.
68. Wolff SN, Herzig RH, Fay JW, et al. High-dose N,N',N''-triethylenethiophosphoramide (thiotepa) with autologous bone marrow transplantation: phase I studies. *Semin Oncol.* 1990;17(1 Suppl 3):2-6.
69. Barredo JC, Devidas M, Lauer SJ, et al. Isolated CNS relapse of acute lymphoblastic leukemia treated with intensive systemic chemotherapy and delayed CNS radiation: a pediatric oncology group study. *J Clin Oncol.* 2006;24(19):3142-9.
70. Soussain C, Hoang-Xuan K, Taillandier L, et al. Intensive chemotherapy followed by hematopoietic stem-cell rescue for refractory and recurrent primary CNS and intraocular lymphoma: Société Française de Greffe de Moëlle Osseuse-Thérapie Cellulaire. *J Clin Oncol.* 2008;26(15):2512-8.
71. Cote GM, Hochberg EP, Muzikansky A, et al. Autologous stem cell transplantation with thiotepa, busulfan, and cyclophosphamide (TBC) conditioning in patients with CNS involvement by non-Hodgkin lymphoma. *Biol Blood Marrow Transplant.* 2012;18(1):76-83.
72. Pui CH, Howard SC. Current management and challenges of malignant disease in the CNS in paediatric leukaemia. *Lancet Oncol.* 2008;9(3):257-68.
73. Pui CH, Thiel E. Central nervous system disease in hematologic malignancies: historical perspective and practical applications. *Semin Oncol.* 2009;36(4 Suppl 2):S2-S16.
74. Surapaneni UR, Cortes JE, Thomas D, et al. Central nervous system relapse in adults with acute lymphoblastic leukemia. *Cancer.* 2002;94(3):773-9.
75. Fielding AK, Richards SM, Chopra R, et al. Outcome of 609 adults after relapse of acute lymphoblastic leukemia (ALL); an MRC UKALL12/ECOG 2993 study. *Blood.* 2007;109(3):944-50.
76. Chamberlain MC, Glantz MJ. Re: Neurologic complications associated with intrathecal liposomal cytarabine given prophylactically in combination with high-dose methotrexate and cytarabine to patients with acute lymphocytic leukemia. *Blood.* 2007;110(5):1698.

77. Hilgendorf I, Wolff D, Junghanss C, et al. Neurological complications after intrathecal liposomal cytarabine application in patients after allogeneic haematopoietic stem cell transplantation. *Ann Hematol.* 2008;87(12):1009-12.

78. Gutiérrez-Aguirre H, García-Rodríguez F, Cantú-Rodríguez O, et al. Effectiveness of dasatinib in relapsed CNS, Ph$^+$ ALL that is refractory to radiochemotherapy plus imatinib: a case report. *Clin Adv Hematol Oncol.* 2011;9(11):875-8.

79. Clarke M, Gaynon P, Hann I, et al. CNS-directed therapy for childhood acute lymphoblastic leukemia: Childhood ALL Collaborative Group overview of 43 randomized trials. *J Clin Oncol.* 2003;21(9):1798-809.

80. Pui CH, Mahmoud HH, Rivera GK, et al. Early intensification of intrathecal chemotherapy virtually eliminates central nervous system relapse in children with acute lymphoblastic leukemia. *Blood.* 1998;92(2):411-5.

81. Conter V, Schrappe M, Aricó M, et al. Role of cranial radiotherapy for childhood T-cell acute lymphoblastic leukemia with high WBC count and good response to prednisone. Associazione Italiana Ematologia Oncologia Pediatrica and the Berlin-Frankfurt-Münster groups. *J Clin Oncol.* 1997;15(8):2786-91.

82. Vilmer E, Suciu S, Ferster A, et al. Long-term results of three randomized trials (58831, 58832, 58881) in childhood acute lymphoblastic leukemia: a CLCG-EORTC report. Children Leukemia Cooperative Group. *Leukemia.* 2000;14(12):2257-66.

83. Linker CA, Levitt LJ, O'Donnell M, et al. Treatment of adult acute lymphoblastic leukemia with intensive cyclical chemotherapy: a follow-up report. *Blood.* 1991;78(11):2814-22.

84. Linker C, Damon L, Ries C, et al. Intensified and shortened cyclical chemotherapy for adult acute lymphoblastic leukemia. *J Clin Oncol.* 2002;20(10):2464-71..

85. Larson RA, Dodge RK, Burns CP, et al. A five-drug remission induction regimen with intensive consolidation for adults with acute lymphoblastic leukemia: cancer and leukemia group B study 8811. *Blood.* 1995;85(8):2025-37.

86. Stock W, Johnson JL, Stone RM, et al. Dose intensification of daunorubicin and cytarabine during treatment of adult acute lymphoblastic leukemia: results of Cancer and Leukemia Group B Study 19802. *Cancer.* 2013;119(1):90-8.

87. Matloub Y, Lindemulder S, Gaynon PS, et al. Intrathecal triple therapy decreases central nervous system relapse but fails to improve event-free survival when compared with intra-thecal methotrexate: results of the Children's Cancer Group (CCG) 1952 study for standard-risk acute lymphoblastic leukemia, reported by the Children's Oncology Group. *Blood.* 2006;108(4):1165-73.

88. McClune B, Buadi FK, Aslam N, et al. Intrathecal liposomal cytarabine for prevention of meningeal disease in patients with acute lymphocytic leukemia and high-grade lymphoma. *Leuk Lymphoma.* 2007;48(9):1849-51.

89. Teuffel O, Kuster SP, Hunger SP, et al. Dexamethasone versus prednisone for induction therapy in childhood acute lymphoblastic leukemia: a systematic review and meta-analysis. *Leukemia.* 2011;25(8):1232-8.

90. Jones B, Freeman AI, Shuster JJ, et al. Lower incidence of meningeal leukemia when prednisone is replaced by dexamethasone in the treatment of acute lymphocytic leukemia. *Med Pediatr Oncol.* 1991;19(4):269-75.

91. Bostrom BC, Sensel MR, Sather HN, et al. Dexamethasone versus prednisone and daily oral versus weekly intravenous mercaptopurine for patients with standard-risk acute lymphoblastic leukemia: a report from the Children's Cancer Group. *Blood.* 2003;101(10):3809-17.

92. Mitchell CD, Richards SM, Kinsey SE, et al. Benefit of dexamethasone compared with prednisolone for childhood acute lymphoblastic leukaemia: results of the UK Medical Research Council ALL97 randomized trial. *Br J Haematol.* 2005;129(6):734-45.

93. Schrappe M, Zimmermann M, Möricke A, et al. (2008). Dexamethasone in induction can eliminate one third of all relapses in childhood acute lymphoblastic leukemia (ALL): results of an international randomized trial in 3655 patients (Trial AIEOP-BFM ALL 2000). [online]

Available from: ash.confex.com/ash/2008/webprogram/Paper6711.html. [Accessed August, 2013].

94. Igarashi S, Manabe A, Ohara A, et al. No advantage of dexamethasone over prednisolone for the outcome of standard- and intermediate-risk childhood acute lymphoblastic leukemia in the Tokyo Children's Cancer Study Group L95-14 protocol. *J Clin Oncol.* 2005;23(27):6489-98.

95. Bertrand Y, Suciu S, Benoit Y, et al. (2008). Dexamethasone (DEX) (6 mg/sm/d) and prednisolone (PRED) (60 mg/sm/d) in induction therapy of childhood ALL are equally effective: results of the 2nd interim analysis of EORTC trial 58951. [online] Available from: ash.confex.com/ash/2008/webprogram/Paper7866.html. [Accessed August, 2013].

96. Larsen E, Raetz EA, Winick NJ, et al. (2012). Outcome in adolescent and young adult (AYA) patients compared with younger patients treated for high-risk B-precursor acute lymphoblastic leukemia (HR-ALL): A report from the Children's Oncology Group study AALL0232. [online] Available from: meetinglibrary.asco.org/content/99179-114. [Accessed August, 2013].

97. Larsen EC, Salzer WL, Devidas M, et al. (2011). Comparison of high-dose methotrexate (HD-MTX) with Capizzi methotrexate plus asparaginase (C-MTX/ASNase) in children and young adults with high-risk acute lymphoblastic leukemia (HR-ALL): A report from the Children's Oncology Group Study AALL0232. [online] Available from: meetinglibrary.asco. org/content/83893-102. [Accessed August, 2013].

98. Gökbuget N, Hoelzer D. High-dose methotrexate in the treatment of adult acute lympho-blastic leukemia. *Ann Hematol.* 1996;72(4):194-201.

99. Wiernik PH, Dutcher JP, Paietta E, et al. Long-term follow-up of treatment and potential cure of adult acute lymphocytic leukemia with MOAD: a non-anthracycline containing regimen. *Leukemia.* 1993;7(8):1236-41.

100. Evensen SA, Brinch L, Tjønnfjord G, et al. Estimated 8-year survival of more than 40% in a population-based study of 79 adult patients with acute lymphoblastic leukaemia. *Br J Haematol.* 1994;88(1):88-93.

101. Hoelzer D, Gökbuget N. Recent approaches in acute lymphoblastic leukemia in adults. *Crit Rev Oncol Hematol.* 2000;36(1):49-58.

102. Ganem G, Kuentz M, Bernaudin F, et al. Central nervous system relapses after bone marrow transplantation for acute lymphoblastic leukemia in remission. *Cancer.* 1989;64(9):1796-804.

103. Singhal S, Powles R, Treleaven J, et al. Central nervous system relapse after bone marrow transplantation for acute leukemia in first remission. *Bone Marrow Transplant.* 1996; 17(4):637-41.

104. Oshima K, Kanda Y, Yamashita T, et al. Central nervous system relapse of leukemia after allogeneic hematopoietic stem cell transplantation. *Biol Blood Marrow Transplant.* 2008; 14(10):1100-7.

105. Hibi S, Tsunamoto K, Todo S, et al. Chimerism analysis on mononuclear cells in the CSF after allogeneic bone marrow transplantation. *Bone Marrow Transplant.* 1997;20(6):503-6.

106. Harker-Murray PD, Thomas AJ, Wagner JE, et al. Allogeneic hematopoietic cell transplantation in children with relapsed acute lymphoblastic leukemia isolated to the central nervous system. *Biol Blood Marrow Transplant.* 2008;14(6):685-92.

107. Glass B, Majolino I, Dreger P, et al. Allogeneic peripheral blood progenitor cells for treatment of relapse after bone marrow transplantation. *Bone Marrow Transplant.* 1997;20(7):533-41.

108. Ruutu T, Corradini P, Gratwohl A, et al. Use of intrathecal prophylaxis in allogeneic haematopoietic stem cell transplantation for malignant blood diseases: a survey of the European Group for Blood and Marrow Transplantation (EBMT). *Bone Marrow Transplant.* 2005;35(2):121-4.

109. Thompson CB, Sanders JE, Flournoy N, et al. The risks of central nervous system relapse and leukoencephalopathy in patients receiving marrow transplants for acute leukemia. *Blood.* 1986;67(1):195-9.

Pharmacogenomics of Acute Lymphoblastic Leukemia Chemotherapy

Stéphanie Dulucq, Maja Krajinovic

INTRODUCTION

Despite great progress in treatment of acute lymphoblastic leukemia (ALL) particularly pediatric ALL, 20% of children and 60% of adults with ALL, relapse or die from their disease or therapy-related toxicity. Variability in treatment response can be: physiologic (age, liver status), pathological (disease severity), environmental (food, coadministration of drugs), or genetic.[1-3]

Pharmacogenetics contributes to understand the variability in treatment responses and identifies genetic polymorphisms that may predict such responses prior to drug administration ultimately leading to individualized treatment based on a patient's genetic profile. Two main approaches can be used: (1) candidate gene studies and (2) whole genome screening.

Identification of pharmacogenetic markers was initially addressed through candidate gene approach that analyzed variations in genes that are essential for drug effects (e.g., those which encode for drug pharmacokinetic and pharmacodynamic determinants), such as for example receptors, ionic channels, transporters, metabolizing enzymes or drug targets. Whereas initial studies analyzed the impact of one polymorphism, more recent studies have analyzed the impact of several polymorphisms of the same gene or even screened polymorphic content of many relevant genes. The approach combining information from several genes in the same pathway is more appropriate since it minimizes the "noise" produced by non-targeted genes.

Progress in molecular biology, particularly the development of ribonucleic acid (RNA) and deoxyribonucleic acid (DNA) microarrays, has allowed addressing the genetic component of variability in treatment response through whole genome approaches. Genome-wide expression profiling can screen all potentially important genes and could identify new resistance mechanisms, as well as new targets for treatment or diagnosis. For example, using such analysis in cells that are defined as resistant or sensitive following an exposure to a given drug, it is possible to identify a set of differently expressed genes which are likely to influence treatment outcomes.[4,5] Subsequently, more targeted analyses are needed to identify variations in differentially expressed genes that alter such expression or modulate clinical outcomes. DNA microarray technology has led to the development of genome-wide association studies (GWAS) allowing the analysis of more than 500,000 polymorphisms at the same time that could thus identify, in large cohorts, additional genes and variations that can affect therapeutic responses. And finally, with the advent of next-generation sequencing (NGS) technologies, the way we think about scientific approaches in basic, applied and clinical research will change. It will be possible to obtain more in-depth view of genomic variations involved in human health and diseases and to identify mutations (both common and rare) leading to the variability in treatment responses.[6]

This chapter will summarize the pharmacogenomic studies in ALL that have highlighted the impact of genetic polymorphisms on treatment responses. Therapy of ALL is based on sequential polychemotherapy (see Chapters 6 and 7), and most of the studies have examined the key components of such treatment protocols: thiopurines, methotrexate (MTX), corticosteroids (CS), and more recently, asparaginase. ALL has a much higher incidence in children than in adults,[7] thus the majority of pharmacogenetic studies have been carried out in childhood ALL patients.

THIOPURINES

Thiopurine S-methyl transferase (TPMT) is a key enzyme in the metabolism of thiopurines (including 6-mercaptopurine, 6-MP). It inactivates 6-MP by transferring a methyl group and prevents the accumulation of its main active cytotoxic metabolites, the thioguanine nucleotides (TGNs) produced by the hypoxanthine phosphoribosyltransferase (HPRT) pathway (Figure 11-1). Risk of severe hematopoietic toxicity depends on intracellular TGN levels in inverse proportion to TPMT activity.[4] Up to 30 polymorphisms in the TPMT gene have been identified to date. They are defined by DNA base substitutions leading to amino acid replacements and reduction in enzyme activity. The most frequent variants (listed in Table 11-1) are TPMT*2 (defined by G to C substitution at position 238 of the gene), TPMT*3A (defined by c.460G > A and c.719A > G nucleotide transitions), and TPMT*3C (defined by c.719A > G).[3,4,8] Approximately 10% of the population is heterozygous for non-functional variants, resulting in intermediate enzyme activity, whereas 1 in 300 people inherit two non-functional alleles, resulting in very low or no enzyme activity.[4] Numerous studies demonstrating a clear correlation between TPMT genotype and 6-MP intolerance prompted the Food and Drug Administration (FDA) to recommend TPMT testing in patients with clinical evidence of myelosuppression.[9] Reduction to 10% of standard 6-MP doses is recommended for individuals who are homozygous for variant TPMT alleles. Heterozygous individuals might also benefit from dose reduction.[10] Recently, the Clinical Pharmacogenetics Implementation Consortium, published guidelines

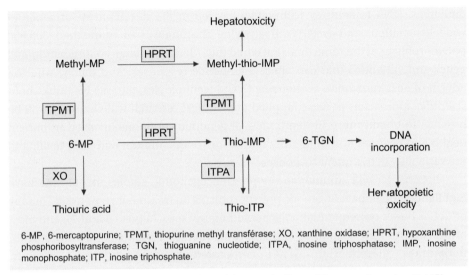

6-MP, 6-mercaptopurine; TPMT, thiopurine methyl transférase; XO, xanthine oxidase; HPRT, hypoxanthine phosphoribosyltransferase; TGN, thioguanine nucleotide; ITPA, inosine triphosphatase; IMP, inosine monophosphate; ITP, inosine triphosphate.

Figure 11-1 Schematic representation of the metabolism of 6-mercaptopurine (6-MP).

and strongly recommends determination of TPMT genotypes before 6-MP administration to adapt initial drug doses.[11]

Conversely, patients with high TPMT activity are at a higher risk of hepatotoxicity due to accumulation of methylated metabolites and are also at higher risk of relapse due to low TGN levels. TPMT genotyping does not permit to identify these patients and complementary clinical laboratory tests, such as TPMT activity dosage or TGN levels may be helpful.[11-14]

In addition to influencing hematologic toxicity, TPMT variants seem to be associated with a higher risk to develop secondary acute myeloid leukemia (AML) following ALL treatment[15] or secondary brain tumors in children receiving concurrent thiopurine and radiation therapy.[16]

Other enzymes involved in 6-MP metabolism may also influence 6-MP response. Xanthine oxidase (XO) is an alternative pathway to TPMT for 6-MP inactivation (Figure 11-1). Several polymorphisms have been recently described in the XO gene in the Japanese population.[17] The T-1756 to C substitution seems to affect XO promoter activity,[17] while several polymorphisms in coding regions leading to amino-acid substitutions change enzyme activity.[17] Although these polymorphisms may potentially affect 6-MP related toxicity, no such association was found in ALL patients.[18]

Inosine triphosphate pyrophosphatase (ITPA) catalyzes the conversion of inosine triphosphate (ITP) into inosine monophosphate (IMP), thereby preventing the accumulation of ITP in normal cells. In ITPA deficient patients treated with thiopurines, accumulation of ITP can occur, resulting in drug related toxicity.[19] Two polymorphisms are associated with ITPA deficiency: c.94C > A (Pro32Thr) in exon 2 and IVS2 + 21A > C near the splice donor site of intron 2. Compound heterozygous patients possess 10% of enzyme activity.[20,21] In childhood ALL, a significant association exists between intronic A to C polymorphism and thrombocytopenia[18] and between the c.94 C > A variant and febrile neutropenia.[22] Nevertheless, controversial results has been obtained regarding the latter single nucleotide polymorphism (SNP) because studies separately analyzed TPMT and ITPA genotypes, and these two enzymes affect the methylated metabolites [6-methylmercaptopurine nucleotide (6-MMPN)] concentration in opposite ways.[22,23] The lowest 6-MMPN levels are observed in patients with TMPT variant and wild type ITPA, whereas the highest 6-MMPN are observed in patients with wild type TPMT and ITPA variant.[22,24] Indeed if 6-MP doses are adjusted for TPMT genotype, then coding ITPA c.94 C > A variation has a significant influence on the risk of febrile neutropenia in pediatric ALL patients.[22,24]

METHOTREXATE

Methotrexate (MTX), a folate antagonist, competitively inhibits dihydrofolate reductase (DHFR) which catalyzes reduction of dihydrofolate (DHF) into tetrahydrofolate (THF), resulting in depletion of reduced folate (Figure 11-2). Two reduced folates play a key role in nucleic acid synthesis: N_5, N_{10}-methylene THF, which allows deoxythymidylate synthesis and N_{10}-formyl THF, required for purine synthesis. MTX treatment induces inhibition of nucleic acid formation ultimately leading to cell death.[24]

Reduced Folate Carrier

Methotrexate efficacy depends on its concentration inside cells. MTX enters the cells via the reduced folate carrier (RFC), which is also responsible for the cellular uptake of reduced folates. Decrease in expression or impaired function of RFC has been reported to affect MTX sensitivity.[25,26] A G80A polymorphism in RFC1 gene leads to His27Arg replacement in the first transmembrane domain of the RFC protein, which is considered to play a key role in folate-antifolate binding.[27] Initially, an *in vitro* study, did not find any difference in MTX uptake in transfected cells between two alleles of this polymorphism.[28] A more recent study, however, demonstrated increased MTX uptake in cells from healthy controls with the AA genotype.[29] In childhood ALL patients, the presence of allele A or AA genotypes was associated with a higher degree of gastrointestinal and bone marrow toxicity during consolidation and maintenance treatment,[30-33] consistent with the observation of higher MTX levels in individuals with the A allele.[32,33] The analysis addressing relationship of G80A with ALL outcome produced somewhat ambiguous results. Whereas some groups

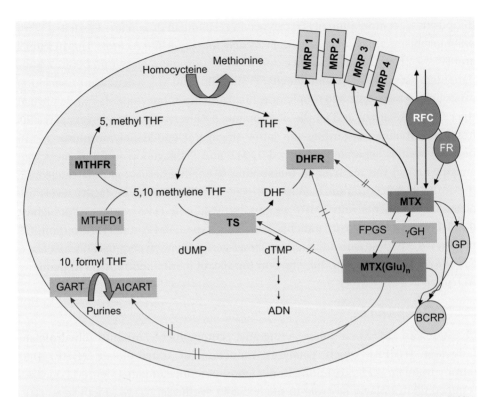

Enzymes and transporters whose genetic polymorphisms are described in the text are given in bold character. DHF, dihydrofolate; THF, tetrahydrofolate; DHFR, dihydrofolate reductase; dUMP, deoxyuridine monophosphate; dTMP, deoxythymidine monophosphate; TS, thymidylate synthase; FGPS, folylpolyglutamate synthase; γGH, gamma-glutamyl hydrolase; MTX(Glu)n, methotrexate polyglutamate; MTHFR, methylene tetrahydrofolate reductase; RFC, reduced folate carrier; MRP; multidrug resistance associated proteins; GP, P-glycoprotein; BCRP, breast cancer resistance protein; GART, glycinamide ribonucleotide formyltransferase; AICART, aminoimidazole carboxamide ribonucleotide formyltransferase; MTHFD, methylene tetrahydrofolate deshydrogenase.

Figure 11-2 The effect of methotrexate on the folate cycle. *Modified from* Krajinovic M, Moghrabi A. Pharmacogenetics of methotrexate. *Pharmacogenomics.* 2004;5:819-34.

reported absence of association with disease outcome,[34,35] others found association of either A[33] or G allele[32] or GG genotype[36] with increased risk of relapse. Different reasons may account for this discrepancy including profound difference in total MTX doses between treatment protocols, diet, folate intake and folate homeostasis, chromosome 21 copy number,[32] and confounding effects of other polymorphisms. Indeed, it was reported that relative importance of G80A substitution is less relevant when analyzed simultaneously with other variations of MTX pathway, particularly in genes affecting MTX efflux.[37]

SLCOB1

SLCOB1 is a hepatic organic anion transporter polypeptide (OATP) whose key role in MTX disposition was revealed by GWAS.[38] SLCOB1 gene is located on chromosome 12 and mediates uptake of MTX[39-41] and many others compounds like bilirubin or medications, like statins and irinotecan. A non-synonymous 521T > C polymorphism, resulting in a Val174Ala substitution, has been associated with MTX disposition.[38,42] The 521C allele is associated with decreased transporter function *in vitro*.[40] Patients with this allele had lower MTX clearance and higher MTX plasma concentration[38,42] consistent with previous studies analyzing other SLCOB1 substrates.[43] The same variant was associated with gastrointestinal toxicity in childhood ALL patients.[42] Fifteen other polymorphisms located across the gene and organized in about 20 haplotypes have been described.[44] Particular haplotypes (*5, *15, *23, and *31) predicted to harbor damaging SNPs, were associated with a lower MTX clearance whereas haplotypes *14 and *35 were associated with higher MTX clearance.[44] Interestingly, rare variations obtained by next generation sequencing were also analyzed in the same study.[44] Those predicted to be functionally damaging were more likely to be found among patients with the lowest MTX clearance. All variants (both common and rare) accounted for about 10% of interpatient variability in MTX clearance.[44]

N$_5$, N$_{10}$-Methylene Tetrahydrofolate Reductase

Decrease of reduced folate pool due to MTX treatment increases homocysteine levels and decreases methionine synthesis. Among enzymes involved in regulation of homocysteine levels, the N$_5$, N$_{10}$-methylene tetrahydrofolate reductase (MTHFR) catalyzes the reduction of the N$_5$, N$_{10}$-methylene THF to N$_5$-methyl THF which provides a methyl group for homocyteine methylation[45] (Figure 11-2). Reduced levels of N$_5$, N$_{10}$-methylene THF facilitate the action of MTX, whereas increased levels can antagonize its effects. Two common polymorphisms in MTHFR gene with functional impact have been described: 677C > T (Ala220Val)[46] and 1298A > C(Glu429Ala).[47] The 677C > T polymorphism leads to altered catalytic domain whereas the 1298A > C polymorphism affects the regulatory domain. Decreased enzymatic activity is observed in patients who are homozygous for 677T or 1298C alleles, and to a lesser extent in heterozygous individuals.[46,47] In ALL, the 677T allele seems to have an impact on MTX efficacy in childhood ALL whereas an impact on drug-related toxicity has been more often seen in adult ALL patients. The presence of 677T was associated with an increased risk of relapse in several cohorts of childhood ALL patients[48-52] or with reduced overall survival in both pediatric and adult ALL.[53-55] Homozygosity for the same allele was associated with an increased risk of hepatotoxicity or myelosuppression in adult ALL. Many studies conducted in childhood ALL patients did not see an association of 677T allele with MTX-related toxicity,[48,56-58] even if a decreased MTX clearance and/or high MTX serum concentration were noted in patients with 677TT genotype.[30,51,58] Nevertheless, in two recent studies, children with unfavorable MTHFR genotype more frequently developed myelosuppression[50,51] and had higher creatinine levels.[50] Potential explanations for the difference in MTX toxicity across studies may include differences in MTX dose and administration schedule, concurrent medications, folate status, diet, and a different mechanism leading to drug-related toxicity.

Dihydrofolate Reductase

Altered levels of DHFR are found at diagnosis in childhood ALL, particularly in patients with a shorter event-free survival (EFS).[59-61] Changes in the level of DHFR expression and consequently in the sensitivity to MTX can also be due to genetic polymorphisms. A comprehensive study of the minor promoter polymorphisms in DHFR gene identified 15 variations that were in linkage disequilibrium.[62] Three polymorphisms (-1610 C > G/T, -680 C > A, -317 A > G) were identified as sufficient to define all haplotypes (tagSNPs). Reduction in EFS was associated with -317A and -1610C variants and haplotype *1 defined by these alleles. Haplotype *1 was associated with higher DHFR expression.[62] More recently, additional study of the major promoter/noncoding transcript region, adjacent to previously studied regulatory region, was performed.[63] Three tag polymorphisms [35C > T, 308G > A and a length polymorphism composed of two sequence motifs (insertion/deletion 9pb at position 63 and variable number of 9pb element at position 91)] further diversified the haplotype *1 into five subtypes. Lower EFS was associated with the 308A allele and haplotype *1b, particularly in high-risk patients. Haplotype *1b was the only subtype associated with higher mRNA levels likely explaining the worse prognosis for *1b carriers.[63] Another polymorphism, defined by a insertion/deletion (indel) of 19-bp sequence in the first intron of DHFR gene, was suggested to modulate DHFR expression.[64] This polymorphism was associated with an increased risk of hepatotoxicity in adult ALL.[55] Homozygosity for the wild type allele was in contrast associated with thrombocytopenia in childhood ALL,[50] whereas others did not find such an association.[62] 19-bp indel is in linkage disequilibrium (LD) with the promoter polymorphisms and is shared between several promoter haplotypes,[62] whose different frequency across studies might explain some of the discrepancies seen.

Thymidylate Synthase

Thymidylate synthase (TS) is a key enzyme in the nucleotide biosynthetic pathway that catalyzes conversion of deoxyuridylate to deoxythymidylate (Figure 11-2). Several enzymes of purine and pyrimidine synthesis, including TS are inhibited by MTX polyglutamates.[24] A repeat polymorphism was identified in the enhancer element of the 5'untranslated region (UTR) region.[65] This polymorphism contains variable numbers of a 28-bp repeat element with the double (2R) and triple repeat (3R) alleles being the most frequent. Expression level of TS gene is linked to number of repeats. Patients who are homozygous for the triple repetition (3R3R) have higher TS mRNA levels compared to 2R2R patients.[66,67] Higher risk of relapse has been reported for 3R3R childhood ALL patients,[68-70] and for those with 3R4R genotype.[52] Another study demonstrated that low-risk 3R3R patients had a predisposition for central nervous system (CNS) relapse, whereas high-risk patients with a combined TS 3R3R and glutathione-S-transferase non null genotype had an increased risk of hematologic relapse.[34]

Another polymorphism defined by a deletion (del) of 6-bp was identified in 3'UTR region of *TS* gene.[71] *In vitro*, this polymorphism leads to reduced mRNA stability.[72] Thus, the presence of this polymorphism should oppose the impact of 3R variant or increase that of the 2R allele. A childhood ALL study showed a lower frequency of haplotype 2R6bpdel in children with an event. The same study also observed reduced EFS in patients with genotype 3R3R only if they did not have the 6-bp deletion.[69]

Drug-related toxicity studies suggest that patients with low-activity genotypes are more sensitive to MTX. In fact, a higher incidence of osteonecrosis of the hip has been demonstrated in ALL patients with 2R2R genotype[73] as well as higher incidence of leukopenia and thrombocytopenia.[58]

Cyclin D1

Cyclin D1 (CCND1) is a key protein which regulates the G1 phase of the cell cycle. CCND1 has an important role in the phosphorylation and the functional inactivation of the retinoblastoma protein (pRb). The phosphorylation state of pRb can be affected by the increased expression of CCND1, thus resulting in higher E2F levels and increased transcription of MTX targets like DHFR and TS (Figure 11-3). This in turn can reduce the sensitivity of leukemia cells to MTX.[74,75] A polymorphism defined by an A to G substitution (870A > G) has been described in the splicing donor site between exon and intron 4. It modulates the mRNA ratio of isoform (a) and isoform (b).[76] The 870G allele leads to the synthesis of a shorter mRNA, corresponding to isoform (a) whereas the 870A allele codes for mRNA with a longer half-life, keeping the pRb phosphorylated for a longer time. Patients with genotype 870AA had reduced EFS[77,78] and less drug-related toxicity, as estimated by myelosuppression and hepatotoxicity.[56] Since CCND1 can upregulate DHFR and TS, the combined effect of genetic polymorphisms in these genes is more pronounced and leads to a further reduction in EFS in childhood ALL patients.[62] Nevertheless, CCND1 can modulate response to several drugs[79] and it is possible that the observed impact is due to the response modulation of other drugs used in ALL treatment.[45]

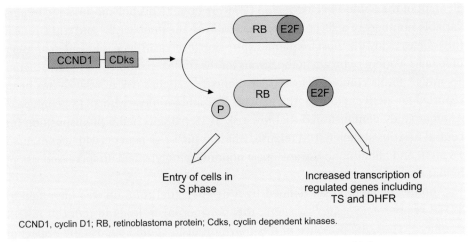

CCND1, cyclin D1; RB, retinoblastoma protein; Cdks, cyclin dependent kinases.

Figure 11-3 Action of Cyclin D1 on cell cycle and transcription of folate genes.

CORTICOSTEROIDS

Polymorphisms Relevant for Corticosteroid Effects and ALL Outcome

Prednisone and dexamethasone are key components of ALL treatment. About 10% of children show glucocorticoid resistance[80] at diagnosis, which can further increase, even to 70% at relapse.[81] Moreover, certain patients may suffer from CS-related toxicity. In about 20% of children treated for ALL, a decrease in bone mineral density is reported, resulting in osteoporosis and avascular bone necrosis.[82] CS act through binding to a specific cytoplasmic glucocorticoid receptor (GR). The GR/CS complex is transported to the nucleus, where it binds to glucocorticoid responsive elements in DNA, allowing for the transcriptional control of responsive genes (Figure 11-4). Different levels of GR isoforms, each with different functional properties[83,84] were reported to mediate resistance to CS in hematologic malignancies. Likewise, some studies found an association between GR expression levels and CS resistance *in vitro*.[85-87] However, other groups reported an absence of such association in primary ALL cells.[88,89] Several studies have analyzed the impact of GR gene polymorphisms.[90-92] One group reported an association of 646C > G substitution in intron 2 of GR gene (also known as Bcl-1 polymorphism) with GR isoform ratio and ALL outcome.[91,92]

Interleukin-10 (IL-10) is an anti-inflammatory cytokine that modulates the transcriptional activity of the GR. Overproduction of IL-10 seems to upregulate the binding capacity for dexamethasone.[93,94] A polymorphism (-1082 A > G) in the regulatory region of the IL-10 gene leads to an increased expression of IL-10.

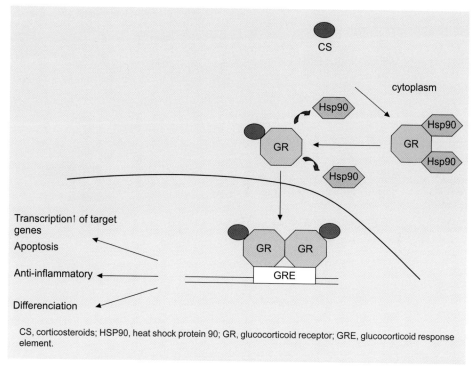

CS, corticosteroids; HSP90, heat shock protein 90; GR, glucocorticoid receptor; GRE, glucocorticoid response element.

Figure 11-4 Glucocorticoid mechanism of action.

Pediatric ALL patients who are homozygous for allele G had an improved response to prednisone.[94] IL-15 is a pro-inflammatory cytokine that promotes T-cell proliferation and upregulates cytokine secretion, cell adhesion, and migration.[95] Higher expression of IL-15 was found in lymphoblasts of patients with CNS relapse or those presenting with CNS disease.[96] Interestingly, recent GWAS[97] conducted in childhood ALL patients identified polymorphisms in IL-15 gene that are associated with minimal residual disease (MRD) status at the end of remission induction (Table 11-1).

Some of drugs used in ALL treatment, including CS, are metabolized by gluthatione-S-transferases (GSTs). Several GST subfamilies are described with multiple polymorphisms modulating enzyme activity. GSTM1 and GSTT1 null genotypes result from homozygous gene deletion leading to the loss of GST activity. These genotypes[98,99] could represent a therapeutic advantage or may confer higher risk of drug-related toxicity.[100] A lower incidence of relapse was found, at least in some studies, in pediatric ALL patients with GSTM1/GSTT1 null genotypes.[101-103] Likewise, an improved prednisone response has been associated with homozygous GSTT1 deletion.[101,104]

Table 11-1 The Summary of the Polymorphisms Associated with Clinical Outcomes in ALL

Genes	rsID	Genetic variation / Frequency of minor allele in different ethnicities	Function	Population	Drug*	Association	References
TPMT	1800462	*2 :c.238G>C Ala80Pro Caucasians: 0.5% Africans: 0.3% Asians: 0%	Reduced	Childhood	Thiopurines	Toxicity (myelosuppression, secondary malignancies)	3, 4, 8, 10, 11, 15, 16
	1800460 - 1142345	*3A: c.460G>A;c.719A>G Ala154Thr;Tyr240Cys Caucasians:4–7% Africans: 0% Southwest Asians: 1–2%	Reduced	Childhood	Thiopurines	Toxicity (myelosuppression, secondary malignancies)	3, 4, 8, 10, 11, 15, 16
	1800460	*3B c.460G>A Ala154Thr Caucasians: 0–3% Africans: 0 Asians: 0%	Reduced	Childhood	Thiopurines	Toxicity (myelosuppression, secondary malignancies)	3, 4, 8, 10, 11, 15, 16
	1142345	*3C: c.719A>G Tyr240Cys Caucasians:1–3% Africans: 3–7% Eastern Asians: 1–3%	Reduced	Childhood	Thiopurines	Toxicity (myelosuppression, secondary malignancies)	3, 4, 8, 10, 11, 15, 16
ITPA	1127354	c.94C>A, Pro32Thrg Caucasians:7–8% Africans: 3–5% Asians: 11–15%	Reduced	Childhood	Thiopurines	Febrile neutropenia (adjusted for TPMT genotypes)	13, 20–23

Continued

Continued

Genes	rsID	Genetic variation / Frequency of minor allele in different ethnicities	Function	Population	Drug*	Association	References
	7270101	IVS2 + 21A>C Caucasians: 13% Africans: 11% Asians: 0%	Reduced	Childhood	Thiopurines	Thrombocytopenia (Not adjusted for TPMT genotypes)	13, 14, 18, 20, 21
DHFR	1650694	-1610C>G/T Caucasians: 35/11%	Increased	Childhood	MTX	Reduced EFS	62
	408626	-317A>G Caucasians: 42%	Increased	Childhood	MTX	Reduced EFS	62
	1105525	308 G>A Caucasians: 12%	Increased	Childhood	MTX	Reduced EFS (HR patients)	63
	70991108	Ins/Del 19bp (intron1 + 57) Caucasians: 50%	Altered	Adult	MTX	Hepatotoxicity	55, 158
				Childhood	MTX	Thrombocytopenia in homozygous WT	50, 158
MTHFR	1801133	c.677C>T Ala220Val Caucasians: 34% Africans: 8% Eastern Asians: 42%	Reduced	Childhood	MTX	Increased risk of relapse Reduced OS Myelosuppression	48-52
				Adult	MTX	Increased risk of hepatotoxicity and myelosuppression Reduced OS	54, 55

Continued

Continued

Genes	rsID	Genetic variation Frequency of minor allele in different ethnicities	Function	Population	Drug*	Association	References
TS	34743033	5'UTR répétition 28pb 2R-97 3R Caucasians: 50–60% Southwest Eastern: 60% Eastern Asians: 80%	Increased	Childhood	MTX	Increased risk of relapse (3R3R), CNS relapse Osteonecrosis, leuko-cytopenia, thrombo-cytopenia (2R2R)	52, 68-70 34 58, 73
	34489327	3'UTR délétion 6pb Caucasians: 60 Africans: 52	Reduced	Childhood	MTX	Better EFS in patients with 2Rdel6pb haplotype	69
CCND1	9344	870A>G Caucasians: 50% Africans: 20% Asians: 39–54%	Alternative Splicing	Childhood	MTX	Reduced EFS and less myelosuppression and hepatotoxicity (AA)	56, 77, 78
RFC1	1051266	80G>A His27Arg Caucasians: 45–55% Africans: 30% Asians: 50%	Increased	Childhood	MTX	Increased gastrointestinal toxicity and myelo-suppression Conflicting result: Increased risk of relapse (GG or AG/AA)	30-33, 36
SLCOB1	4149056	521T>C, Val74Ala Caucasians: 18% Africans: 1.9% Native Amricans: 24%	Reduced	Childhood	MTX	Increased gastrointestinal toxicity	42

Continued

Continued

Genes	rsID	Genetic variation Frequency of minor allele in different ethnicities	Function	Population	Drug*	Association	References
ARID5B	6479778	C>T Caucasians: 50% Africans: 34–50%	Unknown	Childhood		Increased risk of relapse, positive MRD at the end of induction	154
MDR1	1045642	3435C>T Caucasians: 47–55% Africans: 7–20% Asians: 37–52%	Reduced	Childhood	Glucocorticoids, anthracycline, vincristine, etoposide	Better EFS, lower rate of CNS relapse, Increased risk of infection	138, 139, 142
MRP2	3743527	C>T Caucasians: 19% Africans: 4% Asians: 5–18%	Unknown	Childhood	MTX, etoposide, vincristine	Left ventricular dysfunction	146
MRP4	868853	-1393T>C Caucasians: 9% Africans: 37% Asians: 9–19%	Increased	Childhood	MTX, 6-MP	Better EFS	37
	2274407	934C>A Caucasians: 2% Africans: 10–19% Asians: 17–29%	Unknown	Childhood		Lower EFS and higher thrombocytopenia	37
MRP3	9895420	-189A>T Caucasians: 15% Africans: 9%	Increased	Childhood	MTX, etoposide	Reduced EFS (CNS) and lower thrombocytopenia (AT/AA)	149

Continued

Continued

Genes	rsID	Genetic variation Frequency of minor allele in different ethnicities	Function	Population	Drug*	Association	References
GR	41423247	Ivs2 646G>C Caucasians: 36% Africans: 14%	Altered	Childhood	CS	Reduced EFS	91, 92
IL10	1800896	-1082A>G Caucasians: 33–53% Africans: 27–40% Asians: 2–5%	Increased	Childhood	CS	Improved response to prednisone	94
IL15	17007695 and 35964658	T>C A>G Caucasians: 6–9% Africans: 0.4–3% Asians: 37–49%	Unknown	Childhood	CS	MRD status at the end of induction	97
GSTT1		Null genotype Caucasians: 17–20% Africans: 23% Asians: 35–50% Indian: 15%	Deletion	Childhood	Alkylating agents, anthracyclines, CS, etoposide	Lower incidence of relapse, improved prednisone response	101-104
GSTM1		Null genotype Caucasians: 50–53% Africans: 21–27% Asians: 42–62% Indian: 28%	Deletion	Childhood	Alkylating agents, anthracyclines, CS, etoposide	Lower incidence of relapse Higher incidence of severe infection and hepatotoxicity	100, 103, 52
PAI-1	6092	G>A, Ala15Thr Caucasians: 10% Africans: 0% Asians: 9–21%	Unknown	Childhood	CS	Osteonecrosis	109

Continued

Continued

Genes	rsID	Genetic variation / Frequency of minor allele in different ethnicities	Function	Population	Drug*	Association	References
VDR	2228570	FokI T>C Caucasians: 60% Africans: 80% Asians: 55–67%	Unknown	Childhood	CS	Osteonecrosis	73
CRHR1	1876828	G>A Caucasians: 21%	Unknown	Childhood	CS	Osteonecrosis	110
ACP1	12714403 and 10167992	G>A C>T Caucasians: 14–50% Africans: 0–3% Asians: 9–14%	Unknown	Childhood	CS	Osteonecrosis	108
SH3YL1	4241316 and 10193882	T>C and A>T Caucasians: 14–50% Africans: 0–4% Asians: 8–14%	Unknown	Childhood	CS	Osteonecrosis	108
APOB	693	C7673T, XbaI Caucasians: 50% Africans: 19–50% Asians: 35–70%	Unknown	Childhood	CS	CS induced hypertension	113
LEPR	1137101	C870TArg223Gln Caucasians: 45–50% Africans: 19–50% Asians: 11–17%	Unknown	Childhood	CS	CS induced hypertension	113

Continued

Continued

Genes	rsID	Genetic variation / Frequency of minor allele in different ethnicities	Function	Population	Drug*	Association	References
CNTNAP2	2286128	C2226T, Caucasians: 0%, Africans: 9%, Asians: 3–6%	Unknown	Childhood	CS	CS induced hypertension	113
SLC12A3	11643718	G2744A Arg913Gln, Caucasians: 12–14%, Africans: 0%, Asians: 3–12%	Unknown	Childhood	CS	CS induced hypertension	113
ATF5	11554772	1562C>T, Caucasians: 3%, Africans: 7%	Increased	Childhood	Asparaginase	Reduced EFS (E. coli asparaginase)	129
ADRB2	11168070, 11959427, 1042711, 1801704	-468C>G, -376T>C, -47T>C, -20T>C, Caucasians: 41%, Africans: 17%, Asians: 8–12%	Altered	Childhood		worse initial treatment response (GCCC haplotype)	155

*genes are related to a given drug action pathway or are related to complication of the treatment with a given drug.

ALL, acute lymphoblastic leukemia; TPMT, thiopurine-S-methyl transferase; IPTA, inosine triphosphate pyrophosphatase; DHFR, dihydrofolate reductase; MTHFR, methylene tetrahydrofolate reductase; TS, thymidylate synthase; CCND1, cyclin D1; RFC1, reduced folate carrier; SLCOB1, solute carrier organic anion transporter; ARID5B, AT-rich interactive domain protein 5B; MDR, multidrug resistance protein; MRP, multidrug resistance associated protein; GR, glucocorticoid receptor; IL, interleukin; MRD, minimal residual disease; EFS, event-free survival; OS, overall survival; CNS, central nervous system; MTX, methotrexate; CS, corticosteroids; GSTT1, glutathione-S transferase; PAI-1, serine peptidase inhibitor or plasminogen activator inhibitor type 1; VDR, vitamin D receptor; CRHR1, corticotrophin releasing hormone receptor 1; ACP1, acid phosphatase 1; SH3YL1, SH3 domain containing Ysc 84 like; APOB, apolipoprotein B; LEPR, leptine receptor; CNTNAP2, contractin associated protein like 2; SCL12A3, sodium chloride transporter; ATF5, activating transcription factor; ADRB2, β-2 adrenergic receptor.

Polymorphisms and Corticosteroid-Related Toxicity

Osteonecrosis is a severe side effect of CS treatment, and is thought to be in part related to CS-induced hyperlipidemia, hypercoagulability, and hypofibrinolysis.[105,106] Glucocorticoids also cause direct toxicity to osteocytes.[107] Several predictive factors have been associated with symptomatic osteonecrosis, such as age, CS type and dose, treatment protocol, hypercholesterolemia and lower serum albumin levels.[108] The latter suggests that asparaginase treatment may potentiate CS osteonecrosis.[108] Several candidate gene studies have been conducted to identify genetic factors predisposing to this treatment complication. Polymorphisms (rs6092 G > A) in serpin peptidase inhibitor or plasminogen activator inhibitor type 1 (SERPINE 1 or PAI-1)[109] and vitamin D receptor genes (*VDR* FokI C > T polymorphism)[73] have been identified as putatively related to the development of osteonecrosis. PAI-1 inhibits fibrinolysis. Increased serum levels have been associated with increased incidence of thrombophilia and osteonecrosis.[109] The association of VDR and PAI-1 polymorphisms were not confirmed in subsequent replication studies.[73,108] The association of genetic variation (rs1876828 G > A) in corticotropin releasing hormone receptor 1 (CRHR1) gene has been also associated in a sex-specific manner with increased risk of bone density deficits in patients treated with CS and antimetabolites.[110] A recent GWAS study[108] identified several SNPs associated with osteonecrosis in acid phosphatase 1 (ACP1, rs12714403 G > A and rs10167992 C > T) and SH3 domain containing Ysc84-like 1 (SH3YL1, rs4241316 T > C and rs10193882 A > T) genes. These polymorphisms were also associated with higher cholesterol and lower serum albumin, and remained independent predictive factors for osteonecrosis in multivariate analysis[108] (Table 11-1). Particularly interesting is the finding of ACP1 gene polymorphisms since this is consistent with previous association with serum cholesterol and triglyceride levels[111] and involvement in osteoblast differentiation.[112]

Hypertension may as well develop as a side effect of CS treatment. Polymorphisms in several genes, including the leptin receptor (LEPR, Gln233Arg), the sodium chloride transporter (SLC12A3, 2744G > A, Arg913Gln), apolipoprotein B (APOB, XbaI polymorphism) and contactin-associated protein like2 (CNTNAP2, rs22886128) have been identified as a potential modulators of CS-induced hypertension[113] (Table 11-1).

And finally, a higher risk of severe infection and hepatotoxicity was reported in childhood ALL patients with the GSTM1 null genotype.[52,100]

Genome-Wide Expression Profiling

Given the major impact of CS resistance and CS-related toxicity on clinical outcomes and the limited knowledge of the pathways leading to CS-induced apoptosis in ALL, expression profiling has been performed to determine CS-regulated genes in leukemia. Using microarray profiling,[114-116] many differentially regulated genes have been identified. The role of some of them in CS-induced apoptosis was highlighted in subsequent validation experiments. For example, induction of Bim, an apoptotic protein of the Bcl-2 family, appears essential for glucocorticoid-mediated apoptosis[117] and plays important role in glucocorticoid resistance in ALL.[118] Likewise, associations has been found between decreased expression of genes coding for core subunits of the SWItch/Sucrose NonFermentable (SWI/SNF) chromatin-remodeling complex and resistance to CS *in vitro* in primary ALL cells.[119] A functional SNP in the promoter of one of these genes has been also identified.[120] No data are yet available to determine whether polymorphisms of differentially expressed genes affect response to treatment in ALL patients. Further pharmacogenetic studies are needed to assess their impact on ALL outcome and CS-related toxicity.

L-ASPARAGINASE

Asparaginase is used in ALL to induce depletion of asparagine produced by asparagine synthetase (ASNS). As lymphoblasts have low levels of ASNS, they are more sensitive to asparaginase treatment than normal cells. Experiments conducted in leukemia cell lines and patients' lymphoblasts suggest, at least in some studies, that elevated ASNS activity might be a cause of asparaginase resistance.[121-125] ASNS expression can be upregulated by the basic region leucine zipper activating transcription factor (ATF) whose expression is in turn triggered by acid amino acid deprivation.[126] ATF expression (including that of ATF5) differed between leukemia cells that are sensitive or resistance to asparaginase treatment.[127,128] Several polymorphisms located in the regulatory region has been described in ATF5 gene and show LD.[129] Haplotypes *1 and *2 were associated with lower promoter activity whereas haplotypes *3, *4, and *5 conferred a higher promoter activity. The haplotype*5 is tagged by a polymorphism in the 5'UTR region defined by a C to T substitution at the position 1562. The allele 1562T was associated with reduced EFS in two cohorts of childhood ALL treated with *Escherichia coli* asparaginase.[129] A recent GWAS identified among other SNPs, polymorphisms in genes of aspartate metabolism as contributors to asparaginase sensitivity *in vitro*.[130] Among these genes, polymorphisms of arginosuccinate synthase 1 (ASS1) gene were associated with asparaginase sensitivity in primary ALL cells.[130] ASS1 catalyzes the conversion of aspartate and citrulline into arginosuccinate which can serve as a source for de novo asparagine synthesis[131] and has been identified through microarray expression profiling as upregulated in cell lines with resistance to asparaginase.[127]

MULTIDRUG-RESISTANCE PROTEIN AND MULTIDRUG-RESISTANCE-ASSOCIATED-PROTEINS

Bioavailability of many drugs used in ALL treatment (e.g., MTX, 6-MP, CS, anthracyclines, vincristine, etoposide, and cyclophosphamide) depends, also, on the activity and expression of the ATP-binding cassette (ABC) transporters including P-glycoprotein (P-gp) and multidrug-resistance (MDR)-related proteins (MRP).[24,132,133] These transporters use ATP as an energy source to export drugs and are expressed in the membrane of many tissues as intestine, liver, kidney, blood-brain barrier, and hematopoietic cells.

P-gp is encoded by the MDR1 gene. Increased MDR1 expression is associated with a poor prognosis in adult and childhood ALL.[134,135] A 3435C > T polymorphism in exon 26 is associated with reduced P-gp function,[136,137] however, its clinical impact in ALL remains uncertain. Childhood ALL patients with the 3435T allele showed a better EFS and a lower rate of CNS relapse,[138,139] whereas other studies[140,141] reported no impact of this polymorphism on prognosis of childhood or adult ALL. Increased risk of infectious complications was also observed in patients with 3435T allele.[142]

Multidrug-resistance related proteins are encoded by MRP genes and comprise 13 members with 9 major transporters, MRP1 to MRP9, contributing to drug resistance.[143] MTX, vincristine, 6-MP, and doxorubicin used in ALL treatment protocols are all MRP substrates. Several MRPs mediate efflux of each of these drugs.[143] Increased expression of MRP1 and MRP3 was associated with a poor prognosis of adult and childhood ALL.[144,145] The ABCC1 rs3743527TT genotype of C to T substitution was associated with anthracycline-induced left ventricular dysfunction in childhood ALL patients.[146] A C24T polymorphism, located in the regulatory region of the MRP2 gene, has been associated with lower mRNA levels[147] and higher MTX concentration in childhood ALL requiring more frequent leucovorin rescue.[148] No association of this polymorphism with ALL relapse in pediatric patients was reported.[149] Two polymorphisms in MRP4 gene, -1393T > C located in the promoter region and 934C > A leading to Lys304Asn amino-acid substitution, affected MTX levels and EFS probability in childhood ALL patients.[37] The C-1393 allele gene was associated with better EFS, lower MTX plasma levels, and higher promoter activity; whereas in contrast, the A allele at the position 934 correlated with lower EFS and higher frequency of high-grade thrombocytopenia.[37] Likewise, the A-189 allele of the A to T substitution in promoter of MRP3 gene correlated with poorer disease outcome (higher risk of relapse in the CNS), lower frequency of thrombocytopenia, increased promoter activity, and higher MTX plasma levels.[149] Impact of MRP4 polymorphisms were not, however, confirmed in an adult ALL cohort,[150] highlighting differences in pharmacogenetic findings between childhood and adult patients which might be explained, among other factors, by different treatment protocol, disease-related factors, and complexity of MRP effects. Indeed, MRPs are involved in transport of several drugs used in ALL treatment and they are expressed in the membranes of many barrier tissues which may have different consequences on drug disposition. MRPs may also affect folate efflux, thereby leading to expansion of the intracellular folate pool indirectly affecting antifolate resistance.[151]

OTHER GENES WITH POTENTIAL PHARMACOGENETIC IMPLICATIONS IN ALL

Genome-wide association studies have allowed the discovery of other candidate genes that may play roles in modulation of ALL relapse risk. For example, several SNPs of the gene coding for AT-rich interactive domain protein 5B (ARID5B) has been associated with a higher risk of ALL in two GWAS.[152,153] ARID5B is a transcription factor that plays role in embryogenesis and growth regulation. Several polymorphisms that were associated with ALL susceptibility were also associated with poor treatment outcome. For example, children with T allele of rs6479778 C to T substitution had higher risk of relapse; T allele was also associated with a positive MRD at the end of induction therapy.[154]

Genome-wide profiling of treatment-induced changes in expression between childhood ALL patients who relapsed and those who remained in continuous complete remission revealed significant changes in the β-2 adrenergic receptor gene (ADRB2) expression.[155] The ADRB2 has been reported to regulate apoptosis.[156] Subsequent analysis of ADRB2 promoter polymorphisms (–468C > G, –367T > C, –47T > C, –20T > C) and the resulting haplotype has shown their relationship to early treatment response in ALL.[155]

Cross Resistance

Cross-resistance of ALL cells to multiple anticancer agents could lead to worse prognosis. GWAS identified a set of differentially expressed genes in ALL exhibiting cross-resistance to prednisolone, vincristine, asparaginase, and daunorubicin. These genes are involved in different pathways including transcription, transport, and cell cycle maintenance, underlying complexity to predict the resultant sensitivity phenotype.[157] The same study identified a distinct phenotype of discordant resistance to asparaginase and vincristine. For example, overexpression of ribosomal protein genes was associated with an asparaginase resistance but vincristine sensitive phenotype.[157] Association of discordant resistance phenotype with a better disease-free survival was dependant on the treatment protocol used.[157]

SUMMARY

In the last 10 years, many pharmacogenetic studies have been conducted in ALL and a variety of potential markers have been identified. Extraordinary developments in molecular biology and bioinformatics have profoundly changed the genomic landscape and have provided insights into mechanisms of drug action as well as knowledge of how genetic factors shape treatment responses. Further research is nevertheless needed to identify the best predictors of treatment failure or drug side effects since only few pharmacogenetic markers, such as for example variations in TPMT genes have been used in clinical practice, at least in some institutions, to adjust 6-MP dose. The difficulty to identify best predictors is in part caused by variability of ALL treatment protocols that combine several drugs. Although such a combination therapy approach has led to higher efficacy of treatment, each of the drugs can also contribute to treatment resistance and treatment-related toxicity. The latter may lead to interruptions of treatment, leading as well to higher risk of relapse. The effect of each of these drugs is influenced by many genes, whose variations can all contribute to variability seen in treatment responses rendering ALL pharmacogenetics not an easy task. Drug action pathways are not always fully understood and selection of candidate genes is not necessarily obvious or sufficient through rational approaches. Moreover, drugs used in ALL treatment often share similar side effects. Therefore, resistance or sensitive phenotype of ALL cells likely results from a number of polymorphisms that can potentiate, combine or cancel each other's effects. Indeed, the presence of several-relapse predisposing variants has been shown to further increase the risk of relapse in ALL patients.[62] Discrepancies seen across studies could be explained by variety of different factors including protocol regimen, ethnicity, and the severity of the disease. ALL is a heterogeneous disease which harbors different resistance mechanisms as further supported by some genome-wide studies.[121] Recognizing difficulties and shortcomings of current methods, along with promising results obtained thus far and new technological developments in genomics will likely lead to identification of predictive markers that will allow tailoring ALL treatment according to a patient genetic profile thereby resulting in improved treatment outcomes.

REFERENCES

1. Chauncey TR. Drug resistance mechanisms in acute leukemia. *Curr Opin Oncol.* 2001; 13:21-6.
2. Krajinovic M, Labuda D, Sinnett D. Childhood acute lymphoblastic leukemia: genetic determinants of susceptibility and disease outcome. *Rev Environ Health.* 2001;16:263-79.
3. Cheok MH, Lugthart S, Evans WE. Pharmacogenomics of acute leukemia. *Annu Rev Pharmacol Toxicol.* 2006;46:317-53.
4. Cheok MH, Evans WE. Acute lymphoblastic leukaemia: a model for the pharmacogenomics of cancer therapy. *Nat Rev Cancer.* 2006;6:117-29.
5. Holleman A, Cheok MH, den Boer ML, et al. Gene-expression patterns in drug-resistant acute lymphoblastic leukemia cells and response to treatment. *N Engl J Med.* 2004;351:533-42.
6. Metzker ML. Sequencing technologies-the next generation. *Nat Rev Genet.* 2010;11:31-46.
7. Bleyer WA. The impact of childhood cancer on the United States and the world. *CA Cancer J Clin.* 1990;40:355-67.
8. McLeod HL, Krynetski EY, Relling MV, et al. Genetic polymorphism of thiopurine methyltransferase and its clinical relevance for childhood acute lymphoblastic leukemia. *Leukemia.* 2000;14:567-72.
9. Maitland ML, Vasisht K, Ratain MJ. TPMT, UGT1A1 and DPYD: genotyping to ensure safer cancer therapy? *Trends Pharmacol Sci.* 2006;27:432-7.
10. Evans WE, Relling MV. Moving towards individualized medicine with pharmacogenomics. *Nature.* 2004;429:464-8.

11. Relling MV, Gardner EE, Sandborn WJ, et al. Clinical Pharmacogenetics Implementation Consortium guidelines for thiopurine methyltransferase genotype and thiopurine dosing. *Clin Pharmacol Ther.* 2011;89:387-91.

12. Lennard L, Lilleyman JS, Van Loon J, et al. Genetic variation in response to 6-mercaptopurine for childhood acute lymphoblastic leukaemia. *Lancet.* 1990;336:225-9.

13. de Beaumais AT, Jacqz-Aigrain E. Pharmacogenetic determinants of mercaptopurine disposition in children with acute lymphoblastic leukemia. Eur J Clin Pharmacol. *Eur J Clin Pharmacol.* 2012;68:1233-42

14. Hawwa AF, Collier PS, Millership JS, et al. Population pharmacokinetic and pharmacogenetic analysis of 6-mercaptopurine in paediatric patients with acute lymphoblastic leukaemia. *Br J Clin Pharmacol.* 2008;66:826-37.

15. Bo J, Schroder H, Kristinsson J, et al. Possible carcinogenic effect of 6-mercaptopurine on bone marrow stem cells: relation to thiopurine metabolism. *Cancer.* 1999;86:1080-6.

16. Relling MV, Rubnitz JE, Rivera GK, et al. High incidence of secondary brain tumours after radiotherapy and antimetabolites. *Lancet.* 1999;354:34-9.

17. Kudo M, Moteki T, Sasaki T, et al. Functional characterization of human xanthine oxidase allelic variants. *Pharmacogenet Genomics.* 2008;18:243-51.

18. Hawwa AF, Millership JS, Collier PS, et al. Pharmacogenomic studies of the anticancer and immunosuppressive thiopurines mercaptopurine and azathioprine. *Br J Clin Pharmacol.* 2008;66:517-28.

19. Marinaki AM, Ansari A, Duley JA, et al. Adverse drug reactions to azathioprine therapy are associated with polymorphism in the gene encoding inosine triphosphate pyrophosphatase (ITPase). *Pharmacogenetics.* 2004;14:181-7.

20. Arenas M, Duley J, Sumi S, et al. The ITPA c.94C>A and g.IVS2+21A>C sequence variants contribute to missplicing of the ITPA gene. *Biochim Biophys Acta.* 2007;1772:96-102.

21. Sumi S, Marinaki AM, Arenas M, et al. Genetic basis of inosine triphosphate pyrophosphohydrolase deficiency. *Hum Genet.* 2002;111:360-7.

22. Stocco G, Cheok MH, Crews KR, et al. Genetic polymorphism of inosine triphosphate pyrophosphatase is a determinant of mercaptopurine metabolism and toxicity during treatment for acute lymphoblastic leukemia. *Clin Pharmacol Ther.* 2009;85:164-72.

23. Stocco G, Crews KR, Evans WE. Genetic polymorphism of inosine-triphosphate-pyrophosphatase influences mercaptopurine metabolism and toxicity during treatment of acute lymphoblastic leukemia individualized for thiopurine-S-methyl-transferase status. *Expert Opin Drug Saf.* 2010;9:23-37.

24. Assaraf YG. Molecular basis of antifolate resistance. *Cancer Metastasis Rev.* 2007;26:153-81.

25. Gorlick R, Goker E, Trippett T, et al. Defective transport is a common mechanism of acquired methotrexate resistance in acute lymphocytic leukemia and is associated with decreased reduced folate carrier expression. *Blood.* 1997;89:1013-8.

26. Jansen G, Mauritz R, Drori S, et al. A structurally altered human reduced folate carrier with increased folic acid transport mediates a novel mechanism of antifolate resistance. *J Biol Chem.* 1998;273:30189-98.

27. Chango A, Emery-Fillon N, de Courcy GP, et al. A polymorphism (80G->A) in the reduced folate carrier gene and its associations with folate status and homocysteinemia. *Mol Genet Metab.* 2000;70:310-5.

28. Whetstine JR, Gifford AJ, Witt T, et al. Single nucleotide polymorphisms in the human reduced folate carrier: characterization of a high-frequency G/A variant at position 80 and transport properties of the His(27) and Arg(27) carriers. *Clin Cancer Res.* 2001;7:3416-22.

29. Baslund B, Gregers J, Nielsen CH. Reduced folate carrier polymorphism determines methotrexate uptake by B cells and CD4+ T cells. *Rheumatology (Oxford).* 2008;47:451-3.

30. Imanishi H, Okamura N, Yagi M, et al. Genetic polymorphisms associated with adverse events and elimination of methotrexate in childhood acute lymphoblastic leukemia and malignant lymphoma. *J Hum Genet.* 2007;52:166-71.

31. Kishi S, Cheng C, French D, et al. Ancestry and pharmacogenetics of antileukemic drug toxicity. *Blood.* 2007;109:4151-7.

32. Gregers J, Christensen IJ, Dalhoff K, et al. The association of reduced folate carrier 80G > A polymorphism to outcome in childhood acute lymphoblastic leukemia interacts with chromosome 21 copy number. *Blood.* 2010;115:4671-7.

33. Laverdiere C, Chiasson S, Costea I, et al. Polymorphism G80A in the reduced folate carrier gene and its relationship to methotrexate plasma levels and outcome of childhood acute lymphoblastic leukemia. *Blood.* 2002;100:3832-4.

34. Rocha JC, Cheng C, Liu W, et al. Pharmacogenetics of outcome in children with acute lymphoblastic leukemia. *Blood.* 2005;105:4752-8.

35. Kotnik FB, Dolzan V, Grabnar I, et al. Relationship of the reduced folate carrier gene polymorphism G80A to methotrexate plasma concentration, toxicity, and disease outcome in childhood acute lymphoblastic leukemia. *Leuk Lymphoma.* 2010;51:724-6.

36. Ashton LJ, Gifford AJ, Kwan E, et al. Reduced folate carrier and methylenetetrahydrofolate reductase gene polymorphisms: associations with clinical outcome in childhood acute lymphoblastic leukemia. *Leukemia.* 2009;23:1348-51.

37. Ansari M, Sauty G, Labuda M, et al. Polymorphisms in multidrug resistance-associated protein gene 4 is associated with outcome in childhood acute lymphoblastic leukemia. *Blood.* 2009;114:1383-6.

38. Trevino LR, Shimasaki N, Yang W, et al. Germline genetic variation in an organic anion transporter polypeptide associated with methotrexate pharmacokinetics and clinical effects. *J Clin Oncol.* 2009;27:5972-8.

39. Abe T, Unno M, Onogawa T, et al. LST-2, a human liver-specific organic anion transporter, determines methotrexate sensitivity in gastrointestinal cancers. *Gastroenterology.* 2001;120: 1689-99.

40. Tirona RG, Leake BF, Merino G, et al. Polymorphisms in OATP-C: identification of multiple allelic variants associated with altered transport activity among European- and African-Americans. *J Biol Chem.* 2001;276:35669-75.

41. van de Steeg E, van der Kruijssen CM, Wagenaar E, et al. Methotrexate pharmacokinetics in transgenic mice with liver-specific expression of human organic anion-transporting polypeptide 1B1 (SLCO1B1). *Drug Metab Dispos.* 2009;37:277-81.

42. Lopez-Lopez E, Martin-Guerrero I, Ballesteros J, et al. Polymorphisms of the SLCO1B1 gene predict methotrexate-related toxicity in childhood acute lymphoblastic leukemia. *Pediatr Blood Cancer.* 2011;57:612-9.

43. Niemi M. Role of OATP transporters in the disposition of drugs. *Pharmacogenomics.* 2007; 8:787-802.

44. Ramsey LB, Bruun GH, Yang W, et al. Rare versus common variants in pharmacogenetics: SLCO1B1 variation and methotrexate disposition. *Genome Res.* 2012;22:1-8.

45. Krajinovic M, Moghrabi A. Pharmacogenetics of methotrexate. *Pharmacogenomics.* 2004;5: 819-34.

46. Frosst P, Blom HJ, Milos R, et al. A candidate genetic risk factor for vascular disease: a common mutation in methylenetetrahydrofolate reductase. *Nat Genet.* 1995;10:111-3.

47. Weisberg I, Tran P, Christensen B, et al. A second genetic polymorphism in methylenetetrahydrofolate reductase (MTHFR) associated with decreased enzyme activity. *Mol Genet Metab.* 1998;64:169-72.

48. Aplenc R, Thompson J, Han P, et al. Methylenetetrahydrofolate reductase polymorphisms and therapy response in pediatric acute lymphoblastic leukemia. *Cancer Res.* 2005;65: 2482-7.

49. Krajinovic M, Lemieux-Blanchard E, Chiasson S, et al. Role of polymorphisms in MTHFR and MTHFD1 genes in the outcome of childhood acute lymphoblastic leukemia. *Pharmacogenomics J.* 2004;4:66-72.

50. Salazar J, Altes A, Del Rio E, et al. Methotrexate consolidation treatment according to pharmacogenetics of MTHFR ameliorates event-free survival in childhood acute lymphoblastic leukaemia. *Pharmacogenomics J.* 2012;12:379-85.

51. El-Khodary NM, El-Haggar SM, Eid MA, et al. Study of the pharmacokinetic and pharmacogenetic contribution to the toxicity of high-dose methotrexate in children with acute lymphoblastic leukemia. *Med Oncol.* 2012;29:2053-62.

52. Sepe DM, McWilliams T, Chen J, et al. Germline genetic variation and treatment response on CCG-1891. *Pediatr Blood Cancer.* 2012;58:695-700.

53. Pietrzyk JJ, Bik-Multanowski M, Balwierz W, et al. Additional genetic risk factor for death in children with acute lymphoblastic leukemia: a common polymorphism of the MTHFR gene. *Pediatr Blood Cancer.* 2009;52:364-8.

54. Chiusolo P, Reddiconto G, Farina G, et al. MTHFR polymorphisms' influence on outcome and toxicity in acute lymphoblastic leukemia patients. *Leuk Res.* 2007;31:1669-74.

55. Ongaro A, De Mattei M, Della Porta MG, et al. Gene polymorphisms in folate metabolizing enzymes in adult acute lymphoblastic leukemia: effects on methotrexate-related toxicity and survival. *Haematologica.* 2009;94:1391-8.

56. Costea I, Moghrabi A, Laverdiere C, et al. Folate cycle gene variants and chemotherapy toxicity in pediatric patients with acute lymphoblastic leukemia. *Haematologica.* 2006;91: 1113-6.

57. Kishi S, Griener J, Cheng C, et al. Homocysteine, pharmacogenetics, and neurotoxicity in children with leukemia. *J Clin Oncol.* 2003;21:3084-91.

58. Erculj N, Kotnik BF, Debeljak M, et al. Influence of folate pathway polymorphisms on high-dose methotrexate-related toxicity and survival in childhood acute lymphoblastic leukemia. *Leuk Lymphoma.* 2012;53:1096-104.

59. Matherly LH, Taub JW, Ravindranath Y, et al. Elevated dihydrofolate reductase and impaired methotrexate transport as elements in methotrexate resistance in childhood acute lymphoblastic leukemia. *Blood.* 1995;85:500-9.

60. Matherly LH, Taub JW, Wong SC, et al. Increased frequency of expression of elevated dihydrofolate reductase in T-cell versus B-precursor acute lymphoblastic leukemia in children. *Blood.* 1997;90:578-89.

61. Rots MG, Willey JC, Jansen G, et al. mRNA expression levels of methotrexate resistance-related proteins in childhood leukemia as determined by a standardized competitive template-based RT-PCR method. *Leukemia.* 2000;14:2166-75.

62. Dulucq S, St-Onge G, Gagne V, et al. DNA variants in dihydrofolate reductase gene and outcome in childhood ALL. *Blood.* 2008;111:3692-700.

63. Al-Shakfa F, Dulucq S, Brukner I, et al. DNA variants in region for noncoding interfering transcript of dihydrofolate reductase gene and outcome in childhood acute lymphoblastic leukemia. *Clin Cancer Res.* 2009;15:6931-8.

64. Johnson WG, Scholl TO, Spychala JR, et al. Common dihydrofolate reductase 19-base pair deletion allele: a novel risk factor for preterm delivery. *Am J Clin Nutr.* 2005;81:664-8.

65. Horie N, Aiba H, Oguro K, et al. Functional analysis and DNA polymorphism of the tandemly repeated sequences in the 5'-terminal regulatory region of the human gene for thymidylate synthase. *Cell Struct Funct.* 1995;20:191-7.

66. Pullarkat ST, Stoehlmacher J, Ghaderi V, et al. Thymidylate synthase gene polymorphism determines response and toxicity of 5-FU chemotherapy. *Pharmacogenomics J.* 2001;1:65-70.

67. DiPaolo A, Chu E. The role of thymidylate synthase as a molecular biomarker. *Clin Cancer Res.* 2004;10:411-2.

68. Krajinovic M, Costea I, Chiasson S. Polymorphism of the thymidylate synthase gene and outcome of acute lymphoblastic leukaemia. *Lancet.* 2002;359:1033-4.

69. Krajinovic M, Costea I, Primeau M, et al. Combining several polymorphisms of thymidylate synthase gene for pharmacogenetic analysis. *Pharmacogenomics J.* 2005;5:374-80

70. Pietrzyk JJ, Bik-Multanowski M, Skoczen S, et al. Polymorphism of the thymidylate synthase gene and risk of relapse in childhood ALL. *Leuk Res*. 2011;35:1464-6.

71. Ulrich CM, Bigler J, Velicer CM, et al. Searching expressed sequence tag databases: discovery and confirmation of a common polymorphism in the thymidylate synthase gene. *Cancer Epidemiol Biomarkers Prev*. 2000;9:1381-5.

72. Mandola MV, Stoehlmacher J, Zhang W, et al. A 6 bp polymorphism in the thymidylate synthase gene causes message instability and is associated with decreased intratumoral TS mRNA levels. *Pharmacogenetics*. 2004;14:319-27.

73. Relling MV, Yang W, Das S, et al. Pharmacogenetic risk factors for osteonecrosis of the hip among children with leukemia. *J Clin Oncol*. 2004;22:3930-6.

74. Hochhauser D, Schnieders B, Ercikan-Abali E, et al. Effect of cyclin D1 overexpression on drug sensitivity in a human fibrosarcoma cell line. *J Natl Cancer Inst*. 1996;88:1269-75.

75. Li W, Fan J, Hochhauser D, et al. Lack of functional retinoblastoma protein mediates increased resistance to antimetabolites in human sarcoma cell lines. *Proc Natl Acad Sci U S A*. 1995;92:10436-40.

76. Betticher DC, Thatcher N, Altermatt HJ, et al. Alternate splicing produces a novel cyclin D1 transcript. *Oncogene*. 1995;11:1005-11.

77. Costea I, Moghrabi A, Krajinovic M. The influence of cyclin D1 (CCND1) 870A>G polymorphism and CCND1-thymidylate synthase (TS) gene-gene interaction on the outcome of childhood acute lymphoblastic leukaemia. *Pharmacogenetics*. 2003;13:577-80.

78. Hou X, Wang S, Zhou Y, et al. Cyclin D1 gene polymorphism and susceptibility to childhood acute lymphoblastic leukemia in a Chinese population. *Int J Hematol*. 2005;82:206-9.

79. Kornmann M, Danenberg KD, Arber N, et al. Inhibition of cyclin D1 expression in human pancreatic cancer cells is associated with increased chemosensitivity and decreased expression of multiple chemoresistance genes. *Cancer Res*. 1999;59:3505-11.

80. Bhadri VA, Trahair TN, Lock RB. Glucocorticoid resistance in paediatric acute lymphoblastic leukaemia. *J Paediatr Child Health*. 2012;48:634-40.

81. Bailey S, Hall AG, Pearson AD, et al. Glucocorticoid resistance and the AP-1 transcription factor in leukaemia. *Adv Exp Med Biol*. 1999;457:615-9.

82. Bianchi ML. Glucorticoids and bone: some general remarks and some special observations in pediatric patients. *Calcif Tissue Int*. 2002;70:384-90.

83. de Lange P, Segeren CM, Koper JW, et al. Expression in hematological malignancies of a glucocorticoid receptor splice variant that augments glucocorticoid receptor-mediated effects in transfected cells. *Cancer Res*. 2001;61:3937-41.

84. Longui CA, Vottero A, Adamson PC, et al. Low glucocorticoid receptor alpha/beta ratio in T-cell lymphoblastic leukemia. *Horm Metab Res*. 2000;32:401-6.

85. Schmidt S, Irving JA, Minto L, et al. Glucocorticoid resistance in two key models of acute lymphoblastic leukemia occurs at the level of the glucocorticoid receptor. *Faseb J*. 2006;20:2600-2.

86. Geley S, Hartmann BL, Hala M, et al. Resistance to glucocorticoid-induced apoptosis in human T-cell acute lymphoblastic leukemia CEM-C1 cells is due to insufficient glucocorticoid receptor expression. *Cancer Res*. 1996;56:5033-8.

87. Gruber G, Carlet M, Turtscher E, et al. Levels of glucocorticoid receptor and its ligand determine sensitivity and kinetics of glucocorticoid-induced leukemia apoptosis. *Leukemia*. 2009;23:820-3.

88. Tissing WJ, Meijerink JP, Brinkhof B, et al. Glucocorticoid-induced glucocorticoid-receptor expression and promoter usage is not linked to glucocorticoid resistance in childhood ALL. *Blood*. 2006;108:1045-9.

89. Lauten M, Cario G, Asgedom G, et al. Protein expression of the glucocorticoid receptor in childhood acute lymphoblastic leukemia. *Haematologica*. 2003;88:1253-8.

90. Tissing WJ, Meijerink JP, den Boer ML, et al. Genetic variations in the glucocorticoid receptor gene are not related to glucocorticoid resistance in childhood acute lymphoblastic leukemia. *Clin Cancer Res.* 2005;11:6050-6.

91. Fleury I, Primeau M, Doreau A, et al. Polymorphisms in genes involved in the corticosteroid response and the outcome of childhood acute lymphoblastic leukemia. *Am J Pharmacogenomics.* 2004;4:331-41.

92. Labuda M, Gahier A, Gagne V, et al. Polymorphisms in glucocorticoid receptor gene and the outcome of childhood acute lymphoblastic leukemia (ALL). *Leuk Res.* 2010;34:492-7.

93. Franchimont D, Martens H, Hagelstein MT, et al. Tumor necrosis factor alpha decreases, and interleukin-10 increases, the sensitivity of human monocytes to dexamethasone: potential regulation of the glucocorticoid receptor. *J Clin Endocrinol Metab.* 1999;84:2834-9.

94. Lauten M, Matthias T, Stanulla M, et al. Association of initial response to prednisone treatment in childhood acute lymphoblastic leukaemia and polymorphisms within the tumour necrosis factor and the interleukin-10 genes. *Leukemia.* 2002;16:1437-42.

95. Bulfone-Paus S, Bulanova E, Budagian V, et al. The interleukin-15/interleukin-15 receptor system as a model for juxtacrine and reverse signaling. *Bioessays.* 2006;28:362-77.

96. Cario G, Izraeli S, Teichert A, et al. High interleukin-15 expression characterizes childhood acute lymphoblastic leukemia with involvement of the CNS. *J Clin Oncol.* 2007;25:4813-20.

97. Yang JJ, Cheng C, Yang W, et al. Genome-wide interrogation of germline genetic variation associated with treatment response in childhood acute lymphoblastic leukemia. *JAMA.* 2009;301:393-403.

98. Kurose K, Sugiyama E, Saito Y. Population differences in major functional polymorphisms of pharmacokinetics/pharmacodynamics-related genes in Eastern Asians and Europeans: implications in the clinical trials for novel drug development. *Drug Metab Pharmacokinet.* 2012;27:9-54.

99. Nelson HH, Wiencke JK, Christiani DC, et al. Ethnic differences in the prevalence of the homozygous deleted genotype of glutathione S-transferase theta. *Carcinogenesis.* 1995;16: 1243-5.

100. Marino S, Verzegnassi F, Tamaro P, et al. Response to glucocorticoids and toxicity in childhood acute lymphoblastic leukemia: role of polymorphisms of genes involved in glucocorticoid response. *Pediatr Blood Cancer.* 2009;53:984-91.

101. Anderer G, Schrappe M, Brechlin AM, et al. Polymorphisms within glutathione S-transferase genes and initial response to glucocorticoids in childhood acute lymphoblastic leukaemia. *Pharmacogenetics.* 2000;10:715-26.

102. Stanulla M, Schrappe M, Brechlin AM, et al. Polymorphisms within glutathione S-transferase genes (GSTM1, GSTT1, GSTP1) and risk of relapse in childhood B-cell precursor acute lymphoblastic leukemia: a case-control study. *Blood.* 2000;95:1222-8.

103. Borst L, Buchard A, Rosthoj S, et al. Gene dose effects of GSTM1, GSTT1 and GSTP1 polymorphisms on outcome in childhood acute lymphoblastic leukemia. *J Pediatr Hematol Oncol.* 2012;34:38-42.

104. Meissner B, Stanulla M, Ludwig WD, et al. The GSTT1 deletion polymorphism is associated with initial response to glucocorticoids in childhood acute lymphoblastic leukemia. *Leukemia.* 2004;18:1920-3.

105. Smith RW, Margulis RR, Brennan MJ, et al. The influence of ACTH and cortisone on certain factors of blood coagulation. *Science.* 1950;112:295-7.

106. Yamamoto T, Hirano K, Tsutsui H, et al. Corticosteroid enhances the experimental induction of osteonecrosis in rabbits with Shwartzman reaction. *Clin Orthop Relat Res.* 1995;(316):235-43.

107. Yun SI, Yoon HY, Jeong SY, et al. Glucocorticoid induces apoptosis of osteoblast cells through the activation of glycogen synthase kinase 3beta. *J Bone Miner Metab.* 2009;27:140-8.

108. Kawedia JD, Kaste SC, Pei D, et al. Pharmacokinetic, pharmacodynamic, and pharmacogenetic determinants of osteonecrosis in children with acute lymphoblastic leukemia. *Blood.* 2011;117:2340-7.

109. French D, Hamilton LH, Mattano LA, et al. A PAI-1 (SERPINE1) polymorphism predicts osteonecrosis in children with acute lymphoblastic leukemia: a report from the Children's Oncology Group. *Blood.* 2008;111:4496-9.

110. Jones TS, Kaste SC, Liu W, et al. CRHR1 polymorphisms predict bone density in survivors of acute lymphoblastic leukemia. *J Clin Oncol.* 2008;26:3031-7.

111. Bottini N, MacMurray J, Peters W, et al. Association of the acid phosphatase (ACP1) gene with triglyceride levels in obese women. *Mol Genet Metab.* 2002;77:226-9.

112. Zambuzzi WF, Granjeiro JM, Parikh K, et al. Modulation of Src activity by low molecular weight protein tyrosine phosphatase during osteoblast differentiation. *Cell Physiol Biochem.* 2008;22:497-506.

113. Kamdem LK, Hamilton L, Cheng C, et al. Genetic predictors of glucocorticoid-induced hypertension in children with acute lymphoblastic leukemia. *Pharmacogenet Genomics.* 2008;18:507-14.

114. Tissing WJ, den Boer ML, Meijerink JP, et al. Genome wide identification of prednisolone-responsive genes in acute lymphoblastic leukemia cells. *Blood.* 2007;109:3929-35.

115. Schmidt S, Rainer J, Riml S, et al. Identification of glucocorticoid-response genes in children with acute lymphoblastic leukemia. *Blood.* 2006;107:2061-9.

116. Holleman A, den Boer ML, Cheok MH, et al. Expression of the outcome predictor in acute leukemia 1 (OPAL1) gene is not an independent prognostic factor in patients treated according to COALL or St Jude protocols. *Blood.* 2006;108:1984-90.

117. Wang Z, Malone MH, He H, et al. Microarray analysis uncovers the induction of the proapoptotic BH3-only protein Bim in multiple models of glucocorticoid-induced apoptosis. *J Biol Chem.* 2003;278:23861-7.

118. Bachmann PS, Gorman R, Papa RA, et al. Divergent mechanisms of glucocorticoid resistance in experimental models of pediatric acute lymphoblastic leukemia. *Cancer Res.* 2007;67:4482-90.

119. Pottier N, Yang W, Assem M, et al. The SWI/SNF chromatin-remodeling complex and glucocorticoid resistance in acute lymphoblastic leukemia. *J Natl Cancer Inst.* 2008;100:1792-803.

120. Pottier N, Cheok MH, Yang W, et al. Expression of SMARCB1 modulates steroid sensitivity in human lymphoblastoid cells: identification of a promoter SNP that alters PARP1 binding and SMARCB1 expression. *Hum Mol Genet.* 2007;16:2261-71.

121. Stams WA, den Boer ML, Holleman A, et al. Asparagine synthetase expression is linked with L-asparaginase resistance in TEL-AML1-negative but not TEL-AML1-positive pediatric acute lymphoblastic leukemia. *Blood.* 2005;105:4223-5.

122. Aslanian AM, Fletcher BS, Kilberg MS. Asparagine synthetase expression alone is sufficient to induce L-asparaginase resistance in MOLT-4 human leukaemia cells. *Biochem J.* 2001;357:321-8.

123. Hutson RG, Kitoh T, Moraga Amador DA, et al. Amino acid control of asparagine synthetase: relation to asparaginase resistance in human leukemia cells. *Am J Physiol.* 1997;272:C1691-9.

124. Su N, Pan YX, Zhou M, et al. Correlation between asparaginase sensitivity and asparagine synthetase protein content, but not mRNA, in acute lymphoblastic leukemia cell lines. *Pediatr Blood Cancer.* 2008;50:274-9.

125. Gutierrez JA, Pan YX, Koroniak L, et al. An inhibitor of human asparagine synthetase suppresses proliferation of an L-asparaginase-resistant leukemia cell line. *Chem Biol.* 2006;13:1339-47.

126. Al Sarraj J, Vinson C, Thiel G. Regulation of asparagine synthetase gene transcription by the basic region leucine zipper transcription factors ATF5 and CHOP. *Biol Chem.* 2005;386:873-9.

127. Estes DA, Lovato DM, Khawaja HM, et al. Genetic alterations determine chemotherapy resistance in childhood T-ALL: modelling in stage-specific cell lines and correlation with diagnostic patient samples. *Br J Haematol.* 2007;139:20-30.

128. Fine BM, Kaspers GJ, Ho M, et al. A genome-wide view of the in vitro response to l-asparaginase in acute lymphoblastic leukemia. *Cancer Res.* 2005;65:291-9.

129. Rousseau J, Gagne V, Labuda M, et al. ATF5 polymorphisms influence ATF function and response to treatment in children with childhood acute lymphoblastic leukemia. *Blood.* 2011;118:5883-90.

130. Chen SH, Yang W, Fan Y, et al. A genome-wide approach identifies that the aspartate metabolism pathway contributes to asparaginase sensitivity. *Leukemia.* 2011;25:66-74.

131. Mitchell S, Ellingson C, Coyne T, et al. Genetic variation in the urea cycle: a model resource for investigating key candidate genes for common diseases. *Hum Mutat.* 2009;30:56-60.

132. Marie JP. Drug resistance in hematologic malignancies. *Curr Opin Oncol.* 2001;13:463-9.

133. Bradshaw DM, Arceci RJ. Clinical relevance of transmembrane drug efflux as a mechanism of multidrug resistance. *J Clin Oncol.* 1998;16:3674-90.

134. Kourti M, Vavatsi N, Gombakis N, et al. Expression of multidrug resistance 1 (MDR1), multidrug resistance-related protein 1 (MRP1), lung resistance protein (LRP), and breast cancer resistance protein (BCRP) genes and clinical outcome in childhood acute lymphoblastic leukemia. *Int J Hematol.* 2007;86:166-73.

135. Vitale A, Guarini A, Ariola C, et al. Adult T-cell acute lymphoblastic leukemia: biologic profile at presentation and correlation with response to induction treatment in patients enrolled in the GIMEMA LAL 0496 protocol. *Blood.* 2006;107:473-9.

136. Hoffmeyer S, Burk O, von Richter O, et al. Functional polymorphisms of the human multidrug-resistance gene: multiple sequence variations and correlation of one allele with P-glycoprotein expression and activity in vivo. *Proc Natl Acad Sci U S A.* 2000;97:3473-8.

137. Kimchi-Sarfaty C, Oh JM, Kim IW, et al. A "silent" polymorphism in the MDR1 gene changes substrate specificity. *Science.* 2007;315:525-8.

138. Jamroziak K, Mlynarski W, Balcerczak E, et al. Functional C3435T polymorphism of MDR1 gene: an impact on genetic susceptibility and clinical outcome of childhood acute lymphoblastic leukemia. *Eur J Haematol.* 2004;72:314-21.

139. Stanulla M, Schaffeler E, Arens S, et al. GSTP1 and MDR1 genotypes and central nervous system relapse in childhood acute lymphoblastic leukemia. *Int J Hematol.* 2005;81:39-44.

140. Efferth T, Sauerbrey A, Steinbach D, et al. Analysis of single nucleotide polymorphism C3435T of the multidrug resistance gene MDR1 in acute lymphoblastic leukemia. *Int J Oncol.* 2003;23:509-17.

141. Jamroziak K, Balcerczak E, Cebula B, et al. Multi-drug transporter MDR1 gene polymorphism and prognosis in adult acute lymphoblastic leukemia. *Pharmacol Rep.* 2005;57:882-8.

142. Erdelyi DJ, Kamory E, Zalka A, et al. The role of ABC-transporter gene polymorphisms in chemotherapy induced immunosuppression, a retrospective study in childhood acute lymphoblastic leukaemia. *Cell Immunol.* 2006;244:121-4.

143. Sodani K, Patel A, Kathawala RJ, et al. Multidrug resistance associated proteins in multidrug resistance. *Chin J Cancer.* 2012;31:58-72.

144. Steinbach D, Legrand O. ABC transporters and drug resistance in leukemia: was P-gp nothing but the first head of the Hydra? *Leukemia.* 2007;21:1172-6.

145. Plasschaert SL, de Bont ES, Boezen M, et al. Expression of multidrug resistance-associated proteins predicts prognosis in childhood and adult acute lymphoblastic leukemia. *Clin Cancer Res.* 2005;11:8661-8.

146. Semsei AF, Erdelyi DJ, Ungvari I, et al. ABCC1 polymorphisms in anthracycline-induced cardiotoxicity in childhood acute lymphoblastic leukaemia. *Cell Biol Int.* 2012;36:79-86.
147. Haenisch S, Zimmermann U, Dazert E, et al. Influence of polymorphisms of ABCB1 and ABCC2 on mRNA and protein expression in normal and cancerous kidney cortex. *Pharmacogenomics J.* 2007;7:56-65.
148. Rau T, Erney B, Gores R, et al. High-dose methotrexate in pediatric acute lymphoblastic leukemia: impact of ABCC2 polymorphisms on plasma concentrations. *Clin Pharmacol Ther.* 2006;80:468-76.
149. Ansari M, Sauty G, Labuda M, et al. Polymorphism in multidrug resistance-associated protein gene 3 is associated with outcomes in childhood acute lymphoblastic leukemia. *Pharmacogenomics J.* 2012;12:386-94.
150. Bruggemann M, Trautmann H, Hoelzer D, et al. Multidrug resistance-associated protein 4 (MRP4) gene polymorphisms and treatment response in adult acute lymphoblastic leukemia. *Blood.* 2009;114:5400-1.
151. Assaraf YG. The role of multidrug resistance efflux transporters in antifolate resistance and folate homeostasis. *Drug Resist Updat.* 2006;9:227-46.
152. Papaemmanuil E, Hosking FJ, Vijayakrishnan J, et al. Loci on 7p12.2, 10q21.2 and 14q11.2 are associated with risk of childhood acute lymphoblastic leukemia. *Nat Genet.* 2009;41:1006-10.
153. Trevino LR, Yang W, French D, et al. Germline genomic variants associated with childhood acute lymphoblastic leukemia. *Nat Genet.* 2009;41:1001-5.
154. Xu H, Cheng C, Devidas M, et al. ARID5B genetic polymorphisms contribute to racial disparities in the incidence and treatment outcome of childhood acute lymphoblastic leukemia. *J Clin Oncol.* 2012;30:751-7.
155. Pottier N, Paugh SW, Ding C, et al. Promoter polymorphisms in the beta-2 adrenergic receptor are associated with drug-induced gene expression changes and response in acute lymphoblastic leukemia. *Clin Pharmacol Ther.* 2010;88:854-61.
156. Gu C, Ma YC, Benjamin J, et al. Apoptotic signaling through the beta-adrenergic receptor. A new Gs effector pathway. *J Biol Chem.* 2000;275:20726-33.
157. Lugthart S, Cheok MH, den Boer ML, et al. Identification of genes associated with chemotherapy cross resistance and treatment response in childhood acute lymphoblastic leukemia. *Cancer Cell.* 2005;7:375-86.
158. Johnson WG, Stenroos ES, Spychala JR, et al. New 19 bp deletion polymorphism in intron-1 of dihydrofolate reductase (DHFR): a risk factor for spina bifida acting in mothers during pregnancy? *Am J Med Genet A.* 2004;124:339-45.

Hematopoietic Stem Cell Transplantation for Acute Lymphoblastic Leukemia

12

Sandra H Thomas, Stephen J Forman

TREATMENT STRATEGY FOR ALLOGENEIC HEMATOPOIETIC STEM CELL TRANSPLANTATION

Analysis of treatment responses based on molecular, genetic, and clinical data, as well as changes in the approach to treatment, continue to refine the recommendations relating to the timing of transplantation for the treatment of patients with acute lymphoblastic leukemia (ALL), as seen in the recent National Comprehensive Cancer Network (NCCN) Guidelines.[1] The Leucémie Aiguë Lymphoblastique de l'Adulte (LALA)-87 and -94 trials find allogeneic hematopoietic stem cell transplantation (HSCT) in first complete remission (CR1) beneficial for high-risk patients, while the Medical Research Council/Eastern Cooperative Oncology Group (MRC/ECOG) and Hemato-Oncologie voor Volwassenen Nederland (HOVON) trials find it more beneficial for standard-risk patients.[2-5] For patients who relapse, HSCT is the only treatment with the potential for cure, and then primarily in that minority of patients able to achieve a second remission. Thus, it is important to perform human leukocyte antigen (HLA) typing at diagnosis to explore the transplant possibilities either from related donors or through the unrelated donor registries, especially for patients with high-risk features, such as high white count, older age, slow or no achievement of remission, or evidence of minimal residual disease (MRD). For patients who do not receive transplant in CR1, having the donor information on file in the event of relapse saves precious time in planning for treatment in that setting. Early identification of the presence of Philadelphia chromosome (Ph) allows patients the additional beneficial therapeutic options of inclusion of tyrosine kinase inhibitors (TKIs) as part of the induction, consolidation, and maintenance regimen. Figure 12-1 provides a suggested algorithm for the use of transplant in adult patients with ALL. This chapter will discuss the evidence on which this algorithm is based and the likely directions for the future.

ALLOGENEIC HSCT IN FIRST COMPLETE REMISSION

Allogeneic HSCT in CR1 has generally been reserved for patients presenting with poor-risk features, e.g., high white blood cell (WBC) count, adverse cytogenetic status [t(9;22), t(4;11), -7, +8],[6,7] and CD20 positivity.[8,9] Early phase II studies reported

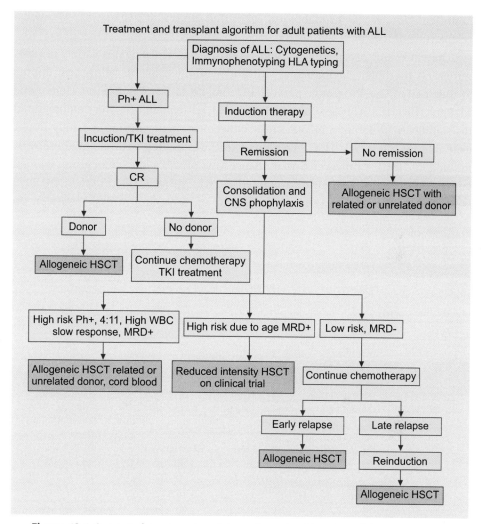

Figure 12-1 Suggested treatment and transplant algorithm for adult patients with acute lymphoblastic leukemia. Patient and disease characteristics and treatment outcomes that may indicate allogeneic transplantation therapy (grey boxes).

better-than-expected disease-free survival (DFS) (40–60%) for patients with high-risk disease following treatment with allogeneic HSCT. Stanford University and City of Hope reported on two series of patients with high-risk features who underwent full intensity allogeneic HSCT in first CR including patients with WBCs more than 25,000/µL, chromosomal translocations t(9;22), t(4;11), t(8;14); age more than 30; extramedullary disease at diagnosis; and/or more than 4 weeks of induction therapy required to achieve CR. One-third of the patients had two or more high-risk features at presentation, yet the probability of event-free survival at 5 years was 64%, with a relapse rate of 15%.[10]

There are four prospective studies reporting outcomes after a variety of post-remission therapies, for patients with and without available allogeneic donors (Table 12-1). The Programa para el Estudio de la Terapéutica en Hemopatía Maligna (PETHEMA) trial analyzed 83 Ph– ALL patients in CR1, but demonstrated no significant difference in outcomes between patients having a family donor available for allogeneic HSCT compared to those treated with chemotherapy or autologous HSCT;[11] however, 5-year relapse rates of 62% in the donor group seemed surprisingly high for patients transplanted in CR1. The MRC UKALLXII/ECOG 2993 study was designed to determine the impact of transplant in firs: remission on

Table 12-1	Randomized Trials in Adult ALL Comparing Allogeneic Transplant to Non-transplant Therapies			
Study	Patients	TRM/NRM	Relapse	Survival
Ribera et al. PETHEMA[11]	N = 156, Ph– age 15–50 years 72 donor 84 no donor	10% donor 2% no donor	@5 years: 62% donor, 51% no donor	DFS @5 years: 37% donor, 46% no donor OS @5 years: 40% donor, 49% no donor
Goldstone et al. MRC-ECOG[4]	N = 1031 age 15–64 years, allo 15–59 years 443 donor, 588 no donor	@2 years High risk: 36% donor, 14% no donor @2 years Std risk: 20% donor, 7% no donor	@10 years High risk: 37% donor, 63% no donor @10 years Std risk: 49% donor, 24% no donor	OS @5 years High risk: 41% donor, 35% no donor OS @5 years Std risk: 62% donor, 52% no donor
Cornelisson et al. HOVON[5]	N = 257 age 15–55 years 96 donor, 161 no donor	@5 years: 16% donor, 3% no donor	@5 years: 24% donor, 55% no donor	DFS @5 years: 60% donor, 42% no donor P = 0.01
Kako et al. JALSG[12]	N = 649 age 15–54 years 241 chemo, 408 allo	NR	NR	OS @10 years High risk: chemo 25%, allo 38% OS @10 years Std risk: chemo 40%, allo 54%

ALL, acute lymphoblastic leukemia; PETHEMA, Programa para el Estudio de la Terapéutica en Hemopatía Maligna; MRC-ECOG, Medical Research Council-Eastern Cooperative Oncology Group; HOVON, Hemato-Oncologie voor Volwassenen Nederland; JALSG, Japan Adult Leukemia Study Group; TRM, treatment-related mortality; NRM, non-relapse mortality; N, number of patients; Ph", Philadelphia chromosome negative; DFS, disease-free survival; OS, overall survival; allo, allogeneic transplant; Std, standard; NR, not reported; chemo, chemotherapy.

Source: Adapted from: Lazarus HM, Advani AS. When, how, and what cell source for hematopoietic cell transplantation in first complete remission adult acute lymphoblastic leukemia? Am Soc Hematolo Educ Program. 2012;382-8.

relapse and survival.[4] In a donor versus no-donor intention-to-treat analysis, they showed that Ph– ALL patients with a sibling donor had an improved 5-year overall survival (OS) (53% vs 45%, p = 0.01) and significantly lower relapse rate (p < 0.001) (Figure 12-2). The survival difference was significant in standard-risk patients, whereas in high-risk (especially older) patients, the reduced relapse risk was offset

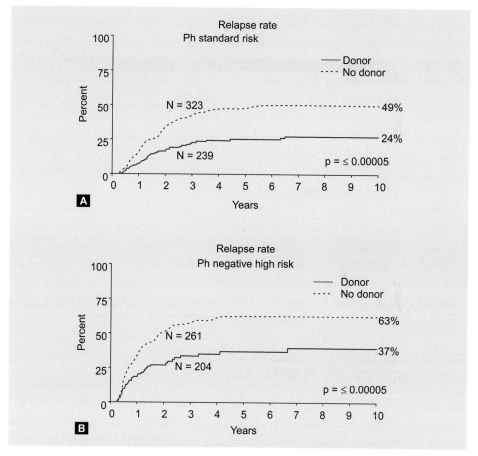

Figure 12-2 Medical Research Council-Eastern Cooperative Oncology Group Relapse Rate is superior in patients with allogeneic donors.[4] In patients with Philadelphia chromosome negative (Ph–) acute lymphoblastic leukemia (ALL), in an intention-to-treat analysis, patients with allogeneic donors (solid line) had significantly lower relapse rates than patients with no donor (dashed line). **A,** Standard-risk Ph– patients with ALL; **B,** High-risk Ph– patients with ALL. *From* Goldstone AH, Richards SM, Lazarus HM, et al. In adults with standard-risk acute lymphoblastic leukemia, the greatest benefit is achieved from a matched sibling allogeneic transplantation in first complete remission, and an autologous transplantation is less effective than conventional consolidation/maintenance chemotherapy in all patients: final results of the International ALL Trial (MRC UKALL XII/ECOG E2993). *Blood.* 2008;111(4):1827-33, *with permission.*

by an increase in non-relapse mortality (NRM). In this study with more than a thousand patients, subjects randomized to chemotherapy had a better 5-year OS (46%) than those randomized to autologous HSCT (37%, p = 0.03). The HOVON study,[5] which reported on two consecutive prospective studies of myeloablative HSCT in ALL for CR1 patients ages 15–55 years, showed significantly better 5-year DFS in the donor group (60% vs 42%, p = 0.01). While NRM was significantly higher in the donor group (16% vs 3%, p = 0.002), patients with a donor had a markedly lower relapse incidence at 5 years (24% vs 55%, p < 0.001), confirming improved disease control for transplanted patients. As in the MRC ECOG study, the benefit was most pronounced in the standard-risk group, although in this study poor-risk patients in the donor group also had a significantly improved outcome. The Japan Adult Leukemia Study Group (JALSG) analyzed two JALSG studies (ALL93 and ALL97) in order to identify the optimal strategy of post-remission therapy in Ph– ALL CR1 patients, ages 15–54 years, with an available HLA-matched sibling donor.[12] Based on 10-year survival probability, allogeneic HSCT was superior to other therapies (48.3% vs 32.6%, respectively) and this superiority was maintained even after adjustment for quality of life.

Taken together, these studies suggest that allogeneic HSCT is superior chemotherapy or autologous HSCT for control of leukemia in Ph– ALL patients in CR1. The survival advantage, however, appears to be greater for standard-risk rather compared to high-risk ALL patients. The lesser impact of allogeneic HSCT in high-risk patients is likely related to the adverse impact of age on outcome, which contributes to increased treatment-related mortality, countering the positive graft-versus-leukemia (GVL) effect in these patients.

MINIMAL RESIDUAL DISEASE AND CONSIDERATION OF TRANSPLANT

Any discussion of allogeneic HSCT at present must consider the impact of MRD testing on traditional definitions of remission and standard versus high-risk groups (Please see Chapter 9 for detailed discussion of MRD monitoring). After consolidation therapy, a high level of MRD at greater than 10^{-4} is associated with a high risk of disease relapse, with a rising level of MRD on treatment also portending relapse.[13,14] In some studies, a high level of MRD after induction and consolidation has been identified as a high-risk feature despite the achievement of a morphologic remission and the absence of high-risk cytogenetics[13,14] and would indicate the need for allogeneic HSCT. Conversely, the identification of patients who are sensitive to chemotherapy and achieve a low level of MRD (non-detectable) may identify a group of patients who do not need transplantation or can wait until there is clear evidence of relapse, including reappearance of MRD.[13,14] It remains to be determined what the benefit of HSCT may be in patients who are in first remission, but have evidence of this new factor defining high-risk disease, i.e., high MRD, compared to those patients who are MRD negative at the time of transplant. Thus, the future of treatment of adult patients with ALL in first remission will be refined to determine those patients who are unlikely to benefit from further chemotherapy and should be considered for transplantation during first remission, and those patients likely to do well with continued chemotherapy.[15] The detection of MRD at the completion of therapy also has implications for the success of transplant when patients with detectable MRD have a greater chance of relapse than those patients who are MRD negative. An important question is whether MRD+ patients should receive additional therapy pre-transplant in order to reduce the disease burden, or perhaps post-transplant to prevent relapse. Such MRD assessment of the patient over the time of treatment could lead to therapeutic changes in treatment in patients who are at high risk for relapse and could also apply to monitoring for patients after HSCT to initiate treatment prior to overt relapse.

HSCT FOR PHILADELPHIA CHROMOSOME POSITIVE ALL

For adults with Ph+ ALL, dismal outcomes after chemotherapy alone have prompted exploration of allogeneic HSCT for treatment of Ph+ disease. Studies have been performed at multiple institutions utilizing a variety of regimens, resulting in cure rates ranging from 30% to 65% based on age and remission status of the cohort.[16,17] Investigators from City of Hope and Stanford University analyzed their combined experience with Ph+ ALL in 79 patients in first CR, transplanted from HLA-identical sibling donors to determine long-term survival and disease control.[18] All patients but one were conditioned with fractionated total body irradiation (TBI) (1320 cGy) and high-dose etoposide (60 mg/kg). The 3-year probability of DFS and relapse was 55% and 18%, respectively, with the latest relapse at 27 months. Beyond first remission, HSCT is curative in a much smaller minority of patients but remains the treatment of choice.

The development of TKIs, imatinib and dasatinib, for the treatment of BCR-ABL positive hematopoietic malignancy has changed the upfront treatment strategy and outcomes and possibly outcomes after HSCT. Dasatinib is a second-generation TKI with enhanced potency against the BCR-ABL protein as well as the ability to block SRC-family kinases. In a phase II clinical trial of newly diagnosed patients with Ph+ ALL treated with hyperfractionated cyclophosphamide, vincristine, doxorubicin, and dexamethasone (hyperCVAD) and dasatinib (100 mg/day), 94% of patients achieved a CR with a 2-year survival of 64%.[19] Improved outcomes for allogeneic HSCT after first-line treatment with imatinib plus chemotherapy have also been reported.[20,21] In Mizuta et al. studies, 54 adult patients who completed induction therapy were treated with allogeneic HSCT and the authors compared their results with 122 patients who had received transplantation in the pre-imatinib era.[21] Relapse risk was significantly lower in the imatinib group (15% vs 50%) (p = 0.002), potentially reflecting a lower burden of residual disease at the time of HSCT, which also allowed a higher percentage of patients to be transplanted in a low-MRD first remission. Imatinib-treated patients also demonstrated superior DFS (58% vs 37%; p < 0.04) with similar NRM (Figure 12-3). Thus, in addition to improving the upfront success of induction therapy and potential long-term outcome of patients with Ph+ ALL, imatinib brings patients to transplantation with lower disease burden, potentially improving the cure rate for such patients.[20,21] A currently accruing national trial (NCT00792948) comparing HyperCVAD and dasatinib to allogeneic transplant followed by post-transplant dasatinib seeks to determine the best upfront approach for patients with Ph+ ALL.

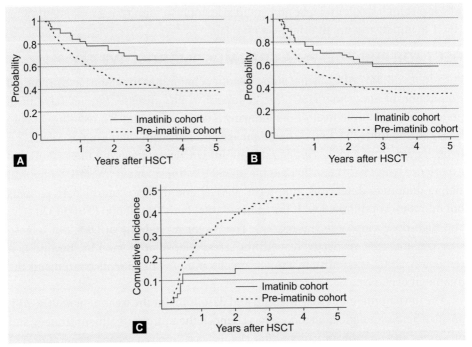

Figures 12-3 Transplantation of Philadelphia chromosome positive patients pre-imatinib and post-imatinib.[21] Outcomes after allogeneic hematopoietic stem cell transplantation of 51 patients who received imatinib-based therapy (solid line) versus 122 historical patients from the pre-imatinib era (dashed line). Median follow-up was 2.6 years for the imatinib cohort and 6.9 years for the pre-imatinib cohort. **A,** Overall survival; **B,** Disease-free survival; **C,** Cumulative incidence of relapse. *From Mizuta S, Matsuo K, Yagasaki F, Yujiri T, Hatta Y, Kimura Y, et al. Pre-transplant imatinib-based therapy improves the outcome of allogeneic hematopoietic stem cell transplantation for BCR-ABL-positive acute lymphoblastic leukemia. Leukemia. 2011;25:41-7, with permission.*

HSCT FOR RELAPSED OR PRIMARY REFRACTORY ALL

Approximately 10–15% of ALL patients are refractory to primary induction chemotherapy, and allogeneic HSCT can achieve remission and long-term disease control in approximately 20% of such patients. Among patients achieving CR after primary therapy, 50% to 70% will relapse. Relapsed ALL in adults is incurable by standard chemotherapy, but remissions are sometimes achieved with reinduction therapy using standard vincristine, prednisone, and anthracycline, or with cytarabine-based regimens, particularly high-dose Ara-C combined with an anthracycline or clofarabine.[22] Reinduction is most successful in patients whose first remission was prolonged. Without HSCT, adult patients with relapsed ALL have an extremely poor prognosis regardless of initial remission duration and transplantation, when feasible, is the only possible curative therapy.[23] Center for International Blood and Marrow Transplant Research (CIBMTR) data indicate that ALL patients transplanted from an HLA-identical sibling donor in second CR have an approximately 35–40% chance of long-term DFS, while those transplanted with disease not in remission have a DFS of only 10–20% (Mary Horowitz, personal communication). Five-year OS is close to 40% for patients with ALL who were able to achieve a second remission, had a donor, and were healthy enough to proceed to allogeneic HSCT (Figure 12-4). As in all series, these data do not account for those patients who suffer a relapse and are unable to undergo transplantation, which represents the majority of patients.[24] The actual cure rate when including all patients whose ALL has relapsed, is less than 20%. There is an urgent need for new therapies that can be used in relapsed

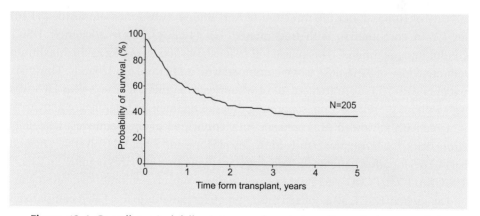

Figure 12-4 Overall survival following second remission allogeneic hematopoietic stem cell transplantation. Probability of survival after allogeneic hematopoietic stem cell transplantation with myeloablative conditioning for acute lymphoblastic leukemia in complete remission 2 in adults 18–50 years of age in the US, 2005–2007. *Courtesy:* CIBMTR Personal communication from Dr. Mary Horowitz, May 2012. *Adapted from* Forman SJ, Rowe JM. The myth of the second remission of acute leukemia in the adult. *Blood.* 2013;121:1077-82, *with permission.*

patients as a bridge to transplant. Some of the most promising novel agents are bi-specific engaging antibodies to CD19 (blinatumomab) drug immunoconjugates, such as inotuzumab, SAR3419, and ponatinib for patients with refractory Ph+ ALL (See Chapter 14 for discussion of novel agents for relapsed ALL). Currently, for adult patients with ALL after a first relapse, therapy that facilitates subsequent treatment with an allogeneic HSCT is the best evidence-based curative option.

REGIMEN DEVELOPMENT FOR ALLOGENEIC HSCT FOR ALL

Historically, the most common conditioning regimen for transplantation of patients with ALL is a myeloablative dose of cyclophosphamide (CY) combined with FTBI. Additional preparative regimens have been developed by substituting various chemotherapeutic agents for CY or TBI.

Investigators at Johns Hopkins University substituted busulfan (BU) for TBI to decrease the long-term side-effects of TBI and to determine the efficacy of high-dose combined alkylating therapy in eliminating leukemic cells.[25,26] This chemotherapy-only regimen has activity against advanced ALL, demonstrating that TBI is not an absolute requirement for successful HSCT. A retrospective analysis from the CIBMTR found that a conventional CY/TBI regimen was superior to a non-TBI-containing BU/CY regimen in pediatric patients. Three-year survival was 55% for CY/TBI versus 40% for BU/CY;[27] however, despite these differences in survival, relapse risk was similar. Studies of another high-dose conditioning regimen, BU and fludarabine with 400 cGy of TBI, reported a low transplant-related mortality of 3% and a projected DFS of 65%.[28]

City of Hope, under the direction of Karl Blume, substituted etoposide (VP16) for CY in combination with fractionated TBI (13.2Gy) in the allogeneic HSCT conditioning regimen.[29] This phase I–II trial established 60 mg/kg as the maximum tolerated dose of VP16 dose when combined with a TBI dose of 1320 rads. Thirty-six patients with ALL were treated, 20 of whom were in relapse. The 3-year DFS was 43% with a 32% relapse rate, suggesting that the regimen had significant activity in patients with advanced ALL, subsequently confirmed by the Southwest Oncology Group trial.[30] A subsequent study from City of Hope and Stanford University showed a 64% DFS for adult patients undergoing transplantation with this regimen in CR1.[10] The UKALL XII/ECOG 2993 Trial,[4] a comparative study of chemotherapy, autologous and allogeneic HSCT, also utilized this regimen for patients in first CR. A comparison of radiation-based transplant regimens consisting of TBI combined with either CY or etoposide chemotherapy suggested that when the TBI dose was greater than 13 Gy, TBI/Cy and TBI-VP16 had similar efficacy.[31] Transplant-related mortality did not differ between the two conditioning regimens.

While a large number of studies evaluating the role of reduced intensity HSCT have been performed for various hematologic malignancies, there are only a few

Table 12-2	Reduced Intensity Transplant Outcomes for ALL			
Study	*Patients*	*TRM/NRM*	*Relapse*	*Survival*
Stein et al. COH[34]	N = 24 (11 CR1)	22% @2 year	21% @2 year	DFS/OS: 62% @2 year
Bachanova et al. UMN[35]	N = 22 (12 CR1; 8 Ph−)	27% @3 year (8% CR1)	36% @3 year	OS: 50% @3 year (81% for CR1)
Cho et al. Korea[36]	N = 37 (30 CR1)	18% @3 year	20% @3 year	DFS: 63% @3 year OS: 64% @3 year
Nishiwaki et al. JMDP/ JSHCT[37]	N = 81 MA, N = 26 RIC (21 CR1)	40% @2 year 36% @2 year	18% @2 year 26% @2 year	DFS/OS: 58% @2 year DFS/OS: 63% @2 year
Mohty et al. EBMT[38]	N = 449 MA (391 CR1); n = 127 RIC (105 CR1)	29% @2 year 21% @2 year	31% @2 year 47% @2 year	LFS: 38% @2 year LFS: 32% @2 year
Marks et al. CIBMTR[39]	N = 1428 MA (747 CR1); n = 93 RIC (55 CR1)	33% @3 year 32% @3 year	26% @3 year 35% @3 year	OS: 51% @3 year OS: 45% @3 year
Kebriaei, MDA[40]	N = 51 (30 CR1), (13 CR2)	32% @1 year	16% @1 year 37% @2 year	OS: 67% @1 year LFS: 54% @1 year
Ram, FHCRC[41]	N = 51	28% @3 year	40% @3 year	OS 34% @3 year 62% for Ph + w/imatinib

ALL, acute lymphoblastic leukemia; COH, City of Hope; UMN, University of Minnesota; JMDP, Japan Marrow Donor Program; JSHCT, Japan Society for Hematopoietic Cell Transplantation; EBMT, European Group for Blood and Marrow Transplantation; CIBMTR, Center for International Blood and Marrow Transplant Research; MDA, MD Anderson; FHCRC, Fred Hutchinson Cancer Research Center; TRM, treatment-related mortality; NRM, non-relapse mortality; N, number of patients; CR, complete remission; DFS, disease-free survival; OS, overall survival; Ph", Philadelphia chromosome negative; MA, myeloablative; RIC, reduced intensity conditioning; LFS, leukemia-free survival.

Source: Adapted and updated based on: Lazarus HM, Advani AS. When, how, and what cell source for hematopoietic cell transplantation in first complete remission adult acute lymphoblastic leukemia? Am Soc Hematology *Educ Program.* 2012;382-8.

conducted in patients with ALL. The consensus has been that for cure of patients with ALL, high dose chemoradiotherapy is required; however, this approach is of limited use in patients over the age of 50. Additionally, the graft-versus-tumor effect appears to be more potent against myeloid malignancies, such as acute myelogenous leukemia (AML) and chronic myelogenous leukemia (CML); and against B cell malignancies of mature B cells, such as low grade non-Hodgkin's lymphoma, CLL, and multiple myeloma, than it is with a more undifferentiated B cell disease, such as pre-B ALL, especially if not in remission.[32,33] Nevertheless, an increasing number of small studies have suggested that there is a role for reduced intensity HSCT even in this disease, particularly in older patients. Table 12-2 summarizes outcomes for several published series of ALL patients with reduced intensity conditioning regimens of varying intensity; DFS ranges from 38% to 63% with only 50% of patients receiving this therapy in CR1.[34-41] In a retrospective analysis of 24 patients with ALL

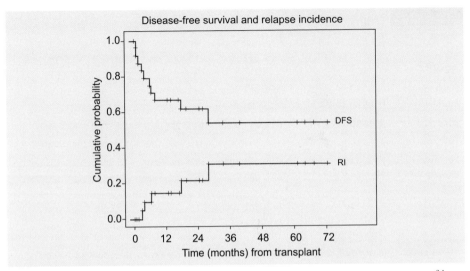

Figure 12-5 Reduced intensity hematopoietic stem cell transplantation outcomes.[34] Median follow-up was 28.5 months for a population of 24 patients. Disease free survival and cumulative incidence of relapse are shown. *From* Stein et al., Reduced-intensity conditioning followed by peripheral blood stem cell transplantation for adult patients with high-risk acute lymphoblastic leukemia. Stein AS, Palmer JM, O'Donnell MR, Kogut NM, Spielberger RT, Slovak ML, et al. Reduced-intensity conditioning followed by peripheral blood stem cell transplantation for adult patients with high-risk acute lymphoblastic leukemia. *Biol Blood Marrow Transplant.* 2009;15(11):1407-14, *with permission.*

who received reduced intensity HSCT, City of Hope reported a DFS of 61.5% and a relapse incidence of 21% at 2 years (Figure 12-5).[34] In a study from Fred Hutchinson Cancer Research Center, patients with Ph+ ALL who received post-transplant imatinib demonstrated DFS of up to 63%.[41] The UKALL XII ECOG 2993 study of adult ALL warns of high toxicity and limited improvement in DFS following myeloablative allogeneic transplant in older adult patients, despite better disease control.[4] This highlights the necessity for clinical trials exploring reduced intensity approaches in older patients with ALL, who would otherwise be candidates for transplantation based on cytogenetics, MRD, and response to initial treatment. Very poor outcomes for older patients ALL treated only with standard chemotherapy make reduced intensity HSCT an important consideration for potentially curative treatment in those patients.

CELL AND DONOR SOURCES FOR HSCT FOR ALL

Peripheral blood stem cells (PBSC) have replaced bone marrow as the most commonly used hematopoietic cell graft in the last decade. A retrospective analysis from the European Group for Blood and Marrow Transplantation (EBMT) compared outcomes for 858 patients with acute leukemia in first remission, of whom 513 received marrow grafts and 345 received PBSC.[42] Similar to findings in other studies, engraftment was faster with PBSC; however, there was also increased risk of chronic graft-versus-host disease (GVHD). Recent reports from the Blood and Marrow Transplant Clinical Trials Network trial observed that in patients undergoing myeloablative transplants, relapse rates were similar in patients who received blood and marrow grafts, but incidence of chronic GVHD was higher in patients who received PBSC.[43] In this series, there was no obvious difference in survival or relapse, but the increased incidence of chronic GVHD in patients who received peripheral blood as the stem cell source should be factored into the decision between available cell sources.

The use of umbilical cord blood (UCB) as a stem cell source is gaining popularity, but there is little available data specifically relating to patients with ALL. In one single-institution trial, transplantation utilizing high-dose conditioning followed by hematopoietic cells derived from either UCBs or unrelated donor cells resulted in comparable outcomes.[44] Several studies have now reported the results of unrelated cord blood grafts, with outcomes that are similar to unrelated adult donor-derived stem cells, but with different patterns of treatment failure.[45,46] At present, the data suggests that this cell source is acceptable for transplant where an unrelated donor cannot be identified and there is an available UCB with an adequate CD34+ cell dose.

Historically, outcomes after transplantation from unrelated donors have been inferior to those observed after matched-sibling transplantations due to increased rates of graft rejection and GVHD, resulting from increased alloreactivity in this setting. Over the past few years, results from several single-center studies have reflected improvements in donor/recipient allele-level molecular matching in class I and II histocompatibility genes, GVHD prophylaxis, and supportive care, particularly viral and fungal infection prophylaxis. OS results for patients with related and unrelated donors are essentially equivalent, with a somewhat lower relapse risk in patients receiving transplant from an unrelated donor,[47-49] making this a very reasonable, and in some cases preferred option, for patients requiring an allogeneic HSCT.

Haploidentical related donor transplant is being evaluated in patients with a variety of hematologic malignancies and has shown promise, especially with the use of post-transplant CY to reduce the alloreactivity of donor T cells. To date, there is limited data about the outcomes in patients undergoing haploidentical transplant for treatment of ALL. In the context of a clinical trial, this would be an option in a patient lacking a suitable matched related, unrelated or cord blood donor source of stem cells.

MANAGEMENT OF ALL RELAPSE AFTER ALLOGENEIC TRANSPLANT

For patients with ALL who relapse following HSCT, prognosis is very poor. A strategy of manipulating the graft-versus-tumor effect is the first line of defense; however this approach is less successful in patients with ALL than it is with AML and CML patients. The EBMT reported on 40 patients with relapsed ALL treated with donor lymphocyte infusion (DLI); of 29 evaluable patients, only one achieved CR.[50] Thus, DLI alone seems unlikely to result in remission and long-term disease-control in patients with relapsed ALL and, if considered, should be a component of a chemotherapy-based treatment program. For patients with Ph+ ALL, TKI therapy, either alone or combined with chemotherapy, can allow some patients to achieve remission, although the duration is often quite short and DLI should be performed before another relapse occurs. The role of donor-derived chimeric antigen receptor (CAR)-transduced CD19-specific T cells is also being explored as a treatment for relapse after transplant. CD19 BiTE antibody has also been utilized to achieve remission after post-transplant relapse without inducing a GVHD flare (See Chapter 14).

GRAFT-VERSUS-LEUKEMIA EFFECT IN ALL

The low response rate to DLI in patients with ALL has called into question the significance of the GVL effect in preventing relapse of this disease. The presence of a GVL effect is based on observations of higher relapse rates after autologous or syngeneic HSCT compared to allogeneic HSCT, the lower incidence of relapse in patients with GVHD, and increased relapse rates in recipients of T-cell-depleted marrow grafts. The most compelling argument for a strong GVL effect in ALL comes from both single-institution and registry data[51,52] showing consistently decreased relapse rates in patients who develop GVHD compared to those patients who do not. The occurrence of acute, chronic, or both forms of GVHD correlates with higher disease-free survival. Other studies have also demonstrated the beneficial impact of GVHD on reducing relapse in patients undergoing allogeneic HSCT for ALL, including Ph+ ALL.[53,54]

Although data support the importance of a GVL effect in mediating a clinically useful anti-leukemic response, the effectiveness of DLI therapy for patients with relapsed ALL has been limited. The unexpectedly poor DLI outcomes may stem from inability of ALL cells to present antigen targets, a low frequency of T-cell precursors reactive with the minor antigens presented by ALL cells, poor susceptibility of ALL targets to lysis, or kinetic differences in the way leukemic cells grow after HSCT. Thus, cytoreduction with chemotherapy prior to infusion of DLI is a better strategy for patients with relapsed ALL. For related reasons, reduced intensity HSCT is of limited effectiveness in patients with ALL who are not in remission. Studies focused on developing CD19-specific CAR-transduced T-cell immunotherapy for ALL may help to augment the GVL activity of donor T cells.

AUTOLOGOUS HSCT FOR ADULT ALL

Autologous transplantation for patients with ALL has been focused primarily on those patients in either first or second remission who lacked a sibling or unrelated allogeneic donor. Some studies have utilized the same conditioning regimens used in allogeneic transplantaion for autologous transplantation, based on the idea that the allogeneic GVL effect is weaker against ALL than against myeloid malignancies and, therefore, the preparative regimen may contribute to the cure. Several groups have reported outcomes for autologous HSCT in large series of adults with ALL in first remission.[55] The most important prognostic factor was the interval between achieving a CR and proceeding to transplant, with those patients transplanted later having the better DFS, but achieving no real advantage over chemotherapy. This effect may represent the drop-out rate for high-risk patients who relapse before transplantation, or possibly the effect of consolidation therapy in reducing tumor burden administered prior to hematopoietic cell transplantation. The European Cooperative Group/MRC report on over 1,000 patients indicated a leukemia-free survival of 36%[4] while the CIBMTR reported a similar plateau at 39%.[56]

The French LALA 87 randomized trial evaluated outcomes of adults with ALL in first remission treated with chemotherapy versus autologous transplantation.[2] Patients under age 40 with HLA-matched siblings were allocated to allogeneic transplantation, while the remaining patients were randomized to receive either consolidation treatment with modest dose chemotherapy or an autologous transplant. There was a significant drop out rate in the autologous arm due to early relapse and the long-term follow-up showed no significant difference in OS between the two groups: 34% OS for autologous HSCT and 29% for chemotherapy. The large MRC UKALL XII/ECOG E2993 trial reported the outcome comparing allogeneic transplant, autologous transplant, or chemotherapy in all adult patients with ALL in first remission.[4] In an intention-to-treat analysis, patients without allogeneic donors were randomly assigned to autologous transplantation versus continued chemotherapy and consolidation/maintenance chemotherapy was superior in both high-risk groups and low-risk groups.

FUTURE CONSIDERATIONS

For 20 years, there have been few, if any, innovations in the treatment of ALL in the adult, especially with regard to development of new agents. However, over the last few years, a number of agents have been in development that may improve treatment outcomes for patients with ALL, including monoclonal antibodies to CD20, CD52 and CD22; new drugs for T cell ALL, such as nelarabine; and TKI drugs imatinib, dasatinib, and nilotinib for the treatment of Ph+ ALL. In addition, the development of novel immune-based approaches, including CD19-specific CAR T cells to treat relapse, are now being tested as part of upfront therapy in the setting of allogeneic or autologous transplant. Blinatumomab and drug immumnoconjugates are being developed that may serve as more effective bridges to transplant by reducing disease burden and decreasing MRD at the time of transplant, and are being explored as part of upfront disease management.

The most important contributions may come from studies defining which patients are most likely to benefit from transplantation early in the course of their disease. Thus, MRD might prove to have a priority predictive value for relapse, reflecting disease chemosensitivity. This would be an important development for all patients. Then, even patients with higher risk disease, if they achieve CR with no detection of MRD, might be spared the risk of transplantation while other patients, even those with low risk disease, who have not achieved an adequate depth of remission, would be better served by early transplantation. Thus, introduction of MRD monitoring over the course of treatment might provide a new strategy for how to advise patients regarding timing of transplantation. Some investigators believe that MRD measurement, as a reflection of sensitivity to therapy, may substitute for, or "trump", all other prognostic features once a patient achieves a remission.

In addition, to address patients with high-risk disease transplantation, regimens are being developed that could include radio-immunotherapy targeted to the CD45 antigen[57] and the use of marrow-directed radiation therapy techniques to augment the radiation dose that can be delivered to the marrow while decreasing doses to sensitive organs.[58,59] Studies are also being conducted to determine the efficacy of utilizing antigen-specific T cells to augment the graft-versus-tumor effect. These cells can be derived from normal donors and could be transduced to recognize the CD19 antigen present on nearly all patients with pre-B ALL.[60] And, finally, given the results of chemotherapy treatment of older patients with ALL, studies of reduced intensity conditioning should be pursued for such patients in order to explore the potential therapeutic role of GVL in this high-risk patient population.

REFERENCES

1. National Comprehensive Cancer Network. NCCN Clinical Practice Guidelines in Oncology for Acute Lymphoblastic Lymphoma Version 2.2012. [online] NCCN website. Available from: www.nccn.org. [Accessed 2012].
2. Sebban C, Lepage E, Vernant JP, et al. Allogeneic bone marrow transplantation in adult acute lymphoblastic leukemia in first complete remission: a comparative study. French Group of Therapy of Adult Acute Lymphoblastic Leukemia. *J Clin Oncol*. 1994;12(12):2580-7.
3. Thomas X, Boiron JM, Huguet F, et al. Outcome of treatment in adults with acute lymphoblastic leukemia: analysis of the LALA-94 trial. *J Clin Oncol*. 2004;22(20):4075-86.
4. Goldstone AH, Richards SM, Lazarus HM, et al. In adults with standard-risk acute lymphoblastic leukemia, the greatest benefit is achieved from a matched sibling allogeneic

transplantation in first complete remission, and an autologous transplantation is less effective than conventional consolidation/maintenance chemotherapy in all patients: final results of the International ALL Trial (MRC UKALL XII/ECOG E2993). *Blood.* 2008;111(4):1827-33.

5. Cornelissen JJ, van der Holt B, Verhoef GE, et al. Myeloablative allogeneic versus autologous stem cell transplantation in adult patients with acute lymphoblastic leukemia in first remission: a prospective sibling donor versus no-donor comparison. *Blood.* 2009;113(6):1375-82.

6. Moorman AV, Harrison CJ, Buck GA, et al. Karyotype is an independent prognostic factor in adult acute lymphoblastic leukemia (ALL): analysis of cytogenetic data from patients treated on the Medical Research Council (MRC) UKALLXII/Eastern Cooperative Oncology Group (ECOG) 2993 trial. *Blood.* 2007;109(8):3189-97.

7. Wetzler M, Dodge RK, Mrózek K, et al. Prospective karyotype analysis in adult acute lymphoblastic leukemia: the cancer and leukemia group B experience. *Blood.* 1999;93(11): 3983-93.

8. Maury S, Huguet F, Leguay T, et al. Adverse prognostic significance of CD20 expression in adults with Philadelphia chromosome-negative B-cell precursor acute lymphoblastic leukemia. *Haematologica.* 2010;95(2):324-8.

9. Thomas DA, O'Brien S, Jorgensen JL, et al. Prognostic significance of CD20 expression in adults with de novo precursor B-lineage acute lymphoblastic leukemia. *Blood.* 2009;113(25):6330-7.

10. Jamieson CH, Amylon MD, Wong RM, et al. Allogeneic hematopoietic cell transplantation for patients with high-risk acute lymphoblastic leukemia in first or second complete remission using fractionated total-body irradiation and high-dose etoposide: a 15-year experience. *Exp Hematol.* 2003;31(10):981-6.

11. Ribera JM, Oriol A, Bethencourt C, et al. Comparison of intensive chemotherapy, allogeneic or autologous stem cell transplantation as post-remission treatment for adult patients with high-risk acute lymphoblastic leukemia. Results of the PETHEMA ALL-93 trial. *Haematologica.* 2005;90(10):1346-56.

12. Kako S, Morita S, Sakamaki H, et al. A decision analysis of allogeneic hematopoietic stem cell transplantation in adult patients with Philadelphia chromosome-negative acute lymphoblastic leukemia in first remission who have an HLA-matched sibling donor. *Leukemia.* 2011;25(2):259-65.

13. Mortuza FY, Papaioannou M, Moreira IM, et al. Minimal residual disease tests provide an independent predictor of clinical outcome in adult acute lymphoblastic leukemia. *J Clin Oncol.* 2002;20(4):1094-104.

14. Brüggemann M, Raff T, Flohr T, et al. Clinical significance of minimal residual disease quantification in adult patients with standard-risk acute lymphoblastic leukemia. *Blood.* 2006;107(3):1116-23.

15. Gökbuget N, Kneba M, Raff T, et al. Adult patients with acute lymphoblastic leukemia and molecular failure display a poor prognosis and are candidates for stem cell transplantation and targeted therapies. *Blood.* 2012;120(9):1868-76.

16. Snyder DS. Allogeneic stem cell transplantation for Philadelphia chromosome-positive acute lymphoblastic leukemia. *Biol Blood Marrow Transplant.* 2000;6(6):597-603.

17. Dombret H, Gabert J, Boiron JM, et al. Outcome of treatment in adults with Philadelphia chromosome-positive acute lymphoblastic leukemia—results of the prospective multicenter LALA-94 trial. *Blood.* 2002;100(7):2357-66.

18. Laport GG, Alvarnas JC, Palmer JM, et al. Long-term remission of Philadelphia chromosome-positive acute lymphoblastic leukemia after allogeneic hematopoietic cell transplantation from matched sibling donors: a 20-year experience with the fractionated total body irradiation-etoposide regimen. *Blood.* 2008;112(3):903-9.

19. Ravandi F, O'Brien S, Thomas D, et al. First report of phase 2 study of dasatinib with hyper-CVAD for the frontline treatment of patients with Philadelphia chromosome-positive (Ph+) acute lymphoblastic leukemia. *Blood.* 2010;116(12):2070-7.

20. Lee S, Kim YJ, Min CK, et al. The effect of first-line imatinib interim therapy on the outcome of allogeneic stem cell transplantation in adults with newly diagnosed Philadelphia chromosome-positive acute lymphoblastic leukemia. *Blood.* 2005;105(9):3449-57.

21. Mizuta S, Matsuo K, Yagasaki F, et al. Pre-transplant imatinib-based therapy improves the outcome of allogeneic hematopoietic stem cell transplantation for BCR-ABL-positive acute lymphoblastic leukemia. *Leukemia.* 2011;25(1):41-7.

22. Gökbuget N, Stanze D, Beck J, et al. Outcome of relapsed adult lymphoblastic leukemia depends on response to salvage chemotherapy, prognostic factors, and performance of stem cell transplantation. *Blood.* 2012;120(10):2032-41.

23. Tavernier E, Boiron JM, Huguet F, et al. Outcome of treatment after first relapse in adults with acute lymphoblastic leukemia initially treated by the LALA-94 trial. *Leukemia.* 2007; 21(9):1907-14.

24. Forman SJ, Rowe JM. The myth of the second remission of acute leukemia in the adult. *Blood.* 2013;121(7):1077-82.

25. Santos GW, Tutschka PJ, Brookmeyer R, et al. Marrow transplantation for acute non-lymphocytic leukemia after treatment with busulfan and cyclophosphamide. *N Engl J Med.* 1983;309(22):1347-53.

26. Tutschka PJ, Copelan EA, Klein JP. Bone marrow transplantation for leukemia following a new busulfan and cyclophosphamide regimen. *Blood.* 1987;70(5):1382-8.

27. Davies SM, Ramsay NK, Klein JP, et al. Comparison of preparative regimens in transplants for children with acute lymphoblastic leukemia. *J Clin Oncol.* 2000;18(2):340-7.

28. Russell JA, Savoie ML, Balogh A, et al. Allogeneic transplantation for adult acute leukemia in first and second remission with a novel regimen incorporating daily intravenous busulfan, fludarabine, 400 CGY total-body irradiation, and thymoglobulin. *Biol Blood Marrow Transplant.* 2007;13(7):814-21.

29. Blume KG, Forman SJ, O'Donnell MR, et al. Total body irradiation and high-dose etoposide: a new preparatory regimen for bone marrow transplantation in patients with advanced hematologic malignancies. *Blood.* 1987;69(4):1015-20.

30. Blume KG, Kopecky KJ, Henslee-Downey JP, et al. A prospective randomized comparison of total body irradiation-etoposide versus busulfan-cyclophosphamide as preparatory regimens for bone marrow transplantation in patients with leukemia who were not in first remission: a Southwest Oncology Group study. *Blood.* 1993;81(8):2187-93.

31. Marks DI, Forman SJ, Blume KG, et al. A comparison of cyclophosphamide and total body irradiation with etoposide and total body irradiation as conditioning regimens for patients undergoing sibling allografting for acute lymphoblastic leukemia in first or second complete remission. *Biol Blood Marrow Transplant.* 2006;12(4):438-53.

32. Valcárcel D, Martino R, Sureda A, et al. Conventional versus reduced-intensity conditioning regimen for allogeneic stem cell transplantation in patients with hematological malignancies. *Eur J Haematol.* 2005;74(2):144-51.

33. Arnold R, Massenkeil G, Bornhäuser M, et al. Nonmyeloablative stem cell transplantation in adults with high-risk ALL may be effective in early but not in advanced disease. *Leukemia.* 2002;16(12):2423-8.

34. Stein AS, Palmer JM, O'Donnell MR, et al. Reduced-intensity conditioning followed by peripheral blood stem cell transplantation for adult patients with high-risk acute lympho-blastic leukemia. *Biol Blood Marrow Transplant.* 2009;15(11):1407-14.

35. Bachanova V, Verneris MR, DeFor T, et al. Prolonged survival in adults with acute lympho-blastic leukemia after reduced-intensity conditioning with cord blood or sibling donor transplantation. *Blood.* 2009;113(13):2902-5.

36. Cho BS, Lee S, Kim YJ, et al. Reduced-intensity conditioning allogeneic stem cell trans-plantation is a potential therapeutic approach for adults with high-risk acute lymphoblastic leukemia in remission: results of a prospective phase 2 study. *Leukemia.* 2009;23(10):1763-70.

37. Nishiwaki S, Inamoto Y, Imamura M, et al. Reduced-intensity versus conventional myeloablative conditioning for patients with Philadelphia chromosome-negative acute lymphoblastic leukemia in complete remission. *Blood.* 2011;117(13):3698-9.

38. Mohty M, Labopin M, Volin L, et al. Reduced-intensity versus conventional myeloablative conditioning allogeneic stem cell transplantation for patients with acute lymphoblastic leukemia: a retrospective study from the European Group for Blood and Marrow Transplantation. *Blood.* 2010;116(22):4439-43.

39. Marks DI, Wang T, Pérez WS, et al. The outcome of full-intensity and reduced-intensity conditioning matched sibling or unrelated donor transplantation in adults with Philadelphia chromosome-negative acute lymphoblastic leukemia in first and second complete remission. *Blood.* 2010;116(3):366-74.

40. Kebriaei P, Basset R, Ledesma C, et al. Clofarabine combined with busulfan provides excellent disease control in adult patients with acute lymphoblastic leukemia undergoing allogeneic hematopoietic stem cell transplantation. Biol Blood Marrow *Transplant.* 2012; 18(12):1819-26.

41. Ram R, Storb R, Sandmaier BM, et al. Non-myeloablative conditioning with allogeneic hematopoietic cell transplantation for the treatment of high-risk acute lymphoblastic leukemia. *Haematologica.* 2011;96(8):1113-20.

42. Ringdén O, Labopin M, Bacigalupo A, et al. Transplantation of peripheral blood stem cells as compared with bone marrow from HLA-identical siblings in adult patients with acute myeloid leukemia and acute lymphoblastic leukemia. *J Clin Oncol.* 2002;20(24):4655-64.

43. Anasetti C, Logan BR, Lee SJ, et al. Peripheral-blood stem cells versus bone marrow from unrelated donors. *N Engl J Med.* 2012 Oct 18;367(16):1487-96.

44. Eapen M, Rocha V, Sanz G, et al. Effect of graft source on unrelated donor haemopoietic stem-cell transplantation in adults with acute leukaemia: a retrospective analysis. *Lancet Oncol.* 2010;11(7):653-60.

45. Atsuta Y, Suzuki R, Nagamura-Inoue T, et al. Disease-specific analyses of unrelated cord blood transplantation compared with unrelated bone marrow transplantation in adult patients with acute leukemia. *Blood.* 2009;113(8):1631-8.

46. Ferrá C, Sanz J, de la Camara R, et al. Unrelated transplantation for poor-prognosis adult acute lymphoblastic leukemia: long-term outcome analysis and study of the impact of hematopoietic graft source. *Biol Blood Marrow Transplant.* 2010;16(7):957-66.

47. Chim CS, Lie AK, Liang R, et al. Long-term results of allogeneic bone marrow transplantation for 108 adult patients with acute lymphoblastic leukemia: favorable outcome with BMT at first remission and HLA-matched unrelated donor. *Bone Marrow Transplant.* 2007;40(4):339-47.

48. Dahlke J, Kröger N, Zabelina T, et al. Comparable results in patients with acute lymphoblastic leukemia after related and unrelated stem cell transplantation. *Bone Marrow Transplant.* 2006;37(2):155-63.

49. Kiehl MG, Kraut L, Schwerdtfeger R, et al. Outcome of allogeneic hematopoietic stem-cell transplantation in adult patients with acute lymphoblastic leukemia: no difference in related compared with unrelated transplant in first complete remission. *J Clin Oncol.* 2004;22(14):2816-25.

50. Kolb HJ, Schattenberg A, Goldman JM, et al. Graft-versus-leukemia effect of donor lymphocyte transfusions in marrow grafted patients. *Blood.* 1995;86(5):2041-50.

51. Horowitz MM, Gale RP, Sondel PM, et al. Graft-versus-leukemia reactions after bone marrow transplantation. *Blood.* 1990;75(3):555-62.

52. Appelbaum FR. Graft versus leukemia (GVL) in the therapy of acute lymphoblastic leukemia (ALL). *Leukemia.* 1997;11:S15-7.

53. Esperou H, Boiron JM, Cayuela JM, et al. A potential graft-versus-leukemia effect after allogeneic hematopoietic stem cell transplantation for patients with Philadelphia chromosome-positive acute lymphoblastic leukemia: results from the French Bone Marrow Transplantation Society. *Bone Marrow Transplant.* 2003;31(10):909-18.

54. Lee S, Cho BS, Kim SY, et al. Allogeneic stem cell transplantation in first complete remission enhances graft-versus-leukemia effect in adults with acute lymphoblastic leukemia: antileukemic activity of chronic graft-versus-host disease. *Biol Blood Marrow Transplant.* 2007;13(9):1083-94.

55. Willemze R, Labar B. Post-remission treatment for adult patients with acute lymphoblastic leukemia in first remission: is there a role for autologous stem cell transplantation? *Semin Hematol.* 2007;44(4):267-73.

56. Bishop MR, Logan BR, Gandham S, et al. Long-term outcomes of adults with acute lympho-blastic leukemia after autologous or unrelated donor bone marrow transplantation: a comparative analysis by the National Marrow Donor Program and Center for International Blood and Marrow Transplant Research. *Bone Marrow Transplant.* 2008;41(7):635-42.

57. Pagel JM, Gooley TA, Rajendran J, Fisher DR, Wilson WA, Sandmaier BM, et al. Allogeneic hematopoietic cell transplantation after conditioning with 131I–anti-CD45 antibody plus fludarabine and low-dose total body irradiation for elderly patients with advanced acute myeloid leukemia or high-risk myelodysplastic syndrome. *Blood.* 2009;114(27):5444-53.

58. Rosenthal J, Wong J, Stein A, Qian D, Hitt D, Naeem H, et al. Phase 1/2 trial of total marrow and lymph node irradiation to augment reduced-intensity transplantation for advanced hematologic malignancies. *Blood.* 2011;117(1):309-15.

59. Wong JY, Liu A, Schultheiss T, Popplewell L, Stein A, Rosenthal J, et al. Targeted total marrow irradiation using three-dimensional image-guided tomographic intensity-modulated radiation therapy: an alternative to standard total body irradiation. *Biol Blood Marrow Transplant.* 2006;12(3):306-15.

60. Forman SJ. Hematopoietic cell transplantation for acute lymphoblastic leukemia in adults. In: Appelbaum FR, Forman SJ, Negrin RS, Blume KG, editors. Thomas' Hematooietic Cell Transplantation: Stem Cell Transplantation. 4th ed. Chichester: Wiley-Blackwell; 2009. p. 791-805.

Late Effects of Acute Lymphoblastic Leukemia Therapy

13

Preeti Chaudhary, Vinod Pullarkat

INTRODUCTION

With improvements in outcomes of acute lymphoblastic leukemia (ALL) therapy, we now face new challenges of understanding and minimizing the late sequelae of therapy. This is particularly true for pediatric ALL given the excellent cure rates and the increased vulnerability of children to many of the treatment side effects. ALL is treated with sequential chemotherapy cycles which include induction, consolidation, intensification, and maintenance phases over a period of 2–3 years and many of the cytotoxic drugs used have long lasting effects. Central nervous system (CNS) prophylaxis/treatment with radiation or chemotherapy is an integral part of ALL therapy and can have long-term adverse outcomes. In addition, patients who undergo allogenic hematopoietic stem cell transplant (HSCT) deal with late toxicities as well which are diverse in nature and severity and range from toxicities secondary to conditioning regimen used for HSCT, infections from prolonged immunosuppression as well as effects of graft-versus-host disease (GVHD). A summary of the more common therapy related complications is provided in tables 13-1 and 13-2.

ENDOCRINE DYSFUNCTION

Growth hormone (GH) production is the most vulnerable hypothalamic pituitary axis to be affected by ALL therapy, particularly cranial radiotherapy (CRT), although it has been described in ALL patients treated with chemotherapy alone.[1-3] Growth deceleration following CRT is usually permanent in contrast to growth failure from chemotherapy which is followed by a period of catch-up growth after completion of treatment.[4] During the maintenance phase of ALL chemotherapy, 6-mercaptopurine and methotrexate (MTX) are mainly responsible for suppressed catch-up growth.[5] Roman et al. have hypothesized that high dose MTX crosses blood brain barrier and may be toxic to the hypothalamus-pituitary axis leading to GH deficiency and growth impairment.[6] Most recently, Vandecruys et al. found modest but significant loss in final heights of 67 childhood ALL survivors treated with chemotherapy alone without CRT irrespective of the age at onset of chemotherapy and GH status at the cessation of treatment.[7] In their study, significant losses in height were noted

Table 13-1 Commonly Occurring Late Effects After ALL Chemotherapy

System/organ	Treatment	Risk factors	Late complications and consequences	Prevention and treatment
Growth hormone deficiency	• IT MTX • High dose systemic MTX • High dose GCs	• Hypothyroidism • Younger age • Premature puberty	• Growth hormone deficiency • Short stature Metabolic syndrome • Osteoporosis • Premature atherosclerosis	Growth hormone replacement
Gonads	High dose cyclophosphamide	• Abdominal radiation • Younger age treatment during peripubertal or post-pubertal period in girls	• Infertility • Reproductive problems	• Hormone replacement • Sperm/oocyte banking
Thyroid Adrenal insufficiency	High dose GCs	Cranial radiation	Growth retardation	• Hormone replacement • Stress doses of steroids when indicated
Cardiovascular	• Anthracyclines (higher risk with doses > 300 mg/m^2) • Cyclophosphamide • Vinca alkaloids	• Age < 4 years • Time since treatment • Female gender • ABCC1 genepolymorphism • Concomitant radiation	Congestive heart failure	Dexrazoxane
Skeleton system	Dexamethasone MTXL-asparaginase	• Pubertal delay • Male sex • Younger age • Poor nutrition • Inactivity • Endocrine glands irradiation	• Low BMD-Osteopenia • Osteoporosis • Osteonecrosis	• Lifestyle modification, calcium and vitamin D supplementation • Bisphosphonates • Hormone replacement • Joint replacement

Continued

Continued

System/organ	Treatment	Risk factors	Late complications and consequences	Prevention and treatment
Neurotoxicity	• GCs • IT MTX high-dose systemic MTX	• Female gender • Treatment at younger age • Longer time since treatment	• Chronic headaches • Seizures • Co-ordination and motor deficits • Neurocognitive deficits • Leukoencephalopathy	
Psychosocial Adjustment disorders	• IT MTX • High dose systemic MTX • High-dose GCs	• Treatment at younger age • Longer time since treatment	• Unemployment • Depression • Unmarried • Post-traumatic stress disorder	Environmental enrichment and appreciate psychological counseling
Secondary malignancies	• Alkylating agents • Topoisomerase II inhibitors		• Secondary AML • MDS • Solid tumors	Surveillance for SN including mammograms, colonoscopy, skin examination

MTX, methotrexate; GCs, glucocorticoids; IT, intrathecal; AML, acute myelogenous leukemia; MDS, myelodysplastic syndrome; SN, secondary neoplasm.

Table 13-2	Commonly Occurring Late Effects After Radiotherapy
Type of radiation	*Associated adverse outcomes*
Cranial radiotherapy	Neurocognitive deficits, precocious or delayed puberty, obesity, hypogonadism, Growth hormone deficiency, thyroid dysfunction, ACTH deficiency, secondary neoplasm
Craniospinal radiation	Growth-stunting effects, ↓Bone mineral density (plus late effects of cranial radiation), late menarche, hypogonadism
Testicular radiation	Infertility, hypogonadism
Total body radiation	Growth hormone deficiency, secondary neoplasm, neurocognitive deficits

ACTH, adrenocorticotropic hormone.

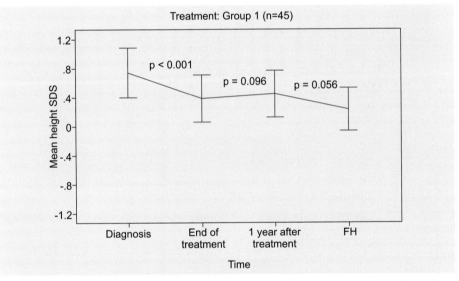

Figure 13-1 Changes in mean height standard deviation score at diagnosis; at the end of treatment; at 1 year after treatment; and at achievement of final height in childhood ALL survivors treated without cranial radiation therapy.[7]

between the time of diagnosis and the end of treatment as well as between 1 year after the end of treatment and achievement of final height. Mean height standard deviation decreased from 0.76±1.15 at the time of diagnosis to 0.23±0.97 at final height (Figure 13-1).

Radiation doses as low as 10 Gy given as total body irradiation (TBI) or CNS prophylaxis (18–24 Gy) can be directly damaging to the hypothalamus-pituitary axis. Heights of more than one fourth of childhood ALL survivors who receive CRT as part of their therapy are below the fifth percentile of population normative values and the poorest growth pattern is noted in children with earlier disease onset.[8-11]

Apart from GH deficiency, premature puberty with early closure of the epiphyses, hypothyroidism, and use of corticosteroids, especially dexamethasone contribute to growth impairment.[12,13] Likewise, final height standard deviation of children who undergo HSCT is significantly lower than their predicted genetic heights based on corrected mid-parental heights.[12,14] Growth impairment is more pronounced in children conditioned for HSCT with TBI as opposed to non-TBI regimens, such as cyclophosphamide and busulfan (CY/BU), boys compared to girls, children transplanted at a younger age (under 10 years of age), patients exposed to CRT prior to conditioning with TBI, and single dose TBI as compared to standard fractionated TBI.[12-15] Some series report the poorest growth pattern during the first year after TBI whereas others report the greatest impairment in growth several years after TBI.[16-19]

Growth hormone deficiency can also lead to the metabolic syndrome with dyslipidemia, insulin resistance, and increased risk of premature cardiovascular mortality.[20,21] These patients should be followed in endocrinology clinics as early detection and treatment with recombinant human GH can have positive impact on cardiovascular risk.[22] However, data on safety of GH use in terms of development of secondary malignancies is scant[23] and not all patients respond to GH replacement. In general, these complications have become less common with the trend toward decreasing the dose of CRT or avoiding it completely from ALL treatment protocols.

Primary hypothyroidism is the other common endocrine abnormality that occurs as a result of CRT or TBI secondary to direct exposure of the thyroid gland to radiation. ALL chemotherapy regimens themselves do not seem to increase the risk of thyroid dysfunction.[24] In patients who receive HSCT, subclinical hypothyroidism is noted in 7–15% of survivors.[25] Autoimmune thyroid disease has been reported in patients who have received allogeneic HSCT from a donor affected with an autoimmune thyroid disorder.[26,27] There is also a high standardized incidence ratio of secondary thyroid carcinoma in the transplanted population.[28]

Cranial radiotherapy or intrathecal (IT) chemotherapy itself does not seem to be detrimental to hypothalamic-pituitary-adrenal axis. However, high-dose glucocorticoid treatment used as part of ALL chemotherapy protocols or for the treatment of GVHD can cause adrenal suppression. These patients should be supplemented with stress doses of corticosteroids during surgical procedures or acute medical illnesses.

OBESITY

Long-term ALL survivors are at risk for being overweight [body mass index (BMI) over 25] or obese (BMI over 30). A multitude of factors contribute to development of obesity in ALL survivors including physical inactivity, GH insufficiency, presence of steroid-related myopathy, vincristine-related neuropathy, and leptin gene receptor polymorphism (Gln223Arg) particularly in women treated with more than or equal to 20 Gy CRT.[29,30] Conflicting data has been reported on the effect of ALL chemotherapy on metabolism. Vaisman et al. demonstrated that MTX and 6-mercaptopurine therapy affects metabolic fuel utilization as well as protein synthesis and turnover thereby altering body composition,[31] whereas, data published by Oeffinger et al. showed that there is no chemotherapeutic agent, either individually or in combination that can be significantly associated with overweight and obesity in ALL survivors during and after treatment.[30] Female gender, young age (under 4 years) at treatment, and patients treated with more than 20 Gy cranial radiation are at notably increased risk for being obese in adulthood.[32] Lifestyle is the unique modifiable factor and, therefore, promotion of a healthy lifestyle among ALL survivors is imperative.

INFERTILITY

In males, primary or secondary hypogonadism as a result of ALL therapy may lead to infertility. Inhibin B levels (which correlate well with decreased sperm concentration), follicle-stimulating hormone, luteinizing hormone (FSH, LH), testosterone levels, as well as sperm analysis have reported to be within normal limits in various long-term follow-up studies of ALL male survivors treated with chemotherapy.[33,34] Therefore, men treated before the age of 18 years can be reassured of preserved fertility. However, those treated with CRT, high dose CY (more than 7.5 gm/m^2) and of younger age (under 9 years) at treatment have abnormal sperm counts, reduced testicular size and are less likely to sire children.[35-37]

The medium term outlook for ovarian function is good for the majority of childhood ALL survivors. The time of onset of menarche and incidence of premature menopause were reported to be similar in ALL survivors compared to their sibling control groups.[38,39] However, females who receive craniospinal radiation therapy particularly CRT doses less than 18 Gy may experience earlier menarche and the spinal component of craniospinal irradiation is a major risk factor for late menarche and ovarian damage as evidenced by elevated gonadotropins levels.[40] Other risk factors for impaired fertility in female ALL survivors include CRT within 2 years of menarche, pelvic radiation, and cumulative doses of CY greater than 7.5 g/m^2.[41,42] Females above the age of 10 who were treated with alkylating agents also have an increased relative risk of preterm delivery.[43] In conclusion, fertility is generally preserved in ALL survivors who do not receive CRT, gonadal irradiation, or high doses of CY. Pregnancy outcomes are similar to those of the general population, except of a higher risk of preterm delivery.

Gonadal failure in ALL survivors who have undergone HSCT is mainly associated with TBI and use of busulfan and high dose CY conditioning.[44,45] Leydig cells are tolerant to irradiation and cytotoxic chemotherapy, and therefore, despite a high incidence of testicular damage and low testicular volumes, according to one series, most male children will experience normal sexual maturation.[46] In the same series, about 25% of postpubertal males treated with CY or CY plus TBI recovered testicular function and pregnancies among partners of male patients were unlikely to be adversely affected by the previous treatment. Recovered male patients had normal LH, FSH, testosterone, and sperm production.[46] On the other hand, there are long-term follow-up studies that have reported testicular failure with azoospermia in about 48–85% of males who undergo HSCT.[46-48] Irradiation and BU/CY conditioning protocols can lead to permanent ovarian damage and recovery is unusual.[46,49] Pregnancy after HSCT for ALL is a rare occurrence. Female HSCT survivors who do get pregnant are at an increased risk for premature delivery, spontaneous abortions, producing low birth babies, and increased rate of cesarean sections.[50] All adolescents and young adults receiving HSCT therapy should be offered sperm and oocyte cryopreservation as a way to preserve future fertility.[51]

CARDIOVASCULAR COMPLICATIONS

Anthracyclines are an integral component of ALL chemotherapy regimens. Cardiac toxicity from doxorubicin therapy is persistent and progressive and seems to be caused by formation of doxorubicin-iron complex that facilitates formation of reactive oxygen species in tissues leading to oxidative damage to myocardiocytes.[52,53] Progressive loss of myocytes, increased apoptosis, and reduced collagen production from doxorubicin toxicity may lead to left-ventricular wall thinning and subsequent enlargement of remaining myocardiocytes.[54] The spectrum of cardiotoxicity ranges from subclinical suppression of myocardial contractility to overt late congestive heart failure, high grade ectopy, pericarditis, myocarditis, acute myocardial infarction, and increased risk of sudden cardiac death.[53] The deficits are worst after higher cumulative doses of doxorubicin (400 mg/m^2), but no dose is considered safe.[55] A single dose of doxorubicin can cause cardiac troponin-T leak, a marker of myocardial injury.[56] There are other risk factors identified for anthracycline induced cardiotoxicity including age at treatment (below 4 years), time since treatment, concomitant therapy (irradiation, cyclophosphamide, vinca alkaloids), gender (female), and most recently genetic variants in the ABCC1 gene have been found to influence anthracycline-induced left ventricular dysfunction.[57,58] Effective preventive and therapeutic strategies, such as pretreatment with cardioprotectants like dexrazoxane, which reduces free-radical injury may help reduce doxorubicin induced cardiac impairment in long-term ALL survivors.[59] The Children's Oncology Group recommends a screening echocardiogram or MUGA at frequencies of every 1, 2, or 5 years, depending on age at exposure, cumulative anthracycline dose, and concomitant radiation exposure.[60]

Adult ALL survivors not receiving cardiotoxic chemotherapy nevertheless are prone to accelerated atherosclerosis and premature cardiovascular disease.[61]

Sulicka et al. have suggested that chronic inflammation and immune dysregulation occurs in adult ALL survivors treated with chemotherapy alone as demonstrated by elevated markers of chronic inflammation, which on a long-term basis can translate into late cardiovascular morbidity.[62] Systemic inflammation may worsen the cardiovascular status of adult ALL survivors who may already have impaired left ventricular structure and function from use of cardiotoxic chemotherapy.[63,64] GH deficiency resulting from damage to hypothalamic-pituitary axis by CRT also contributes to significant metabolic derangements including dyslipidemia and premature coronary artery disease.[65,66]

In a retrospective series, the cumulative incidence of first arterial event after allogeneic HSCT was 7.5% at 15 years as compared with 2.3% after autologous HSCT. The incidence was estimated at 22.1% (95% CI, 12.0–40.9) at 25 years.[67] The exact mechanism by which HSCT accelerates atherosclerosis is unknown; however, the cardiovascular risk factors, such as hypertension, insulin resistance, dyslipidemia, central obesity, and diabetes are more frequent after allogeneic HSCT [68] and all these factors are implicated in the pathophysiology of cardiovascular disease. Other transplant related factors that may contribute to early and increased arterial disease risk is the development of GVHD which has been shown to cause endothelial damage,[69] prolonged administration of high doses of corticosteroids,[70,71] and use of TBI as part of conditioning regimen which not only plays a role in the development of insulin resistance and metabolic syndrome, but also has direct toxic effects on the pericardium, myocardium, endocardium valves, conduction system, and coronary arteries.[72,73] Radiation also induces endothelial cell injury resulting in capillary loss and ischemia at the microcirculatory level.[74] Levels of N-terminal pro-brain natriuretic peptide and high sensitivity-C-reactive protein may provide valuable information on the cardiovascular status of survivors and identify those in greatest need of early screening and risk-factor modification.

SKELETAL DISORDERS

Several long-term follow-up studies have found that survivors of childhood ALL have bone mineral density (BMD) values below the age- and sex-adjusted population mean.[75,76] Risk factors that contribute to low BMD in ALL survivors include treatment with antimetabolites, namely, MTX and glucocorticoids, irradiation of endocrine organs that regulate bone accretion, pubertal delay in children, male sex, younger age at diagnosis, low body weight, poor nutrition, inactivity, and genetic predisposition.[76-79] Later in life, survivors are at risk for severe and early onset osteoporosis from bone mineral deficits. The pathogenesis of bone disease resulting from various chemotherapy regimens used to treat ALL is poorly understood. High dose MTX induces osteopenia by direct inhibition of osteoblast proliferation and activity as well as stimulating osteoclast recruitment resulting in a subsequent decrease in bone formation.[80,81] Bone mineral accretion is attenuated in adult ALL survivors who receive CRT, a known risk factor for impaired GH secretion. GH deficiency is a causative factor for osteoporosis; however, childhood ALL survivors treated without CRT are at increased risk of forearm fractures from endosteal bone loss and cortical bone thinning.[82]

Hematopoietic stem cell transplant recipients are at an even greater risk for developing low BMD, a complication reported in more than 50% of patients after HSCT.[83,84] The rapid rate of bone loss in the first year post SCT is partly attributed to the high levels of interleukin-6 in the immediate post-transplant period.[85] Avoidance of sun exposure to prevent GVHD, low intake of calcium and vitamin D, primary hypogonadism (low estrogen and testosterone), and secondary hyperparathyroidism due to low serum calcium all interfere with bone accrual growth after HSCT. The pathogenesis of bone disease after HSCT has been comprehensively reviewed by Weilbaecher.[86] Glucocorticoids and calcineurin inhibitors used in transplant setting also have negative effects on bone remodeling.[87] Both liver and cardiac transplant recipients have been shown to sustain rapid bone loss with tacrolimus therapy.[88] Corticosteroids directly cause bone damage by inducing apoptosis of osteoblasts and mature osteocytes, and indirectly by increasing the fat content of the marrow leading to fat embolization and vascular compression.[89]

Total body irradiation directly damages bone cells and has been shown to enlarge resorption lacunae, increase osteoclast number, and activity without an increase in bone formation, leading to increased bone resorption and bone porosity [90,91] BMD after HSCT begins to recover after 12 months, returning to near baseline at 48 months in patients who do not have continued exposure to corticosteroids and calcineurin inhibitors.[85] ALL survivors should be advised general interventions to reduce fracture risk including adequate intake of calcium and vitamin D. Dual energy X-ray absorptiometry is recommended at 1 year after transplantation and those patients found to be at an increased risk for bone loss should be treated with antiresorptive agents when indicated. Hormone replacement therapy (estrogen, testosterone, GH, thyroid) has been clearly shown to improve BMD.[92-95] Women who develop osteoporosis from premature menopause may benefit from bisphosphonate therapy to reduce the risk of fractures. It should also be effectively communicated to young adult survivors that tobacco smoking and excessive alcohol intake can unfavorably influence their bone health.[96]

Another devastating skeletal complication of ALL therapy is osteonecrosis (ON). (Figure 13-2). Age greatly influences the risk of developing ON as maturing bones are more susceptible to ON compared to immature bone which may be able to buffer the elevated intraosseous pressure caused by corticosteroid induced marrow fat-cell hypertrophy that ultimately leads to marrow ischemia and necrosis.[97,98] Risk for developing ON is associated with genetic polymorphism of the vitamin D receptor

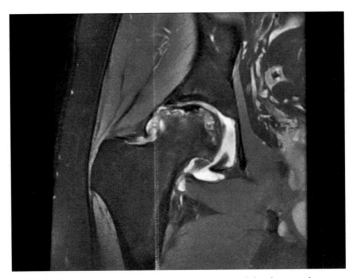

Figure 13-2 Magnetic resonance imaging of the femur of an adult patient who completed acute lymphoblastic leukemia chemotherapy demonstrates avascular necrosis of the femoral head.

(VDR FokI C > T polymorphism) in some populations and may explain the five time increased risk of ON in whites.[99] Details of genetic factors predisposing to ON are provided in chapter 11. Corticosteroids induced ON is significantly more often seen in females than males as they progress through puberty earlier. Dexamethasone is more potent than prednisone in both its antileukemic effects as well as its toxic effects and its use is associated with increased risk of ON.[100] The incidence of ON is directly proportional to the amount of dexamethasone received. Other factors that may contribute to the risk of ON include low serum albumin levels, hypercholesterolemia, use of other chemotherapeutic agents (MTX, L-asparaginase), and the bone-resorbing effects of lymphoblasts themselves.[101-103] HSCT recipients demonstrate a markedly increased relative risk of ON which has been specifically correlated with prolonged use of glucocorticoids used to treat GVHD. However, both TBI and GVHD have been independently associated with ON in multivariate analysis.[104] Weight bearing joints seem to be more commonly affected. Morbidity from progressive joint damage and articular collapse can be considerable often requiring total joint replacement.

NEUROCOGNITIVE DYSFUNCTION

Central nervous system prophylaxis/treatment with CRT and/or chemotherapy has significantly improved survival of ALL patients.[105] IT chemotherapy has nearly replaced CRT in current ALL treatment protocols except for patients who present with

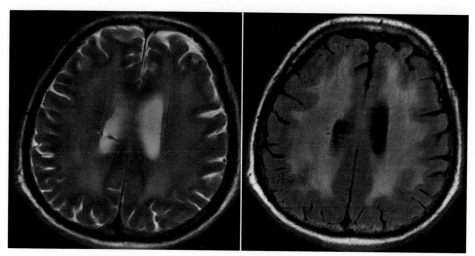

Figure 13-3 FLAIR and T2-weighted magnetic resonance images demonstrate bilateral symmetric extensive areas of signal abnormality throughout the deep white matter in the cerebral hemispheres consistent with methotrexate toxicity. Patient had central nervous system involvement with ALL and was treated with intrathecal as well as systemic methotrexate.

CNS disease or those who are at a high risk of CNS relapse (See Chapter 10). Although chemotherapy alone is associated with less neurotoxicity, long-term neurocognitive and neuropsychologic deficits do occur in these patients; however, these effects are not consistently reported.[106-108] Neurological sequelae include chronic headaches, seizures, co-ordination and motor deficits, auditory-vestibular-visual sensory disturbances, as well as neurocognitive deficits in attention, processing speed, memory, and executive function.[109,110] High-dose systemic MTX, IT chemotherapy, and glucocorticoids are associated with long-term neurotoxicity including white matter injury in the form of leukoencephalopathy (Figure 13-3), mineralizing microangiopathy, dystropic calcification, cerebellar sclerosis, and spinal cord dysfunction.[111,112] Lower performance intelligence quotient has been reported with increasing doses of IT MTX.[113,114] Patients who receive CRT may develop significant impairment in memory, attention, visual spatial skills, task efficiency, and emotional regulation compared to control subjects not exposed to CNS radiation.[115] Cognitive deficits are related to the radiation dose used and are believed to be progressive.[116,117] Other factors that confer a higher risk of neurotoxicity include female gender, treatment at a younger age and a longer time since treatment.[118-120]

Neuropsychological deficits have also been investigated in patients HSCT recipients. Problems with memory can be found in nearly 20% of patients within the first year after HSCT.[121-123] There is also evidence of declining intelligence quotient, achievement, and fine motor skills years after HSCT.[121]

PSYCHOSOCIAL ADJUSTMENT DISORDERS

It has been well recognized now that long-term ALL survivors are at risk for substantial psychosocial morbidity. ALL survivors treated with CNS directed therapy and those who receive HSCT are at a higher risk for compromised psychosocial well-being.[124,125] Employment status, dysfunctional relationships, and poor academic progress are some of the areas affected by leukemia therapy. Fear of disease relapse, late adverse effects of treatment, and impaired social lives has significant adverse effects on overall health-related quality of life. Rates of unemployment and college dropout are significantly higher in ALL survivors when compared to their siblings.[126,127] Treatments with CNS radiation, high-dose systemic MTX, or IT MTX are particularly associated with lower neurocognitive function, executive function, and increased somatic distress.[128-130] ALL survivors report poor emotional health compared to sibling controls and are less often married, have higher rate of depression, and suicidal ideation.[131-133] About 12% of the survivors experience post-traumatic stress disorder often many years after diagnosis.[134]

SECONDARY MALIGNANCIES

Pediatric as well as adult ALL survivors are at an increased risk of secondary hematological and solid organ malignancies from the DNA damaging effects of certain chemotherapeutic agents and radiation.[135,136] Although the risk of developing a secondary neoplasm (SN) is much greater than that observed in the general population, the actual risk for any individual ALL survivor is low, especially for those with no history of radiation exposure.[137-139] The 15-year cumulative incidence of developing an SN after ALL treatment has been estimated between 1.4% and 4.2% and it increases to 14.6% (95% CI: 12.9–16.4) at 30 years.[137,139] The 15-year cumulative risk estimate decreases to 1.2% in ALL survivors not exposed to radiation.[139] Among the chemotherapeutic agents used to treat ALL, alkylating agents and topoisomerase II inhibitors (epipodophyllotoxins and anthracyclines) are associated with secondary acute myeloid leukemia (AML) and myelodysplastic syndrome.[140,141] Monosomies or deletions of chromosome(s) 7 and/or 5 are typical of alkylating agent-induced AML, while balanced translocations involving chromosome bands 11q23 and 21q22 are associated to previous therapy with DNA-topoisomerase II inhibitors.[142] Among the solid tumors, skin and CNS malignancies are the most common. Meningiomas and high grade gliomas account for majority of CNS tumors occurring after ALL therapy. Risk of SN caused by radiation increases with time, and the neoplasms typically appear at least 10–15 years after treatment.[143] The development of meningioma has a long latency period (mean, 25 years) as compared to gliomas which tended to occur within 5 years after treatment.[144] Other SNs include thyroid cancer, breast cancer, sarcoma, lymphoma, and head and neck cancers.[138,145-147] ALL survivors should be counseled regarding general health maintenance, such as using sunscreen, avoiding smoking or excessive alcohol consumption, eating a healthful diet, exercising, and pursuing preventive health services. Survivors with high-risk exposures, such as radiation, may require more careful monitoring, including annual physical examinations with attention to radiation-exposed areas, and early screening for adult malignancies, such as breast and colon cancer. As ALL treatment protocols are moving away from CNS radiation, it is anticipated that the occurrence of SN would decline in future cohorts of ALL survivors.

The incidence of secondary solid tumors in HSCT recipients is estimated to be about 2–6% at 10 years and 6–13% at 15 years.[148-151] Patients who receive TBI or busulfan chemotherapy as part of their conditioning regimen for HSCT are at particularly higher risk for new SN. Rizzo et al. reported a similar second cancer risk in patients who received TBI doses lower than 12 Gy as compared to TBI doses above 12 Gy.[152] This was in contrast to earlier data published by Curtis who found that lower doses of TBI (less than 12 Gy) were associated with a lower risk of second cancer.[148] Solid second cancers tend to occur later as compared to secondary leukemias which have a peak occurrence at 2–6 years after HSCT and post-transplantation lymphoproliferative disease, which manifests within the first few months after HSCT.[153,154] As the cohort of ALL survivors is increasing rapidly, attention should be paid to their risk for SN and appropriate surveillance and screening performed.

PULMONARY, HEPATIC, RENAL, AND INFECTIOUS COMPLICATIONS

Long-term pulmonary, hepatic, and renal complications seen in ALL survivors are mostly related to HSCT. Diffusion disorders and restrictive lung disease have been reported in about one-third of patients within the first year following successful HSCT.[155] Bronchiolitis obliterans (BO), BO organizing pneumonia, and idiopathic pneumonia syndrome are common non-infectious late complications of HSCT. Pulmonary chronic GVHD mostly presents as BO syndrome, a nonspecific inflammatory injury of the small airways. Use of single fraction TBI as conditioning regimen, deranged pulmonary function tests prior to transplant, development of post-transplant pulmonary infections, and GVHD are risk factors for developing late pulmonary toxicity.[156] Liver involvement as part of GVHD is common; however, other factors including risk of chronic hepatitis from hepatitis B and C viruses, herpes viruses, adenoviruses, Epstein-Barr virus, and iron overload resulting from multiple red blood cell transfusions can contribute to long-term liver dysfunction after HSCT.[157,158] There is scant literature on the late renal effects seen in ALL survivors. Chronic kidney disease (CKD) defined as glomerular filtration rate less than 60 mL/min/1.73 m^2 develops in about 15–23% of HSCT recipients.[159,160] Fortunately, only a minority of patients require chronic dialysis.[161] Chronic calcineurin inhibitor nephrotoxicity, chronic GVHD-associated glomerulonephritis, and HSCT associated thrombotic microangiopathy account for most of CKD cases after HSCT. Risk factors for development of CKD following HSCT include female gender, history of hypertension, use of fludarabine, nephrotoxins, and single dose TBI as opposed to hyperfractionated TBI in the conditioning regimen.[159,161] HSCT recipients have significantly deficient immune responses in the first year after transplant. Chronic GVHD, depletion of lymphocytes from the stem cell graft, degree of histocompatibility between donor and recipient, and viral infections particularly herpes viruses are among the many factors that affect rapid reconstitution of immunity in SCT survivors. Risk of both bacterial and viral infections is high in patients receiving active therapy for GVHD, hence antibiotic prophylaxis is recommended against gram positive organisms, *Pneumocystis jiroveci*, and Varicella Zoster virus. Use of live attenuated vaccines is not recommended in patients with active GVHD or within two years of HSCT.[162]

LATE OPHTHALMIC AND DENTAL EFFECTS

Late ophthalmic and dental complications are again mostly seen in ALL transplant survivors. Cataract formation occurs in about 80% at 6–10 years post-HSCT mostly related to the use of single fraction TBI, prolonged administration of corticosteroids and old age.[163] Keratoconjunctivitis sicca is part of the chronic GVHD spectrum, although 10% of the cases can present without GVHD.[164] Long-term posterior segment complications of the eye depend on the conditioning regimen used with ischemic retinopathy mostly noted with BU/CY conditioning and microvascular retinopathy is frequently seen with TBI and cyclosporine use.

Oral health needs of ALL survivors are greater than the general population. The nature and extent of dental problems range from insignificant findings to permanent or prolonged damage to the enamel organ and developing teeth.[165,166] CNS radiation and TBI increases dental injury especially in children under 5 at the time of treatment. Prevalence of hypodontia and microdontia, tapering of the roots of erupted permanent molars or incisors as seen on X-rays, defects in dental root development, and caries is much higher in HSCT survivors when compared with age-matched healthy children.[167,168]

SUMMARY

Therapeutic improvements, particularly in childhood ALL are contributing to an ever increasing population of adult ALL survivors. These patients are at risk for late treatment-related adverse consequences, and long-term surveillance of this population is necessary. Many late effects, such as endocrine abnormalities, are subtle at least at the onset and may require specialized testing for their detection. Appropriate management of late sequelae requires close coordination between hematologists/oncologists and primary care physicians as well as a variety of other specialists. As the risk stratification of ALL improves with better definition of cytogenetic and molecular subsets as well as minimal residual disease monitoring, exposure to certain therapies could be minimized in the good risk patients thereby minimizing late effects. Genomic studies that identify risk for complications may also help define a particular patients risk thereby enabling tailoring of therapy or better surveillance. The Children's Oncology Group has developed comprehensive guidelines for clinical follow-up on survivors of cancer that are available at www. childrensoncologygroup.org/disc/le/pdf/. Early identification and treatment of progressive abnormalities may improve survival and the quality of life of long-term survivors.

REFERENCES

1. Linsenmeier C, Thoennessen D, Negretti L, et al. Total body irradiation (TBI) in pediatric patients. A single-center experience after 30 years of low-dose rate irradiation. *Strahlenther Onkol*. 2010;186(11):614-20.
2. Darzy KH. Radiation-induced hypopituitarism after cancer therapy: who, how and when to test. *Nat Clin Pract Endocrinol Metab*. 2009;5(2):88-99.
3. Haddy TB, Mosher RB, Nunez SB, et al. Growth hormone deficiency after chemotherapy for acute lymphoblastic leukemia in children who have not received cranial radiation. *Pediatr Blood Cancer*. 2006;46(2):258-61.
4. Moell C, Garwicz S, Marky I, et al. Growth in children treated for acute lymphoblastic leukemia with and without prophylactic cranial irradiation. *Acta Paediatr Scand*. 1988;77(5): 688-92.
5. Groot-Loonen JJ, Otten BJ, van t' Hof MA, et al. Chemotherapy plays a major role in the inhibition of catch-up growth during maintenance therapy for childhood acute lymphoblastic leukemia. *Pediatrics*. 1995;96(4 Pt 1):693-5.
6. Roman J, Villaizan CJ, Garcia-Foncillas J, et al. Chemotherapy induced growth hormone deficiency in children with cancer. *Med Pediatr Oncol*. 1995;25(2):90-5.
7. Vandecruys E, Dhooge C, Craen M, et al. Longitudinal linear growth and final height is impaired in childhood acute lymphoblastic leukemia survivors after treatment without cranial irradiation. *J Pediatr*. 2013;163(1):268-73.
8. Schriock EA, Schell MJ, Carter M, et al. Abnormal growth patterns and adult short stature in 115 long-term survivors of childhood leukemia. *J Clin Oncol*. 1991;9(3):400-5.
9. Robison LL, Nesbit ME, Sather HN, et al. Height of children successfully treated for acute lymphoblastic leukemia: a report from the Late Effects Study Committee of Childrens Cancer Study Group. *Med Pediatr Oncol*. 1985;13(1):14-21.
10. Kirk JA, Raghupathy P, Stevens MM, et al. Growth failure and growth-hormone deficiency after treatment for acute lymphoblastic leukaemia. *Lancet*. 1987;1(8526):190-3.
11. Shalet SM, Clayton PE, Morris-Jones PH, et al. Growth in children treated for acute lympho-blastic leukaemia. *Lancet*. 1988;2(8603):164.
12. Cohen A, Rovelli A, Bakker B, et al. Final height of patients who underwent bone marrow transplantation for hematological disorders during childhood: a study by the Working Party for Late Effects–EBMT. *Blood*. 1999;93(12):4109-15.
13. Chemaitilly W, Boulad F, Heller G, et al. Final height in pediatric patients after hyper-fractionated total body irradiation and stem cell transplantation. *Bone Marrow Transplant*. 2007;40(1):29-35.

14. Cohen A, Rovelli A, Van-Lint MT, et al. Final height of patients who underwent bone marrow transplantation during childhood. *Arch Dis Child.* 1996;74(5):437-40.

15. Sklar C, Mertens A, Walter A, et al. Final height after treatment for childhood acute lymphoblastic leukemia: comparison of no cranial irradiation with 1800 and 2400 centigrays of cranial irradiation. *J Pediatr.* 1993;123(1):59-64.

16. Holm K, Nysom K, Rasmussen MH, et al. Growth, growth hormone and final height after BMT: possible recovery of irradiation-induced growth hormone insufficiency. *Bone Marrow Transplant.* 1996;18(1):163-70.

17. Giorgiani G, Bozzola M, Locatelli F, et al. Role of busulfan and total body irradiation on growth of prepubertal children receiving bone marrow transplantation and results of treatment with recombinant human growth hormone. *Blood.* 1995;86(2):825-31.

18. Huma Z, Boulad F, Black P, et al. Growth in children after bone marrow transplantation for acute leukemia. *Blood.* 1995;86(2):819-24.

19. Brauner R, Adan L, Souberbielle JC, et al. Contribution of growth hormone deficiency to the growth failure that follows bone marrow transplantation. *J Pediatr.* 1997;130(5):785-92

20 Nandagopal R, Laverdiere C, Mulrooney D, et al. Endocrine late effects of childhood cancer therapy: a report from the Children's Oncology Group. *Horm Res.* 2008;69(2):65-74.

21. Gurney JG, Ness KK, Sibley SD, et al. Metabolic syndrome and growth hormone deficiency in adult survivors of childhood acute lymphoblastic leukemia. *Cancer.* 2006;107(6):1303-12.

22. Follin C, Thilén U, Osterberg K, et al. Cardiovascular risk, cardiac function, physical activity, and quality of life with and without long-term growth hormone therapy in adult survivors of childhood acute lymphoblastic leukemia. *J Clin Endocrinol Metab.* 2010;95(8):3726-35.

23. Sklar CA, Mertens AC, Mitby P, et al. Risk of disease recurrence and second neoplasms in survivors of childhood cancer treated with growth hormone: a report from the Childhood Cancer Survivor Study. *J Clin Endocrinol Metab.* 2002;87(7):3136-41.

24. Van Santen HM, Vulsma T, Dijkgraaf MG, et al. No damaging effect of chemotherapy in addition to radiotherapy on the thyroid axis in young adult survivors of childhood cancer. *J Clin Endocrinol Metab.* 2003;88(8):3657-63.

25. Thomas O, Mahe M, Campion L, et al. Long-term complications of total body irradiation in adults. *Int J Radiat Oncol Biol Phys.* 2001;49(1):125-31.

26. Aldouri MA, Ruggier R, Epstein O, et al. Adoptive transfer of hyperthyroidism and autoimmune thyroiditis following allogeneic bone marrow transplantation for chronic myeloid leukaemia. *Br J Haematol.* 1990;74(1):118-9.

27. Berisso GA, Van Lint MT, Bacigalupo A, et al. Adoptive autoimmune hyperthyroidism following allogeneic stem cell transplantation from an HLA-identical sibling with Graves' disease. *Bone Marrow Transplant.* 1999;23(10):1091-2.

28. Cohen A, Rovelli A, Merlo DF, et al. Risk for secondary thyroid carcinoma after hematopoietic stem cell transplantation: an EBMT Late Effects Working Party study. *J Clin Oncol.* 2007;25(17):2449-54.

29. Ross JA, Oeffinger KC, Davies SM, et al. Genetic variation in the leptin receptor gene and obesity in survivors of childhood acute lymphoblastic leukemia: a report from the Childhood Cancer Survivor Study. *J Clin Oncol.* 2004;22(17):3558-62.

30. Oeffinger KC, Mertens AC, Sklar CA, et al. Obesity in adult survivors of childhood acute lymphoblastic leukemia: a report from the Childhood Cancer Survivor Study. *J Clin Oncol.* 2003;21(7):1359-65.

31. Vaisman N, Stallings VA, Chan H, et al. Effect of chemotherapy on the energy and protein metabolism of children near the end of treatment for acute lymphoblastic leukemia. *Am J Clin Nutr.* 1993;57(5):679-84.

32. Meacham LR, Gurney JG, Mertens AC, et al. Body mass index in long-term adult survivors of childhood cancer. A report of the Childhood Cancer Survivor Study. *Cancer.* 2005;103(8):1730-9.

33. Marquis A, Kuehni CE, Strippoli MP, et al. Spermanalysis of patients after successful treatment of childhood acute lymphoblastic leukemia with chemotherapy. *Pediatr Blood Cancer.* 2010;55(1):208-10.

34. van Casteren NJ, van der Linden GH, Hakvoort-Cammel FG, et al. Effect of childhood cancer treatment on fertility markers in adult male long-term survivors. *Pediatr Blood Cancer.* 2009; 52(1):108-12.

35. Byrne J, Fears TR, Mills JL, et al. Fertility of long-term male survivors of acute lymphoblastic leukemia diagnosed during childhood. *Pediatr Blood Cancer.* 2004;42(4):364-72.

36. Siimes MA, Rautonen J. Small testicles with impaired production of sperm in adult male survivors of childhood malignancies. *Cancer.* 1990;65(6):1303-6.

37. Uderzo C, Locasciulli A, Marzorati R, et al. Correlation of gonadal function with histology of testicular biopsies at treatment discontinuation in childhood acute leukemia. *Med Pediatr Oncol.* 1984;12(2):97-100.

38. Chemaitilly W, Mertens AC, Mitby P, et al. Acute ovarian failure in the childhood cancer survivor study. *J Clin Endocrinol Metab.* 2006;91(5):1723-8.

39. Chow EJ, Friedman DL, Yasui Y, et al. Timing of menarche among survivors of childhood acute lymphoblastic leukemia: a report from the Childhood Cancer Survivor Study. *Pediatr Blood Cancer.* 2008;50(4):854-8.

40. Hamre MR, Robison LL, Nesbit ME, et al. Effects of radiation on ovarian function in long-term survivors of childhood acute lymphoblastic leukemia: a report from the Childrens Cancer Study Group. *J Clin Oncol.* 1987;5(11):1759-65.

41. Green DM, Kawashima T, Stovall M, et al. Fertility of female survivors of childhood cancer: a report from the childhood cancer survivor study. *J Clin Oncol.* 2009;27(16):2677-85.

42. Byrne J, Fears TR, Mills JL, et al. Fertility in women treated with cranial radiotherapy for childhood acute lymphoblastic leukemia. *Pediatr Blood Cancer.* 2004;42(7):589-97.

43. Mueller BA, Chow EJ, Kamineni A, et al. Pregnancy outcomes in female childhood and adolescent cancer survivors: a linked cancer birth registry analysis. *Arch Pediatr Adolesc Med.* 2009;163(10):879-86.

44. Mertens AC, Ramsay NK, Kouris S, et al. Patterns of gonadal dysfunction following bone marrow transplantation. *Bone Marrow Transplant.* 1998;22(4):345-50.

45. Teinturier C, Hartmann O, Valteau-Couanet D, et al. Ovarian function after autologous bone marrow transplantation in childhood: high-dose busulfan is a major cause of ovarian failure. *Bone Marrow Transplant.* 1998;22(10):989-94.

46. Sanders JE, Hawley J, Levy W, et al. Pregnancies following high-dose cyclophosphamide with or without high-dose busulfan or total-body irradiation and bone marrow transplantation. *Blood.* 1996;87(7):3045-52.

47. Howell SJ, Shalet SM. Spermatogenesis after cancer treatment: damage and recovery. *J Natl Cancer Inst Monogr.* 2005;(34):12-7.

48. Anserini P, Chiodi S, Spinelli S, et al. Semen analysis following allogeneic bone marrow transplantation. Additional data for evidence-based counselling. *Bone Marrow Transplant.* 2002;30(7):447-51.

49. Wallace WH, Thompson AB, Kelsey TW. Radiosensitivity of the human oocyte. *Hum Reprod.* 2003;18(1):117-21.

50. Sanders JE, Buckner CD, Amos D, et al. Ovarian function following marrow transplantation for aplastic anemia or leukaemia. *J Clin Oncol.* 1988;6(5):813-8.

51. Quinn B, Kelly D. Sperm banking and fertility concerns: enhancing practice and the support available to men with cancer. *Eur J Oncol Nurs.* 2000;4(1):55-8.

52. Lipshultz SE, Lipsitz SR, Sallan SE, et al. Chronic progressive cardiac dysfunction years after doxorubicin therapy for childhood acute lymphoblastic leukemia. *J Clin Oncol.* 2005; 23(12):2629-36.

53. Gianni L, Zweiger JL, Levy A, et al. Characterization of the cycle iron-mediated electron transfer from Adriamycin to molecular oxygen. *J Biol Chem.* 1985;260(11):6820-6.

54. Muszyńska A, Wolczyński S, Pałka J. The mechanism for anthracycline-induced inhibition of collagen biosynthesis. *Eur J Pharmacol.* 2001;411(1-2):17-25.

55. Mertens AC, Liu Q, Neglia JP, et al. Cause-specific late mortality among 5-year survivors of childhood cancer: the Childhood Cancer Survivor Study. *J Natl Cancer Inst.* 2008;100(19): 1368-79.

56. Herman EH, Zhang J, Lipshultz SE, et al. Correlation between serum levels of cardiac troponin-T and the severity of the chronic cardiomyopathy induced by doxorubicin. *J Clin Oncol.* 1999:2237-43.

57. Semsei AF, Erdelyi DJ, Ungvari I, et al. ABCC1 polymorphisms in anthracycline-induced cardiotoxicity in childhood acute lymphoblastic leukaemia. *Cell Biol Int.* 2012;36(1):79-86.

58 Tukenova M, Guibout C, Oberlin O, et al. Role of cancer treatment in long-term overall and cardiovascular mortality after childhood cancer. *J Clin Oncol.* 2010;28(8):1308-15.

59. Lipshultz SE, Rifai N, Dalton VM, et al. The effect of dexrazoxane on myocardial injury in doxorubicin-treated children with acute lymphoblastic leukemia. *N Engl J Med.* 2004;351(2): 145-53.

60. Mills J, Bonner A, Francis K. The development of constructivist grounded theory. *Int J Qual Methods.* 2006;5:25-35.

61. Lipshultz SE, Landy DC, Lopez-Mitnik G, et al. Cardiovascular status of childhood cancer survivors exposed and unexposed to cardiotoxic therapy. *J Clin Oncol.* 2012;30(10):1050-7.

62. Sulicka J, Surdacki A, Mikołajczyk T, et al. Elevated markers of inflammation and endothelial activation and increased counts of intermediate monocytes in adult survivors of childhood acute lymphoblastic leukemia. *Immunobiology.* 2013;218(5):810-6.

63. Lipshultz SE, Miller TL, Scully RE, et al. Changes in cardiac biomarkers during doxorubicin treatment of pediatric patients with high-risk acute lymphoblastic leukemia: Associations with Longterm Echocardiographic Outcomes. *J Clin Oncol.* 2012;30(10):1042-9.

64. Ratnasamy C, Kinnamon DD, Lipshultz SE, et al. Associations between neurohormonal and inflammatory activation and heart failure in children. *Am Heart J.* 2008;155(3):527-33.

65. Talvensaari KK, Lanning M, Tapanainen P, et al. Long-term survivors of childhood cancer have an increased risk of manifesting the metabolic syndrome. *J Clin Endocrinol Metab.* 1996;81(8):3051-5.

66. Verhelst J, Abs R. Cardiovascular risk factors in hypopituitary GH-deficient adults. *Eur J Endocrinol.* 2009;161(Suppl 1):S41-9.

67. Tichelli A, Bucher C, Rovó A, et al. Premature cardiovascular disease after allogeneic hematopoietic stem-cell transplantation. *Blood.* 2007;110(9):3463-71.

68. Baker KS, Ness KK, Steinberger J, et al. Diabetes, hypertension and cardiovascular events in survivors of hematopoietic cell transplantation: a report from the bone marrow transplant survivor study. *Blood.* 2007;109(4):1765-72.

69. Biedermann BC, Sahner S, Gregor M, et al. Endothelial injury mediated by cytotoxic T lymphocytes and loss of microvessels in chronic graft versus host disease. *Lancet.* 2002; 359(9323):2078-83.

70. Wei L, MacDonald TM, Walker BR. Taking glucocorticoids by prescription is associated with subsequent cardiovascular disease. *Ann Intern Med.* 2004;141(10):764-70.

71. Souverein PC, Berard A, Van Staa TP, et al. Use of oral glucocorticoids and risk of cardiovascular and cerebrovascular disease in a population based case-control study. *Heart.* 2004;90(8):859-65.

72. Chow EJ, Simmons JH, Roth CL, et al. Increased cardiometabolic traits in pediatric survivors of acute lymphoblastic leukemia treated with total body irradiation. *Biol Blood Marrow Transplant.* 2010;16(12):1674-81.

73 Lipshulz SE, Sallan SE. Cardiovascular abnormalities in long-term survivors of childhood malignancy [Editorial]. *J Clin Oncol.* 1993;11(7):1199-203.

74. Leiper AD. Late effects of total body irradiation. *Arch Dis Child.* 1995;72(5):382-5.

75. Arikoski P, Komulainen J, Voutilainen R, et al. Reduced bone mineral density in long-term survivors of childhood acute lymphoblastic leukemia. *J Pediatr Hematol Oncol.* 1998; 20(3):234-40.

76. Brennan BM, Rahim A, Adams JE, et al. Reduced bone mineral density in young adults following cure of acute lymphoblastic leukaemia in childhood. *Br J Cancer.* 1999;79(11-12): 1859-63.

77. Kaste SC, Jones-Wallace D, Rose SR, et al. Bone mineral decrements in survivors of childhood acute lymphoblastic leukemia: frequency of occurrence and risk factors for their development. *Leukemia.* 2001;15(5):728-34.

78. Munnings F. Osteoporosis: what is the role of exercise? *Phys Sports Med.* 1992;20:127-38.

79. Gilsanz V, Gibbens DT, Roe TF, et al. Vertebral bone density in children: effect of puberty. *Radiology.* 1988;166(3):847-50.

80. Winding B, Jorgensen H, Christiansen C. Osteoporosis in patients with a history of breast cancer: causes and diagnosis. In: Body JJ, editor. Tumor Bone Diseases and Osteoporosis in Cancer Patients. New York: Marcel Dekker; 1999.

81. Weilbaecher KN. Mechanisms of osteoporosis after hematopoietic cell transplantation. *Biol Blood Marrow Transplant.* 2000;6(2A):165-74.

82. Brennan BM, Mughal Z, Roberts SA, et al. Bone mineral density in childhood survivors of acute lymphoblastic leukemia treated without cranial irradiation. *J Clin Endocrinol Metab.* 2005;90(2):689-94.

83. Casteneda S, Carmona L, Carvajal I, et al. Reduction of bone mass in women after bone marrow transplantation. *Calcif Tissue Int.* 1997;60(4):343-7.

84. Eberling P, Thomas D, Erbas B, et al. Mechanisms of bone loss following allogeneic and autologous hemopoietic stem cell transplantation. *J Bone Miner Res.* 1999;14(3):342-50.

85. Schulte CM, Beelen DW. Bone loss following hematopoietic stem cell transplantation: a long-term follow-up. *Blood.* 2004;103(10):3635-43.

86. Weilbaecher KN. Mechanisms of osteoporosis after hematopoietic cell transplantation. *Biol Blood Marrow Transplant.* 2000;6(2A):165-74.

87. Epstein S. Post-transplantation bone disease: the role of immunosuppressive agents and the skeleton. *J Bone Miner Res.* 1996;11(1):1-7.

88. Monegal A, Navasa M, Guanabens N, et al. Bone mass and mineral metabolism in liver transplant patients treated with FK506 or cyclosporine A. *Calcif Tissue Int.* 2001;68(2):83-6.

89. Mattano L. The skeletal remains: porosis and necrosis of bone in the marrow transplantation setting. *Pediatr Transplant.* 2003;7(Suppl 3):71-5.

90. Dyess C, Carter D, Kirchner J, et al. A morphometric comparison of the changes in the laryngeal skeleton associated with invasion by tumor and by external-beam radiation. *Cancer.* 1987;59(6):1117-22.

91. Takahashi S, Sugimoto M, Kotoura Y, et al. Long-term changes in the haversian systems following high-dose irradiation: an ultrastructural and quantitative histomorphological study. *J Bone Joint Surg Am.* 1994;76(5):722-38.

92. Riggs BL, Khosla S, Melton LJ. Sex steroids and the construction and conservation of the adult skeleton. *Endocr Rev.* 2002;23(3):279-302.

93. Monson JP, Drake WM, Carroll PV, et al. Influence of growth hormone on accretion of bone mass. *Horm Res.* 2002;58(Suppl 1):52-6.

94. Wuster C, Harle U, Rehn U, et al. Benefits of growth hormone treatment on bone metabolism, bone density and bone strength in growth hormone deficiency and osteoporosis. *Growth Horm IGF Res.* 1998;8(Suppl A):87-94.

95. Drake WM, Carroll PV, Maher KT, et al. The effect of cessation of growth hormone (GH) therapy on bone mineral accretion in GH deficient adolescents at the completion of linear growth. *J Clin Endocrinol Metab.* 2003;88(4):1658-63.

96. Kaste SC, Rai SN, Fleming K, et al. Changes in bone mineral density in survivors of childhood acute lymphoblastic leukemia. *Pediatr Blood Cancer.* 2006;46(1):77-87.

97. Bockman RS, Weinerman SA. Steroid-induced osteoporosis. *Orthop Clin North Am.* 1990; 21(1):97-107.

98. Haajanen J, Saarinen O, Laasonen L, et al. Steroid treatment and aseptic necrosis of the femoral head in renal transplant recipients. *Transplant Proc.* 1984;16(5):1316-9.

99. Relling MV, Yang W, Das S, et al. Pharmacogenetic risk factors for osteonecrosis of the hip among children with leukemia. *J Clin Oncol.* 2004;22(19):3930-6.

100. Gaynon PS, Lustig RH. The use of glucocorticoids in acute lymphoblastic leukemia of childhood: molecular, cellular, and clinical considerations. *J Pediatr Hematol Oncol.* 1995; 17(1):1-12.

101. Ragab AH, Frech RS, Vietti TJ. Osteoporotic fractures secondary to methotrexate therapy of acute leukemia in remission. *Cancer.* 1970;25(3):580-5.

102. Ribeiro RC, Pui C-H, Schell MJ. Vertebral compression fracture as a presenting feature of acute lymphoblastic leukemia in children. *Cancer.* 1988;61(3):589-92

103. Kawedia JD, Kaste SC, Pei D, et al. Pharmacokinetic, pharmacodynamic, and pharmaco-genetic determinants of osteonecrosis in children with acute lymphoblastic leukemia. *Blood.* 2011;117(8):2340-7.

104. Faraci M, Calevo MG, Lanino E, et al. Osteonecrosis after allogeneic stem cell transplantation in childhood: a case-control study in Italy. *Haematologica.* 2006;91(8):1096-9.

105. Pinkel D. Five-year follow-up of "total therapy" of childhood lymphocytic leukemia. *JAMA.* 1971;216(4):648-52.

106. Harila MJ, Winqvist S, Lanning M, et al. Progressive neurocognitive impairment in young adult survivors of childhood acute lymphoblastic leukemia. *Pediatr Blood Cancer.* 2009; 53(2):156-61.

107. Peterson CC, Johnson CE, Ramirez LY, et al. A meta-analysis of the neuropsychological sequelae of chemotherapy-only treatment for pediatric acute lymphoblastic leukemia. *Pediatr Blood Cancer.* 2008;51(1):99-104.

108. Janzen LA, Spiegler B. Neurodevelopmental sequelae of pediatric acute lymphoblastic leukemia and its treatment. *Dev Disabil Res Rev.* 2008;14(3):185-95.

109. Goldsby RE, Liu Q, Nathan PC, et al. Late-occurring neurologic sequelae in adult survivors of childhood acute lymphoblastic leukemia: a report from the Childhood Cancer Survivor Study. *J Clin Oncol.* 2010;28(2):324-31.

110. Campbell LK, Scaduto M, Sharp W, et al. A meta-analysis of the neurocognitive sequelae of treatment for childhood acute lymphocytic leukemia. *Pediatr Blood Cancer.* 2007;49(1): 65-73.

111. Cole PD, Kamen BA. Delayed neurotoxicity associated with therapy for children with acute lymphoblastic leukemia. *Ment Retard Dev Disabil Res Rev.* 2006;12(3):174-83.

112. Price R. Therapy-related central nervous system diseases in children with acute lymphocytic leukemia. In: Mastrangelo R, Poplack DG, Riccardi R, editors. Central Nervous System Leukemia Prevention and Treatment. Boston: Martinus Nijhoff; 1983. pp. 71-83.

113. Buizer AI, De Sonneville LM, van den Heuvel-Eibrink MM, et al. Visuomotor control in survivors of childhood acute lymphoblastic leukemia treated with chemotherapy only. *J Int Neuropsychol Soc.* 2005;11(5):554-65.

114. Iuvone L, Mariotti P, Colosimo C, et al. Long-term cognitive outcome, brain computed tomography scan, and magnetic resonance imaging in children cured for acute lymphoblastic leukemia. *Cancer.* 2002;95(12):2562-70.

115. Kadan-Lottick NS, Zeltzer LK, Liu Q, et al. Neurocognitive functioning in adult survivors of childhood non-central nervous system cancers. *J Natl Cancer Inst.* 2010;102(12):881-93.

116. Silber JH, Radcliffe J, Peckham V, et al. Whole-brain irradiation and decline in intelligence: the influence of dose and age on IQ score. *J Clin Oncol.* 1992;10(9):1390-6.

117. Cousens P, Waters B, Said J, et al. Cognitive effects of cranial irradiation in leukaemia: a survey and meta-analysis. *J Child Psychol Psychiatry*. 1988;29(6):839-52.

118. Waber DP, Tarbell NJ, Kahn CM, et al. The relationship of sex and treatment modality to neuropsychologic outcome in childhood acute lymphoblastic leukemia. *J Clin Oncol*. 1992;10(5):810-7.

119. Silber JH, Radcliffe J, Peckham V, et al. Whole-brain irradiation and decline in intelligence: the influence of dose and age on IQ score. *J Clin Oncol*. 1992;10(9):1390-6.

120. Rubenstein CL, Varni JW, Katz ER. Cognitive functioning in long-term survivors of childhood leukemia: a prospective analysis. *J Dev Behav Pediatr*. 1990;11(6):301-5.

121. Cool VA. Long-term neuropsychological risks in pediatric bone marrow transplant: what do we know? *Bone Marrow Transplant*. 1996;18(Suppl 3):S45-9.

122. Thuret I, Michel G, Carla H, et al. Long-term side effects in children receiving allogeneic bone marrow transplantation in first complete remission of acute leukaemia. *Bone Marrow Transplant*. 1995;15(3):337-41.

123. Smedler AC, Nilsson C, Bolme P. Total body irradiation: a neuropsychological risk factor in pediatric bone marrow transplant recipients. *Acta Paediatr*. 1995;84(3):325-30.

124. Eiser C. Beyond survival: quality of life and follow-up after childhood cancer. *J Pediatr Psychol*. 2007;32(9):1140-50.

125. Andrykowski MA, Bishop MM, Hahn EA, et al. Long-term health-related quality of life, growth, and spiritual well-being after hematopoietic stem-cell transplantation. *J Clin Oncol*. 2005;23(3):599-608.

126. Pang JW, Friedman DL, Whitton JA, et al. Employment status among adult survivors in the Childhood Cancer Survivor Study. *Pediatr Blood Cancer*. 2008;50(1):104-10.

127. Seitzman RL, Glover DA, Meadows AT, et al. Self-concept in adult survivors of childhood acute lymphoblastic leukemia: a cooperative Children's Cancer Group and National Institutes of Health study. *Pediatr Blood Cancer*. 2004;42(3):230-40.

128. Pakakasama S, Veerakul G, Sosothikul D, et al. Late effects in survivors of childhood acute lymphoblastic leukemia: a study from Thai Pediatric Oncology Group. *Int J Hematol*. 2010; 91(5):850-4.

129. Kadan-Lottick NS, Dinu I, Wasilewski-Masker K, et al. Osteonecrosis in adult survivors of childhood cancer: a report from the Childhood Cancer Survivor Study. *J Clin Oncol*. 2008; 26(18):3038-45.

130. Mulhern RK, Fairclough D, Ochs J. A prospective comparison of neuropsychologic performance of children surviving leukemia who received 18-Gy, 24-Gy, or no cranial irradiation. *J Clin Oncol*. 1991;9(8):1348-56.

131. Zebrack BJ, Zeltzer LK, Whitton J, et al. Psychological outcomes in long-term survivors of childhood leukemia, Hodgkin's disease and non-Hodgkin's lymphoma: a report from the Childhood Cancer Survivor Study. *Pediatrics*. 2002;110(1 Pt 1):42-52.

132. Harila MJ, Salo J, Lanning M, et al. High health-related quality of life among long-term survivors of childhood acute lymphoblastic leukemia. *Pediatr Blood Cancer*. 2010;55(2):331-6.

133. Recklitis CJ, Diller LR, Li X, et al. Suicide ideation in adult survivors of childhood cancer: a report from the Childhood Cancer Survivor Study. *J Clin Oncol*. 2010;28(4):655-61.

134. Hobbie WL, Stuber M, Meeske K, et al. Symptoms of posttraumatic stress in young adult survivors of childhood cancer. *J Clin Oncol*. 2000;18(24):4060-6.

135. Baker A, Cachia P, Ridge S, et al. FMS mutations in patients following cytotoxic therapy for lymphoma. *Leuk Res*. 1995;19(5):309-18.

136. Byrne J. Long-term genetic and reproductive effects of ionizing radiation and chemotherapeutic agents on cancer patients and their offspring. *Teratology*. 1999;59(4):210-5.

137. Hijiya N, Hudson MM, Lensing S, et al. Cumulative incidence of secondary neoplasms as a first event after childhood acute lymphoblastic leukemia. *JAMA*. 2007;297(11):1207-15.

138. Mody R, Li S, Dover DC, et al. Twenty-five-year follow-up among survivors of childhood acute lymphoblastic leukemia: a report from the Childhood Cancer Survivor Study. *Blood.* 2008;111(12):5515-23.

139. Löning L, Zimmermann M, Reiter A, et al. Secondary neoplasms subsequent to Berlin-Frankfurt-Munster therapy of acute lymphoblastic leukemia in childhood: significantly lower risk without cranial radiotherapy. *Blood.* 2000;95(9):2770-5.

140. Mills J, Bonner A, Francis K. The development of constructivist grounded theory. *Int J Qual Methods.* 2006;5:25-35.

141. Lopes LF, Camargo BD, Bianchi A. Late effects of childhood cancer treatment. *Rev Assoc Med Bras.* 2000;46(3):277-84.

142. Leone G, Fianchi L, Pagano L, et al. Incidence and susceptibility to therapy-related myeloid neoplasms. *Chem Biol Interact.* 2010;184(1-2):39-45.

143. Nathan PC, Wasilewski-Masker K, Janzen LA. Long-term outcomes in survivors of childhood acute lymphoblastic leukemia. *Hematol Oncol Clin North Am.* 2009;23(5):1065-82.

144. Banerjee J, Paakko E, Harila M, et al. Radiation-induced meningiomas: a shadow in the success story of childhood leukemia. *Neuro Oncol.* 2009;11(5):543-9.

145. Bhatia S, Sather HN, Pabustan OB, et al. Low incidence of second neoplasms among children diagnosed with acute lymphoblastic leukemia after 1983. *Blood.* 2002;99(12):4257-64.

146. Borgmann A, Zinn C, Hartmann R, et al. Secondary malignant neoplasms after intensive treatment of relapsed acute lymphoblastic leukaemia in childhood. *Eur J Cancer.* 2008;44(2): 257-68.

147. Pui CH, Cheng C, Leung W, et al. Extended follow-up of long term survivors of childhood acute lymphoblastic leukemia. *N Engl J Med.* 2003;349(7):640-9.

148. Curtis RE, Rowlings PA, Deeg HJ, et al. Solid cancers after bone marrow transplantation. *N Engl J Med.* 1997;336(13):897-904.

149. Bhatia S, Louie AD, Bhatia R, et al. Solid cancers after bone marrow transplantation. *J Clin Oncol.* 2001;19(2):464-71.

150. Baker KS, DeFor TE, Burns LJ, et al. New malignancies after blood or marrow stem cell transplantation in children and adults: incidence and risk factors. *J Clin Oncol.* 2003;21(7): 1352-8.

151. Kolb HJ, Socie G, Duell T, et al. Malignant neoplasms in long-term survivors of bone marrow transplantation. Late Effects Working Party of the European Cooperative Group for Blood and Marrow Transplantation and the European Late Effect Project Group. *Ann Intern Med.* 1999;131(10):738-44.

152. Rizzo JD, Curtis RE, Socié G, et al. Solid cancers after allogeneic hematopoietic cell transplantation. *Blood.* 2009;113(5):1175-83.

153. Ahmad I, Cau NV, Kwan J, et al. Preemptive management of Epstein-Barr virus reactivation after hematopoietic stem-cell transplantation. *Transplantation.* 2009;87(8):1240-5.

154. Landgren O, Gilbert ES, Rizzo JD, et al. Risk factors for lymphoproliferative disorders after allogeneic hematopoietic cell transplantation. *Blood.* 2009;113(20):4992-5001.

155. Piesiak P, Gorczynska E, Brzecka A, et al. Pulmonary function impairment in patients undergoing allogeneic hematopoietic cell transplantation. *Adv Exp Med Biol.* 2013;755:143-8.

156. Gore EM, Lawton CA, Ash RC, et al. Pulmonary function changes in long-term survivors of bone marrow transplantation. *Int J Radiat Oncol Biol Phys.* 1996;36(1):67-75.

157. Locasciulli A, Testa M, Valsecchi MG, et al. The role of hepatitis C and B virus infections as risk factors for severe liver complications following allogeneic BMT: a prospective study by the Infectious Disease Working Party of the European Blood and Marrow Transplantation Group. *Transplantation.* 1999;68(10):1486-91.

158. Koreth J, Antin JH. Iron overload in hematologic malignancies and outcome of allogeneic hematopoietic stem cell transplantation. *Haematologica.* 2010;95(3):364-6.

159. Cohen EP, Lawton CA, Moulder JE. Bone marrow transplant nephropathy: radiation nephritis revisited. *Nephron.* 1995;70(2):217-22.

160. Kersting S, Hene RJ, Koomans HA, et al. Chronic kidney disease after myeloablative allogeneic hematopoietic stem cell transplantation. *Biol Blood Marrow Transplant.* 2007; 13(10):1169-75.

161. Delgado J, Cooper N, Thomson K, et al. The importance of age, fludarabine, and total body irradiation in the incidence and severity of chronic renal failure after allogeneic hematopoietic cell transplantation. *Biol Blood Marrow Transplant.* 2006;12(1):75-83.

162. CDC, Infectious Disease Society of America, and the American Society of Blood and Marrow Transplantation. Guidelines for preventing opportunistic infections among hematopoietic cell transplant recipients: Recommendations of CDC, the Infectious Disease Society of America, and the American Society of Blood and Marrow Transplantation. *Cytotherapy.* 2001;3(1):41-54.

163. Tichelli A, Gratwohl A, Egger T, et al. Cataract formation after bone marrow transplantation. *Ann Intern Med.* 1993;119(12):1175-80.

164. Kim SK. Update on ocular graft versus host disease. *Curr Opin Ophthalmol.* 2006;17(4):344-8.

165. Pajari U, Lanning M. Developmental defects of teeth in survivors of childhood ALL are related to the therapy and age at diagnosis. *Med Pediatr Oncol.* 1995;24(5):310-4.

166. Dahllof G, Barr M, Bolme P, et al. Disturbances in dental development after total body irradiation in bone marrow transplant recipients. *Oral Surg Oral Med Oral Pathol.* 1988; 65(1):41-4.

167. Cole BO, Welbury RR, Bond E, et al. Dental manifestations in severe combined immuno-deficiency following bone marrow transplantation. *Bone Marrow Transplant.* 2000;25(9): 1007-9.

168. Uderzo C, Fraschini D, Balduzzi A, et al. Long term effects of bone marrow transplantation on dental status in children with leukaemia. *Bone Marrow Transplant.* 1997;20(10):865-9.

14 Novel Agents for the Treatment of Acute Lymphoblastic Leukemia

Justin M Watts, Patrick W Burke, Dan Douer, Martin S Tallman

INTRODUCTION

Overall outcome in adult acute lymphoblastic leukemia (ALL) has not changed significantly over the past 25 years.[1,2] Although clinical trials in adult ALL have used a variety of chemotherapeutic induction, consolidation, and maintenance strategies with different combinations of agents, overall survival (OS) has remained approximately 35–40%.[3-10] For this reason, in the absence of a clear standard of care, current National Comprehensive Cancer Network (NCCN) guidelines recommend a clinical trial as first-line treatment in adult patients with newly diagnosed ALL.[11] Attempting to optimize treatment for adults with ALL has been both an iterative and integrative process. Moreover, it has become increasingly clear that three different age groups should be considered separately in adult ALL: (1) adolescents and young adults (15–39 years old), (2) adults aged 40 to 60–65 years, and (3) older adults (above 60–65 years old).[11] These three age groups each merit consideration of an age-specific therapeutic strategy, as age affects both disease biology (such as increasing rates of Ph-positive ALL in the elderly) as well as treatment tolerability and outcome.[12] Lastly, it bears mentioning that allogeneic hematopoietic cell transplantation (HCT) has no clearly defined role in non-relapsed adult ALL. All of the above factors shape the way oncologists view current therapy of adult ALL and underlie the need for novel agents and new strategies.

Adult ALL regimens are moving away from repeated cycles of intensive, myelosuppressive chemotherapy as the backbone of treatment. For example, despite intensification of induction with high-dose cytarabine and very high-dose mitoxantrone, the ALL-2 regimen was not superior to other regimens in terms of OS,[9,13] and two other studies have shown no improvement in ALL outcome with anthracycline intensification.[5,14] Furthermore, myeloablative therapy followed by autologous stem cell rescue has been associated with worse outcome in adult ALL.[7] As opposed to simply intensifying therapy, new treatment regimens have adopted several strategies used in pediatric ALL, such as increased use of non-myelosuppressive agents (steroids, vincristine), increased use of asparaginase for prolonged asparagine depletion, and extensive central nervous system prophylaxis with intrathecal and high-dose systemic methotrexate.[15] These "pediatric inspired" protocols follow the Berlin-Frankfurt-Munster (BFM) model, which incorporates a two-phase induction and subsequent planned "reinduction" with traditional cytotoxic agents, and have been shown to be safe in young and middle-aged adults and may improve survival.[16-20]

The lack of a standard of care for the treatment of adult ALL, the apparent benefit of prolonged, less myelosuppressive post-remission and maintenance therapy, and the neutral or negative effects of increasing the intensity of cytotoxic therapy during induction and consolidation, together present a unique opportunity for the development of targeted biological agents in ALL. Several such targeted agents have already been explored in the early relapse/minimal residual disease (MRD) setting and in overt relapsed/refractory disease as a bridge to allogeneic HCT, and the next (and more difficult) step is incorporating their use into frontline treatment regimens for newly diagnosed ALL. The first such "targeted" agent to be used in ALL was rituximab in patients with CD20-positive B-precursor ALL; however, the impact of rituximab, and of unconjugated monoclonal antibodies in general, appears to be minimal in adult ALL.[21-24] Conversely, the use of small molecule tyrosine kinase inhibitors (TKIs) in adults—especially older adults—with Ph-positive ALL has revolutionized the management and outcome of these patients and serves as a model for integrating targeted therapy into existing treatment regimens. While adults with Ph-positive ALL historically have a poor prognosis, the addition of TKIs to frontline chemotherapy has improved survival in all age groups and several studies now show OS rates above 50%.[25-30] After remission is achieved with induction chemotherapy combined with a TKI, consolidative allogeneic HCT may further improve outcome in adults with Ph-positive ALL, but this is still under investigation. In this chapter, we have discussed novel targeted immunotherapeutic strategies and small molecule inhibitors in Ph-negative ALL, including: blinatumomab, chimeric antigen receptor-modified T cells (CARs), anti-CD22 antibodies and antibody-conjugates, and NOTCH1 pathway and DOT1L inhibitors (Table 14-1).

BLINATUMOMAB

Blinatumomab is a single-chain antibody construct that has dual specificity for CD3 and CD19, thereby directing CD3-positive T cells to CD19-positive B cells and ALL cells for cell killing.[31] Blinatumomab represents a new class of therapeutic antibodies, known as bispecific T-cell engaging or "BiTE" antibodies, and has shown substantial ability to promote B-cell aplasia. Since cytotoxic T cells lack Fcγ receptors, conventional monoclonal antibodies, lacking the dual specificity of BiTE antibodies, are unable to bring T cells and B-lineage ALL cells into close proximity for the same degree of highly potent tumor-cell killing (mechanism of cell death is apoptosis).

Table 14-1	Targets and Agents in ALL (Not Including Tyrosine-kinase inhibitors for Ph-positive ALL)			
Drug/therapy	*Mechanism*	*Development*	*Results*	*References*
Rituximab	Anti-CD20 monoclonal antibody	Phase II; combined with frontline chemotherapy in B-ALL	Modest survival benefit	23, 24
Blinatumomab	Bispecific T-cell engager (BiTE) antibody targeting CD19 and CD3	Phase II; relapsed B-ALL	Durable CRs in +MRD; CR+CRh = 17/25 (68%) in overt relapse	33, 34
CARs	Chimeric antigen receptor-modified T cells	Phase I; relapsed/ refractory ALL, other B-cell malignancies	Impressive early response rates	36, 37
Epratuzumab	Anti-CD22 monoclonal antibody (rapidly internalized)	Phase I/II; refractory B-ALL (children only)	Minimal single agent activity	40
Inotuzumab ozogamicin	Anti-CD22; conjugate: calicheamicin	Phase II/III; relapsed/ refractory B-ALL	CR+CRp = 8/20 (40%)*	42
Moxetumomab Pasudotox (HA22)	Anti-CD22; conjugate: truncated pseudo-monasexotoxin A	Phase I; refractory B-ALL (children only)	CR 24%	44
NOTCH1 pathway inhibitor	Small molecule inhibitor of gamma-secretase	Phase I trials ongoing in T-ALL	Results pending	–
DOT1L inhibitor	Inhibits DOT1L, a histone H3K79 methyltransferase	Phase I trials ongoing in AML and adult ALL	Preclinical data against MLL-rearranged ALL	56

*Seven of the eight responders became MRD negative.

CR, complete response; CRh, CR with partial hematologic response; CRp, pathologic complete response; MRD, minimal residual disease; MLL, mixed lineage leukemia; ALL, adult acute lymphoblastic leukemia; AML, acute myeloid leukemia.

Topp and colleagues have conducted two phase II clinical trials of single-agent blinatumomab in adult ALL.[32,33] In the first trial, blinatumomab was administered to 20 adults with MRD or early molecular relapse after standard chemotherapy.[32] The drug was cycled as a 28-day continuous infusion followed by a 14-day treatment-free interval. Sixteen of the twenty patients achieved a complete molecular response (MRD-negative), and relapse-free survival (RFS) at a median follow-up of 405 days was 78%, with 8 of the 16 MRD-negative patients undergoing allogeneic HCT. A recently published update of this study showed that the hematologic RFS was 61% at a median follow-up of 33 months.[34] Of the 9 total patients who received an allogeneic HCT, hematologic RFS was 65%. Lastly, 4 out of the 6 Ph-negative patients who achieved MRD-negativity and did not receive any further therapy are in ongoing complete hematologic and molecular remission, showing that blinatumomab monotherapy can induce a durable complete remission (CR) in patients with MRD-relapsed/refractory disease.

In the second trial, 25 adults with overt hematologic relapse of B-precursor ALL were treated with blinatumomab.[33] Seventeen of the twenty-five patients (68%) achieved both a CR/CR with partial hematologic response (CRh) and an MRD-response (MRD level $<10^{-4}$) within the first two cycles. The average duration of response was 7.1 months for the first 18 patients. The most common treatment-related adverse events were fever, headache, and tremor. More severe neurologic toxicity, namely, confusion and seizure activity was also seen in 5 patients, which was managed with corticosteroids.

Overall, blinatumomab has shown remarkable activity in these two clinical trials, demonstrating high CR rates in patients with MRD and in those with overt disease relapse when used as a single-agent. Furthermore, the drug appears to have an acceptable side effect and tolerability profile, including no grade 4 adverse events.[33] The data are more mature in the MRD setting, where blinatumomab resulted in durable CRs in many patients, including some who did not undergo allogeneic HCT.[34] Limitations to blinatumomab include a modestly cumbersome drug administration schedule, since it requires a 28-day continuous infusion, mandatory drug cassette changes every 48 hours and an on-site sterile facility for drug preparation. Despite these logistical hurdles, blinatumomab is one of the most promising new agents for the treatment of B-lineage ALL, and the next step in its development is incorporation into frontline treatment programs.

CHIMERIC ANTIGEN RECEPTOR-MODIFIED T CELLS

An alternative approach to immunotherapy with BiTE antibodies is cellular therapy with genetically modified autologous T cells. In the laboratory, a patient's own T cells can be bioengineered to target specific antigens expressed by tumor cells. A viral vector is used to transduce a chimeric antigen receptor (CAR) gene construct that encodes tumor-specific single fragment length antibodies (scFvs) fused to the signal transduction component (zeta chain) of the T-cell receptor and T-cell costimulatory domains (CD28 and/or 4-1BB).[35] Autologous T cells are harvested by leukapheresis following which patients receive conditioning chemotherapy prior to reinfusion of the CAR-gene product. CAR-modified T cells are designed to specifically target malignant and normal B cells expressing the targeted antigen (CD19 or CD20), and the costimulatory signaling domains are essential for expansion and persistence of the T-cell clone.

This ingenious method of targeting tumor cells has shown early promise in B-cell malignancies including precursor-B ALL. Two recent phase I clinical trials demonstrated impressive clinical response in patients with advanced chronic lymphocytic leukemia (CLL) and precursor-B ALL, although the side effect profile is still being delineated in subsequent studies.[36,37] One of these trials treated only one patient,[37] but the other treated a total of nine patients: eight with CLL and one with relapsed ALL.[36] The patient with ALL achieved remission with salvage chemotherapy prior to receiving the autologous T cells, and, as expected, developed sustained B-cell aplasia after receiving the engineered T cells and subsequently underwent allogeneic HCT. Apart from the expected toxicities of tumor lysis syndrome and lymphopenia, nine of the ten patients treated on these two trials tolerated the therapy well. In addition, largely due to the inclusion of one or two T cell-derived costimulatory domains, CARs have been shown to proliferate, survive, and persist in patients as memory T cells, possibly providing a sustained anti-leukemia effect.[38] CAR-modified T cells are currently under active investigation in larger cohorts of adult ALL patients.

Like blinatumomab, CAR technology redirects a patient's own T cells to attack tumor-specific antigens. Both have shown clinical efficacy in significantly reducing tumor burden in B-cell malignancies, often with dramatic and/or sustained effect, and both appear to have acceptable safety profiles. CARs offer the advantage of a potentially sustained anti-tumor response without repeated cycles of therapy; however, the procedure requires extensive laboratory support and expertise, and patients must undergo leukapheresis and conditioning therapy with lymphotoxic agents, such as cyclophosphamide, to deplete the endogenous T-cell niche. These factors make cell therapy more difficult to integrate into frontline treatment regimens and may limit its widespread use. Blinatumomab, on the other hand, does not require *ex vivo* engineering of T cells, and the drug's short half-life lessens toxicity concerns to some degree. However, each cycle of blinatumomab consists of a very long continuous infusion, and continued anti-tumor activity may require repeated cycles of therapy, which could also be burdensome for the patient and treating institution. Both of these T-cell recruiting strategies have similar side effect profiles, including tumor lysis syndrome and cytokine release syndromes (both are primarily a problem in patients with a high disease burden) as well as neurotoxicity, such as seizure. These serious complications can be managed successfully with steroids in most patients. Regardless of these potential limitations, both BiTE antibody and CAR-modified T-cell technologies probably represent the most promising advancement in the treatment of B-cell malignancies in the past decade.

ANTI-CD22-DIRECTED THERAPY

Cluster of differentiation (CD22) is more frequently expressed on B-lineage ALL cells than CD20, making it an attractive target. In addition, unlike CD20, CD22 is rapidly internalized into the cell upon ligand binding, which is ideal for the development of anti-CD22 antibodies that are conjugated with a drug toxin.[39] Unconjugated epratuzumab, a humanized monoclonal antibody against CD22, has been studied in children with marrow relapse of CD22-positive ALL, and it showed favorable activity and an acceptable toxicity profile when used in combination with reinduction chemotherapy.[40] Epratuzumab also exists in a conjugated form with SN-38, a topoisomerase I inhibitor with activity at low nanomolar concentrations.[41] Epratuzomab-SN-38 uses a linker that allows the chemotherapy-conjugate to slowly dissociate into the serum, but before toxic levels are reached the antibody-drug conjugate is rapidly internalized into cells expressing CD22. Preclinical studies have shown that epratuzumab-SN-38 can be combined with an unconjugated anti-CD20 antibody (veltuzumab) for enhanced anti-tumor activity against B-cell leukemia and lymphoma cell lines without increased toxicity.

Another anti-CD22 antibody-drug conjugate is inotuzumab ozogamicin (IO), which links an anti-CD22 monoclonal antibody to calicheamicin, an ultra-toxic (sub-nanomolar activity) natural compound that induces breaks in double-stranded deoxyribonucleic acid causing apoptosis. A recent phase II study demonstrated that fractionated doses of IO given on a weekly schedule resulted in an overall response rate of 50% and a tolerable side effect profile in patients with relapsed/refractory ALL.[42] Of the ten responders, seven became MRD negative. Although the duration of CR induced by IO was relatively short, the drug was well-tolerated in this group of heavily pretreated patients and may serve as an effective bridge to allogeneic HCT in some patients. Although calicheamicin has been associated with hepatic veno-occlusive disease (VOD)/sinusoidal obstruction syndrome (SOS) in patients with acute myeloid leukemia (AML) who received gemtuzumab ozogamicin (especially after allogeneic HCT),[43] only 2 out of 20 patients treated with weekly IO developed severe, reversible liver function abnormalities and none developed clinical VOD (4 of the 20 patients underwent allogeneic HCT). In addition to IO, moxetumomab pasudotox is another anti-CD22 antibody connected to an ultra-toxic drug conjugate that has shown single-agent activity in relapsed/refractory ALL.[44]

NOTCH1 PATHWAY INHIBITION

The NOTCH1 signaling pathway regulates the development of normal T lymphocytes from hematopoietic progenitor cells. NOTCH1 encodes a transmembrane receptor, and, upon ligand binding, the intracellular domain of this receptor is cleaved by a gamma-secretase. The NOTCH1 fragment/intracellular domain then translocates to the nucleus where it activates several transcription factors (e.g., MYC), which are involved in T cell proliferation and differentiation. More than 50% of patients with T-cell acute lymphoblastic leukemia (T-ALL) have activating NOTCH1 mutations, which allow for increased cleavage of the intracellular signaling domain by gamma-secretase.[45] In an attempt to disable this pathway, gamma-secretase inhibitors (GSI) have been developed that prevent cleavage of the intracellular signaling domain, the final step of NOTCH1 activation. There are several phase I clinical trials currently studying GSIs in T-ALL and lymphoma, and the major dose-limiting toxicity appears to be diarrhea. Furthermore, there is evidence that T-ALL may be sensitive to NOTCH1 pathway inhibition even in the absence of activating NOTCH1 mutations, suggesting that even NOTCH1-unmutated T-cell malignancies are driven, at least in part, by perturbations in the NOTCH1 pathway.[46,47]

DOT1L INHIBITORS

Chromosomal translocations causing rearrangements of the mixed lineage leukemia (MLL) gene on chromosome 11q23 are present in 5–10% of adult ALL cases.[48-50] In one large, multinational clinical trial, 9% of patients with adult ALL had 11q23 abnormalities, mostly t(4;11), and these patients had a very poor outcome.[49] MLL gene rearrangements are also seen in AML (5%) and infant leukemia (70%), and MLL abnormalities, including partial tandem duplications, are typically associated with a poor prognosis in leukemia.[50-53] Patients with therapy-related acute leukemia after exposure to cytotoxic agents (particularly topoisomerase II poisons) also commonly have 11q23/MLL translocations.[54]

The MLL gene normally encodes for a histone methyltransferase, a protein responsible for the methylation of histone H3 and regulation of downstream transcriptional activation. In MLL-mediated leukemias, a fusion protein is created consisting of a partial MLL gene product and its translocation partner (common partner genes include AF9 and ENL). These aberrant fusion proteins are able to recruit another histone methyltransferase named DOT1L, which, together with the MLL fusion gene product, results in ectopic methylation of histone H3K79 and subsequent increased expression of leukemogenic genes. DOT1L activity appears to be required for the persistence of MLL-mediated leukemias,[55] and attempts to target it have been successful in preclinical models.[56] In the laboratory, a DOT1L inhibitor has been developed that decreases H3K79 methylation, decreases expression of target genes, and induces apoptosis in MLL-mutated leukemia cell lines.[56] This study also showed in vivo activity of the DOT1L inhibitor against MLL-mediated leukemia in xenografted mouse models. This is the first new agent to putatively target MLL-rearranged leukemias, and DOT1L inhibitors are currently being tested in phase I clinical trials in both AML and adult ALL.

OTHER TARGETED AGENTS

NOTCH1 pathway inhibitors and DOT1L inhibitors are two novel small molecule inhibitors under development in ALL that are already in phase I clinical trials. Novel agents that target other pathways involved in ALL leukemogenesis are also being developed, some of which are already in clinical use for other indications. For example, TKIs (e.g., dasatinib) targeting BCR/ABL have also been used effectively against other rearrangements of the BCR gene, such as the NUP214/ABL1 oncogene that is present in 5% patients with T-ALL.[57] Preclinical studies have shown that the mTOR inhibitor everolimus, currently used in solid tumors and also being investigated in mantle cell lymphoma, has synergistic interactions with chemotherapy and other agents in precursor-B ALL.[58] Fingolimod, a drug used to treat multiple sclerosis, can target PP2A mutations in Ph-positive ALL.[59] JAK1 mutations are a relatively frequent event in T-ALL, and JAK inhibitors may be useful in this disease.[60]

Recently, a very interesting new target has been identified in ALL on the cell membrane. It is cytokine receptor-like factor 2 (CRLF2), which normally heterodimerizes with IL-7R, forming the thymic stromal lymphopoietin receptor (TSLR). When activated, TSLR effects the survival and maturation of B and T lymphocytes and enhances cytokine production.[61,62] Rearrangement of the CRLF2 gene results in high expression of CRLF2 on the leukemia cell membrane, potentially promoting B-cell leukemogenesis. This mutation was found in 14% of children with high-risk ALL, was associated with an unfavorable outcome, and was found more commonly in Latinos. Translocations involving CRLF2 have also been associated with decreased survival in adult ALL.[63]

SUMMARY

Novel targeted agents are changing the landscape of adult ALL therapy. Small molecule TKI therapy in Ph-positive ALL and, more recently, blinatumomab in CD19-positive precursor-B ALL have likely had the greatest clinical impact to date. Both are highly active drugs as single agents and are capable of inducing CR in patients with MRD-positivity or overt disease relapse. In addition to using these agents to treat relapsed or refractory disease, how to best combine these with frontline chemotherapy and allogeneic HCT to maximize the cure rate in patients with newly diagnosed ALL is under active investigation. Several investigational therapies in ALL, such as CARs, anti-CD22 antibody-drug conjugates, and NOTCH1 and DOT1L inhibitors are promising new treatment strategies in the early stages of development.

As we better define molecular subsets of ALL and identify new membranous and signal transduction pathway targets, more new agents should continue to become available. Whether or not immunologic or cellular therapy and small molecular inhibitors will replace traditional cytotoxic chemotherapy as the mainstay of ALL treatment remains to be seen, but it seems certain that these agents will at least significantly reduce patient exposure to cytotoxic agents, with the ultimate goal of simultaneously improving patient survival. Moreover, reduced exposure to cytotoxic chemotherapy is critical for improving patient quality-of-life, improving the treatment of elderly patients and those with major medical comorbidities, and reducing the risk of long-term chemotherapy-induced side effects including secondary malignancies, particularly since many adult ALL patients are adolescents or younger adults. Fortunately, all of the recent developments in new technologies and novel agents suggest that we are entering a new and exciting era in the treatment of adult ALL.

REFERENCES

1. Bassan R, Hoelzer D. Modern therapy of acute lymphoblastic leukemia. *J Clin Oncol.* 2011; 29(5):532-43.
2. Pulte D, Gondos A, Brenner H. Improvement in survival in younger patients with acute lymphoblastic leukemia from the 1980s to the early 21st century. *Blood.* 2009;113(7):1408-11.
3. Gökbuget N, Arnold R, Buechner T, et al. Intensification of induction and consolidation improves only subgroups of adult ALL: analysis of 1200 patients in GMALL study 05/03. *Blood.* 2001;98:802a-802b (abstract 3337).
4. Larson RA, Dodge RK, Burns CP, et al. A five-drug remission induction regimen with intensive consolidation for adults with acute lymphoblastic leukemia: cancer and leukemia group B study 8811. *Blood.* 1995;85(8):2025-37.
5. Stock W, Johnson JL, Stone RM, et al. Dose intensification of daunorubicin and cytarabine during treatment of adult acute lymphoblastic leukemia: results of Cancer and Leukemia Group B Study 19802. *Cancer.* 2013;119(1):90-8.
6. Rowe JM, Buck G, Burnett AK, et al. Induction therapy for adults with acute lymphoblastic leukemia: results of more than 1500 patients from the international ALL trial: MRC UKALL XII/ECOG E2993. *Blood.* 2005;106(12):3760-7.
7. Goldstone AH, Richards SM, Lazarus HM, et al. In adults with standard-risk acute lymphoblastic leukemia, the greatest benefit is achieved from a matched sibling allogeneic transplantation in first complete remission, and an autologous transplantation is less effective than conventional consolidation/maintenance chemotherapy in all patients: final results of the International ALL Trial (MRC UKALL XII/ECOG E2993). *Blood.* 2008;111(4):1827-33.
8. Linker C, Damon L, Ries C, et al. Intensified and shortened cyclical chemotherapy for adult acute lymphoblastic leukemia. *J Clin Oncol.* 2002;20(10):2464-71.
9. Weiss MA, Heffner L, Kalaycio M, et al. A randomized trial demonstrating the superiority of cytarabine with high-dose mitoxantrone compared to a standard vincristine/prednisone-based regimen as induction therapy for adult patients with ALL. *J Clin Oncol.* 2005;23:(abstract 6516).
10. Kantarjian H, Thomas D, O'Brien S, et al. Long-term follow-up results of hyperfractionated cyclophosphamide, vincristine, doxorubicin, and dexamethasone (Hyper-CVAD), a dose-intensive regimen, in adult acute lymphocytic leukemia. *Cancer.* 2004;101(12):2788-801.
11. Alvarnas JC, Brown PA, Aoun P, et al. Acute lymphoblastic leukemia. *J Natl Compr Canc Netw.* 2012;10(7):858-914.
12. Larson RA. Management of acute lymphoblastic leukemia in older patients. *Semin Hematol.* 2006;43(2):126-33.
13. Lamanna N, Heffner LT, Kalaycio M, et al. Treatment of adults with acute lymphoblastic leukemia: do the specifics of the regimen matter? Results of a prospective randomized trial. *Cancer.* 2013;119(6):1186-94.
14. Thomas D, O'Brien S, Faderl S, et al. Anthracycline dose intensification in adult acute lymphoblastic leukemia: lack of benefit in the context of the fractionated cyclophosphamide, vincristine, doxorubicin, and dexamethasone regimen. *Cancer.* 2010;116(19):4580-9.
15. Wood WA, Lee SJ. Malignant hematologic diseases in adolescents and young adults. *Blood.* 2011;117(22):5803-15.

16. Ribera JM, Oriol A, Sanz MA, et al. Comparison of the results of the treatment of adolescents and young adults with standard-risk acute lymphoblastic leukemia with the Programa Espanol de Tratamiento en Hematologia pediatric-based protocol ALL-96. *J Clin Oncol.* 2008;26(11):1843-9.

17. Huguet F, Leguay T, Raffoux E, et al. Pediatric-inspired therapy in adults with Philadelphia chromosome-negative acute lymphoblastic leukemia: the GRAALL-2003 study. *J Clin Oncol.* 2009;27(6):911-8.

18. Goekbuget N, Baumann A, Beck J, et al. PEG-asparaginase in adult acute lymphoblastic leukemia (ALL): efficacy and feasibility analysis with increasing dose levels. *Blood.* 2008;112 (abstract 302).

19. DeAngelo DJ, Dahlberg S, Silverman LB, et al. A multicenter phase II study using a dose intensified pediatric regimen in adults with untreated acute lymphoblastic leukemia. *Blood.* 2007;110:181a (abstract 587).

20. Douer D, Watkins K, Mark L, et al. Sustained and prolonged asparagine depletion by multiple doses of intravenous pegylated asparaginase in the treatment of adults with newly diagnosed acute lymphoblastic leukemia. *Blood.* 2008;112 (abstract 1928).

21. Angiolillo AL, Yu AL, Reaman G, et al. A phase II study of Campath-1H in children with relapsed or refractory acute lymphoblastic leukemia: a Children's Oncology Group report. *Pediatr Blood Cancer.* 2009;53(6):978-83.

22. Stock W, Yu D, Sanford B, et al. Incorporation of alemtuzumab into front-line therapy of adult acute lymphoblastic leukemia (ALL) is feasible: a phase I/II study from the Cancer and Leukemia Group B (CALGB 10102). *Blood.* 2005;106 (abstract 145).

23. Hoelzer D, Huettmann A, Kaul F, et al. Immunochemotherapy with rituximab improves molecular CR rate and outcome in CD20+ B-lineage standard and high risk patients; Results of 263 CD20+ patients studied prospectively in GMALL study 07/2003. *Blood.* 2010;116 (abstract 170).

24. Thomas DA, O'Brien S, Faderl S, et al. Chemoimmunotherapy with a modified hyper-CVAD and rituximab regimen improves outcome in de novo Philadelphia chromosome-negative precursor B-lineage acute lymphoblastic leukemia. *J Clin Oncol.* 2010;28(24):3880-9.

25. Lee S, Kim YJ, Min CK, et al. The effect of first-line imatinib interim therapy on the outcome of allogeneic stem cell transplantation in adults with newly diagnosed Philadelphia chromosome-positive acute lymphoblastic leukemia. *Blood.* 2005;105(9):3449-57.

26. Thomas DA, Faderl S, Cortes J, et al. Treatment of Philadelphia chromosome-positive acute lymphocytic leukemia with hyper-CVAD and imatinib mesylate. *Blood.* 2004;103(12):4396-407.

27. Yanada M, Takeuchi J, Sugiura I, et al. High complete remission rate and promising outcome by combination of imatinib and chemotherapy for newly diagnosed BCR-ABL-positive acute lymphoblastic leukemia: a phase II study by the Japan Adult Leukemia Study Group. *J Clin Oncol.* 2006;24:460-6.

28. Ravandi F, O'Brien S, Thomas D, et al. First report of phase 2 study of dasatinib with hyper-CVAD for the frontline treatment of patients with Philadelphia chromosome-positive (Ph+) acute lymphoblastic leukemia. *Blood.* 2010;116(12):2070-7.

29. Wassmann B, Pfeifer H, Goekbuget N, et al. Alternating versus concurrent schedules of imatinib and chemotherapy as front-line therapy for Philadelphia-positive acute lymphoblastic leukemia (Ph+ ALL). *Blood.* 2006;108(5):1469-77.

30. Ravandi F, Kebriaei P. Philadelphia chromosome-positive acute lymphoblastic leukemia. *Hematol Oncol Clin North Am.* 2009;23:1043-63.

31. Nagorsen D, Baeuerle PA. Immunomodulatory therapy of cancer with T cell-engaging BiTE antibody blinatumomab. *Exp Cell Res.* 2011;317(9):1255-60.

32. Topp MS, Kufer P, Gokbuget N, et al. Targeted therapy with the T-cell-engaging antibody blinatumomab of chemotherapy-refractory minimal residual disease in B-lineage acute lymphoblastic leukemia patients results in high response rate and prolonged leukemia-free survival. *J Clin Oncol.* 2011;29(18):2493-8.

33. Topp M, Goekbuget N, Zugmaier G, et al. Effect of anti-CD19 BiTE blinatumomab on complete remission rate and overall survival in adult patients with relapsed/refractory B-precursor ALL. *J Clin Oncol.* 2012;30 (abstract 6500).

34. Topp MS, Gökbuget N, Zugmaier G, et al. Long-term follow-up of hematological relapse-free survival in a phase 2 study of blinatumomab in patients with minimal residual disease (MRD) of B-precursor acute lymphoblastic leukemia (ALL). *Blood.* 2012;120(26):5185-7.

35. Brentjens RJ. CARs and cancers: questions and answers. *Blood.* 2012;119(17):3872-3.

36. Brentjens RJ, Riviere I, Park JH, et al. Safety and persistence of adoptively transferred autologous CD19-targeted T cells in patients with relapsed or chemotherapy refractory B-cell leukemias. *Blood.* 2011;118(18):4817-28.

37. Porter DL, Levine BL, Kalos M, et al. Chimeric antigen receptor-modified T cells in chronic lymphoid leukemia. *N Engl J Med.* 2011;365(8):725-33.

38. Till BG, Jensen MC, Wang J, et al. CD20-specific adoptive immunotherapy for lymphoma using a chimeric antigen receptor with both CD28 and 4-1BB domains: pilot clinical trial results. *Blood.* 2012;119(17):3940-50.

39. Poe JC, Fujimoto Y, Hasegawa M, et al. CD22 regulates B lymphocyte function in vivo through both ligand-dependent and ligand-independent mechanisms. *Nat Immunol.* 2004; 5(10):1078-87.

40. Raetz EA, Cairo MS, Borowitz MJ, et al. Chemoimmunotherapy reinduction with epratuzumab in children with acute lymphoblastic leukemia in marrow relapse: a Children's Oncology Group Pilot Study. *J Clin Oncol.* 2008;26(22):3756-62.

41. Sharkey RM, Govindan SV, Cardillo TM, et al. Epratuzumab-SN-38: a new antibody-drug conjugate for the therapy of hematologic malignancies. *Mol Cancer Ther.* 2012;11(1): 224-34.

42. Jabbour E, O'Brien SM, Thomas DA, et al. Inotuzumab ozogamycin (IO), a CD22 mono-clonal antibody conjugated to calecheamicin, given weekly, for refractory-relapse acute lymphocytic leukemia (R-R ALL). *J Clin Oncol.* 2012;30 (abstract 6501).

43. Cohen AD, Luger SM, Sickles C, et al. Gemtuzumab ozogamicin (mylotarg) monotherapy for relapsed AML after hematopoietic stem cell transplant: efficacy and incidence of hepatic veno-occlusive disease. *Bone Marrow Transplant.* 2002;30(1):23-8.

44. Wayne AS, Bhojwani D, Silverman LB, et al. A novel anti-CD22 immunotoxin, moxetumomab pasudotox: Phase I study in pediatric acute lymphoblastic leukemia (ALL). *Blood.* 2011;118 (abstract 248).

45. Van Vlierberghe P, Ferrando A. The molecular basis of T cell acute lymphoblastic leukemia. *J Clin Invest.* 2012;122(10):3398-406.

46. Clappier E, Collette S, Grardel N, et al. NOTCH1 and FBXW7 mutations have a favorable impact on early response to treatment, but not on outcome, in children with T-cell acute lymphoblastic leukemia (T-ALL) treated on EORTC trials 58881 and 58951. *Leukemia.* 2010;24(12):2023-31.

47. Mansour MR, Sulis ML, Duke V, et al. Prognostic implications of NOTCH1 and FBXW7 mutations in adults with T-cell acute lymphoblastic leukemia treated on the MRC UKALLXII/ ECOG E2993 protocol. *J Clin Oncol.* 2009;27(26):4352-6.

48. Wetzler M, Dodge RK, Mrozek K, et al. Prospective karyotype analysis in adult acute lymphoblastic leukemia: the cancer and leukemia Group B experience. *Blood.* 1999; 93(11):3983-93.

49. Moorman AV, Harrison CJ, Buck GA, et al. Karyotype is an independent prognostic factor in adult acute lymphoblastic leukemia (ALL): analysis of cytogenetic data from patients treated on the Medical Research Council (MRC) UKALLXII/Eastern Cooperative Oncology Group (ECOG) 2993 trial. *Blood.* 2007;109(8):3189-97.

50. Tamai H, Inokuchi K. 11q23/MLL acute leukemia: update of clinical aspects. *J Clin Exp Hematop.* 2010;50(2):91-8.

51. Mrozek K, Heinonen K, Lawrence D, et al. Adult patients with de novo acute myeloid leukemia and t(9; 11)(p22; q23) have a superior outcome to patients with other translocations involving band 11q23: a cancer and leukemia group B study Blood. 1997;90(11):4532-8.

52. Schoch C, Schnittger S, Klaus M, et al. AML with 11q23/MLL abnormalities as defined by the WHO classification: incidence, partner chromosomes, FAB subtype, age distribution, and prognostic impact in an unselected series of 1897 cytogenetically analyzed AML cases. Blood. 2003;102(7):2395-402.

53. Grimwade D, Hills RK, Moorman AV, et al. Refinement of cytogenetic classification in acute myeloid leukemia: determination of prognostic significance of rare recurring chromosomal abnormalities among 5876 younger adult patients treated in the United Kingdom Medical Research Council trials. Blood. 2010;116(3):354-65.

54. Kayser S, Dohner K, Krauter J, et al. The impact of therapy-related acute myeloid leukemia (AML) on outcome in 2853 adult patients with newly diagnosed AML. Blood. 2011;117(7): 2137-45.

55. Nguyen AT, Taranova O, He J, et al. DOT1L, the H3K79 methyltransferase, is required for MLL-AF9-mediated leukemogenesis. Blood. 2011;117(25):6912-22.

56. Daigle SR, Olhava EJ, Therkelsen CA, et al. Selective killing of mixed lineage leukemia cells by a potent small-molecule DOT1L inhibitor. Cancer Cell. 2011;20(1):53-65.

57. Deenik W, Beverloo HB, van der Poel-van de Luytgaarde SC, et al. Rapid complete cytogenetic remission after upfront dasatinib monotherapy in a patient with a NUP214-ABL1-positive T-cell acute lymphoblastic leukemia. Leukemia. 2009;23(3):627-9.

58. Saunders P, Cisterne A, Weiss J, et al. The mammalian target of rapamycin inhibitor RAD001 (everolimus) synergizes with chemotherapeutic agents, ionizing radiation and proteasome inhibitors in pre-B acute lymphocytic leukemia. Haematologica. 2011;96(1):69-77.

59. Neviani P, Santhanam R, Oaks JJ, et al. FTY720, a new alternative for treating blast crisis chronic myelogenous leukemia and Philadelphia chromosome-positive acute lymphocytic leukemia. J Clin Invest. 2007;117(9):2408-21.

60. Jeong EG, Kim MS, Nam HK, et al. Somatic mutations of JAK1 and JAK3 in acute leukemias and solid cancers. Clin Cancer Res. 2008;14(12):3716-21.

61. Harvey RC, Mullighan CG, Chen IM, et al. Rearrangement of CRLF2 is associated with mutation of JAK kinases, alteration of IKZF1, Hispanic/Latino ethnicity, and a poor outcome in pediatric B-progenitor acute lymphoblastic leukemia. Blood. 2010;115(26):5312-21.

62. Mullighan CG. New strategies in acute lymphoblastic leukemia: translating advances in genomics into clinical practice. Clin Cancer Res. 2011;17(3):396-400.

63. Moorman AV, Schwab C, Ensor HM, et al. IGH@ translocations, CRLF2 deregulation, and microdeletions in adolescents and adults with acute lymphoblastic leukemia. J Clin Oncol. 2012;30(25):3100-8.

Index

Page numbers followed by *f* refer to figure